Aeroallergen and Food Immunotherapy

Editors

LINDA S. COX
ANNA H. NOWAK-WĘGRZYN

IMMUNOLOGY AND ALLERGY CLINICS OF NORTH AMERICA

www.immunology.theclinics.com

Consulting Editor
STEPHEN A. TILLES

February 2016 • Volume 36 • Number 1

ELSEVIER

1600 John F. Kennedy Boulevard • Suite 1800 • Philadelphia, Pennsylvania, 19103-2899
http://www.theclinics.com

IMMUNOLOGY AND ALLERGY CLINICS OF NORTH AMERICA Volume 36, Number 1
February 2016 ISSN 0889-8561, ISBN-13: 978-0-323-41694-8
Editor: Jessica McCool
Developmental Editor: Kristen Helm

Immunology and Allergy Clinics of North America (ISSN 0889–8561) is published quarterly by Elsevier Inc., 360 Park Avenue South, New York, NY 10010-1710. Months of issue are February, May, August, and November. Periodicals postage paid at New York, NY and additional mailing offices. Subscription prices are $320.00 per year for US individuals, $508.00 per year for US institutions, $100.00 per year for US students and residents, $395.00 per year for Canadian individuals, $220.00 per year for Canadian students, $644.00 per year for Canadian institutions, $445.00 per year for international individuals, $644.00 per year for international institutions, $220.00 per year for international students. To receive student/resident rate, orders must be accompanied by name of affiliated institution, date of term, and the *signature* of program/residency coordinator on institution letterhead. Orders will be billed at individual rate until proof of status is received. Foreign air speed delivery is included in all *Clinics* subscription prices. All prices are subject to change without notice. **POSTMASTER**: Send address changes to *Immunology and Allergy Clinics of North America,* Elsevier Health Sciences Division, Subscription Customer Service, 3251 Riverport Lane, Maryland Heights, MO 63043. **Customer Service: 1-800-654-2452 (U.S. and Canada); 314-447-8871 (outside U.S. and Canada). Fax: 314-447-8029. E-mail: journalscustomerservice-usa@elsevier.com (for print support); journalsonlinesupport-usa@elsevier.com (for online support).**

Reprints. For copies of 100 or more, of articles in this publication, please contact the Commercial Reprints Department, Elsevier Inc., 360 Park Avenue South, New York, New York 10010-1710. Tel. 212-633-3874, Fax: 212-633-3820, E-mail: reprints@elsevier.com.

Immunology and Allergy Clinics of North America is covered in MEDLINE/PubMed (Index Medicus), Current Contents/Life Sciences, Science Citation Index, ISI/BIOMED, Chemical Abstracts, and EMBASE/Excerpta Medica.

Contributors

CONSULTING EDITOR

STEPHEN A. TILLES, MD
Executive Director, ASTHMA Inc. Clinical Research Center; Partner, Northwest Asthma and Allergy Center; Clinical Professor of Medicine, University of Washington, Seattle, Washington

EDITORS

LINDA S. COX, MD
Department of Medicine, Nova Southeastern University Davie Florida, Ft. Lauderdale, Florida

ANNA H. NOWAK-WĘGRZYN, MD
Associate Professor of Pediatrics, Division of Pediatric Allergy, Department of Pediatrics, Jaffe Food Allergy Institute, Icahn School of Medicine at Mount Sinai, New York, New York

AUTHORS

CEZMI A. AKDIS, MD
Professor of Immunology, Allergology, Swiss Institute of Allergy and Asthma Research, University of Zurich, Davos, Switzerland

MÜBECCEL AKDIS, PD, MD, PhD
Swiss Institute of Allergy and Asthma Research, University of Zurich, Davos, Switzerland

BRUCE G. BENDER, PhD
Professor of Pediatrics and Psychiatry; Head, Division of Pediatric Behavioral Health; Co-Director, Center for Health Promotion, National Jewish Health, Denver, Colorado

M. CECILIA BERIN, PhD
Associate Professor, Pediatric Allergy and Immunology, Mindich Child Health and Development Institute, Immunology Institute, Icahn School of Medicine at Mount Sinai, New York, New York

JEAN BOUSQUET, MD, PhD
MACVIA-LR, European Innovation Partnership on Active and Healthy Ageing Reference Site, University Hospital of Montpellier, Montpellier, France

ALLISON J. BURBANK, MD
Department of Rheumatology, Allergy, and Immunology, University of North Carolina at Chapel Hill, Chapel Hill, North Carolina

DAVIDE CAIMMI, MD
Division of Allergy, Department of Pulmonology, Hôpital Arnaud de Villeneuve, University Hospital of Montpellier; MACVIA-LR, European Innovation Partnership on Active and Healthy Ageing Reference Site, University Hospital of Montpellier, Montpellier, France

MOISES A. CALDERON, MD, PhD
Director, Clinical Trials Unit, Section of Allergy and Clinical Immunology, Royal Brompton and Harefield Hospital NHS Trust, National Heart and Lung Institute, Imperial College London, London, United Kingdom; Professor of Internal Medicine and Allergy, Faculty of Medicine, University of Costa Rica, San Jose, Costa Rica

GIORGIO WALTER CANONICA, MD
Allergy and Respiratory Diseases, IRCCS San Martino-IST, University of Genoa, Genoa, Italy

JULIE CHESNÉ, PhD
Center of Allergy and Environment (ZAUM), Technical University of Munich and Helmholtz Center, Munich, Germany

PETER SOCRATES CRETICOS, MD
Associate Professor of Medicine, Division of Allergy and Clinical Immunology, Johns Hopkins Medicine, Baltimore, Maryland; Clinical Director, Creticos Research Group, Crownsville, Maryland

PASCAL DEMOLY, MD, PhD
Division of Allergy, Department of Pulmonology, Hôpital Arnaud de Villeneuve, University Hospital of Montpellier, Montpellier, France; Sorbonne Universités, UPMC Paris 06, UMR-S 1136, IPLESP, Equipe EPAR, Paris, France

JULIA ESSER VON-BIEREN, PhD
Center of Allergy and Environment (ZAUM), Technical University of Munich and Helmholtz Center, Munich, Germany

DAVID M. FLEISCHER, MD
Section of Allergy, Department of Pediatrics, Children's Hospital Colorado, University of Colorado Denver School of Medicine, Aurora, Colorado

ROBERT G. HAMILTON, PhD, D.ABMLI
Johns Hopkins Dermatology, Allergy and Clinical Immunology Reference Laboratory, Johns Hopkins Asthma and Allergy Center, Johns Hopkins University School of Medicine, Baltimore, Maryland

JÖRG KLEINE-TEBBE, MD
Allergy and Asthma Center Westend, Outpatient Clinic Hanf, Ackermann and Kleine-Tebbe, Berlin, Germany

UMUT CAN KUCUKSEZER, PhD
Associate Professor, Department of Immunology, Institute of Experimental Medicine, Istanbul University, Istanbul, Turkey

THOMAS M. KÜNDIG, MD
Department of Dermatology, University Hospital Zurich, Zurich, Switzerland

STEPHANIE A. LEONARD, MD
Assistant Clinical Professor, Division of Pediatric Allergy and Immunology, Department of Pediatrics, Rady Children's Hospital San Diego, University of California, San Diego, San Diego, California

RICHARD F. LOCKEY, MD
Distinguished University Health Professor, Professor of Medicine, Pediatrics and Public Health, Joy McCann Culverhouse Chair of Allergy and Immunology, Director, Division of Allergy and Immunology, Department of Internal Medicine, University of South Florida Morsani College of Medicine, Tampa, Florida

MELINA MAKATSORI, MD
Physician, Section of Allergy and Clinical Immunology, Royal Brompton and Harefield
Hospital NHS Trust, National Heart and Lung Institute, Imperial College London, London,
United Kingdom

PAOLO M. MATRICARDI, MD
AG Molecular Allergology and Immunomodulation, Department of Pediatric Pneumology
and Immunology, Charité Medical University, Berlin, Germany

PHILIPPE MOINGEON, PhD
Research and Development, Stallergenes SAS, Antony, France

HAROLD S. NELSON, MD
Professor of Medicine, National Jewish Health and University of Colorado Denver School
of Medicine, Denver, Colorado

ANNA H. NOWAK-WĘGRZYN, MD
Associate Professor of Pediatrics, Division of Pediatric Allergy, Department of Pediatrics,
Jaffe Food Allergy Institute, Icahn School of Medicine at Mount Sinai, New York,
New York

CEVDET OZDEMIR, MD
Associate Professor, Department of Pediatric Allergy, Memorial Atasehir Hospital,
Memorial Health Group, Istanbul, Turkey

GIOVANNI PASSALACQUA, MD
Allergy and Respiratory Diseases, IRCCS San Martino-IST, University of Genoa, Genoa,
Italy

CARSTEN B. SCHMIDT-WEBER, PhD
Center of Allergy and Environment (ZAUM), Technical University of Munich and Helmholtz
Center, Munich, Germany

GABRIELA SENTI, MD
Clinical Trials Center, University Hospital Zurich, Zurich, Switzerland

WAYNE G. SHREFFLER, MD, PhD
Associate Professor of Pediatrics, Center for Immunology and Inflammatory Diseases,
Food Allergy Center, MassGeneral Hospital for Children, Massachusetts General
Hospital, Harvard Medical School, Boston, Massachusetts

SAYANTANI SINDHER, MD
Division of Allergy and Immunology, Department of Pediatrics, The Children's Hospital of
Philadelphia, Perelman School of Medicine at University of Pennsylvania, Philadelphia,
Pennsylvania

PUJA SOOD, MD
Department of Pediatrics, University of Maryland Children's Hospital, Baltimore,
Maryland

JONATHAN M. SPERGEL, MD, PhD
Division of Allergy and Immunology, Department of Pediatrics, The Children's Hospital of
Philadelphia, Perelman School of Medicine at University of Pennsylvania, Philadelphia,
Pennsylvania

BRIAN P. VICKERY, MD
Assistant Professor of Pediatrics, University of North Carolina, Chapel Hill, North Carolina

ROBERT A. WOOD, MD
Professor of Pediatrics, Johns Hopkins University School of Medicine, Baltimore, Maryland

Contents

> Allergen immunotherapy (AIT) was introduced in clinical practice more
> than 100 years ago. The clinical effectiveness in allergic rhinitis (and
> asthma) and in hymenoptera allergy was apparent early on but it was
> not until the mid-1900s that randomized placebo-controlled trials proved
> its efficacy. In the 1980s, sublingual immunotherapy (SLIT) was accepted
> in official guidelines. The availability of safer routes, such as SLIT, promp-
> ted increasing investigation of AIT for food allergy. The introduction of
> molecular-based diagnosis introduced the possibility of better targeted
> prescription of AIT. Other approaches are being explored, such as immu-
> nogenic peptides, recombinant allergens, and adjuvants.

> Subcutaneous immunotherapy and sublingual immunotherapy are effec-
> tive for allergic rhinitis and allergic asthma and with some support for
> use in selected patients with atopic dermatitis. The sequence of immuno-
> logic responses is the same, irrespective of the route of administration,
> and similar disease modification has been demonstrated. However, there
> are differences between the two approaches. The most important is the
> greatly reduced likelihood of sublingual immunotherapy producing sys-
> temic reactions. There are major drawbacks for sublingual immunotherapy
> in regard to dosing. Finally, there is the question of relative clinical efficacy,
> with the currently available data favoring subcutaneous immunotherapy.

> Current allergy immunotherapy protocols suffer from two main problems:
> long treatment duration and systemic allergic side effects of the allergen
> administrations. The immunologic effects of allergen administration could

be enhanced and the number of allergen administrations and treatment duration reduced by choosing a tissue for administration that contains a high density of antigen-presenting cells. Local side effects could be reduced by choosing a route characterized by a low density of mast cells, and systemic side effects could be reduced by administration to nonvascularized tissues, so that inadvertent systemic distribution of the allergen and consequent systemic allergic side effects are minimized.

Oral tolerance refers to a systemic immune nonresponsiveness to antigens first encountered by the oral route, and a failure in development of this homeostatic process can result in food allergy. Clinical tolerance induced by allergen immunotherapy is associated with alterations in immune mechanisms relevant to the allergic response, including reduction of basophil reactivity, induction of IgG4, loss of effector Th2 cells, and induction of Tregs. The relative contribution of these immune changes to clinical tolerance to foods, and the duration of these immune changes after termination of immunotherapy, remains to be identified.

There is a need for newer therapeutic agents that improve the safety of allergen immunotherapy, provide ease of delivery to patients that fosters compliance and allows access to a greater proportion of the allergic population who could benefit from this disease-modifying treatment, and achieve an acceptable therapeutic benefit for patients committing to the treatment. The advances in sublingual allergen immunotherapy are encouraging, as this offers patients a noninjectable form of treatment of inhalant allergies. The continued research and development of the novel therapeutic constructs discussed in this article holds the promise of accomplishing the aforementioned goals in the future.

One key approach to increase the efficacy and the safety of immunotherapy is the use of adjuvants. However, many of the adjuvants currently in use can cause adverse events, raising concerns regarding their clinical use, and are geared toward productive immune responses but not necessarily tolerogenic responses. Thus, novel adjuvants for immunotherapy are needed and are being developed. Their potential to boost appropriate tolerogenic adaptive immune responses to allergens while limiting side effects is essential. This review provides an overview of adjuvants currently in clinical use or under development and discusses their therapeutic effect in enhancing allergen-induced tolerance.

In baked form, cow's milk and egg are less allergenic and tolerated by a majority of milk- and egg-allergic children. Not only may including baked milk and egg in the diets of children who are tolerant improve nutrition and promote more social inclusion but there is also evidence that inclusion may accelerate the resolution of unheated milk and egg allergy. Further research is needed to identify biomarkers that can predict baked milk or egg reactivity; however, data suggest casein- and ovomucoid-specific

achieve full benefit. Numerous studies reveal that fewer than 10% of patients complete a full course and that most abandon treatment in the first year. The development and testing of interventions to improve AIT are emerging. Data from adherence interventions in other chronic conditions provide guidance to allergists/immunologists. Evidence-based communication strategies—patient-centered care, motivational interviewing, and shared-decision making—underscore the importance of taking time to establish trust, understand patient concerns and priorities, and involve the patient in decisions regarding AIT.

IMMUNOLOGY AND ALLERGY CLINICS OF NORTH AMERICA

Foreword

Allergen Immunotherapy—An Old Friend Coming of Age

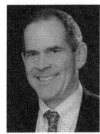

Stephen A. Tilles, MD
Consulting Editor

Introduced a century ago and practiced in essentially the same way ever since, treating patients with allergen immunotherapy has withstood both scientific rigor and competition from a slew of more "sophisticated" potential magic bullets. With the continuing rise in prevalence of allergic diseases, including an astounding increase in food allergy in the past 2 decades, our old friend is alive, well, and as relevant as ever.

Optimizing and diversifying immunotherapy approaches have progressed rapidly in recent years, including evaluating alternative allergen forms and routes of exposure. These include several FDA-approved sublingual aeroallergen immunotherapy products and ongoing FDA clinical trials evaluating epicutaneous and oral immunotherapy products for food allergy, intradermal peptide immunotherapy to aeroallergens, and intranodal immunotherapy to aeroallergens. In addition, there has been continued interest in improving the convenience, duration, and durability of subcutaneous immunotherapy, including coadministration of adjuvants such as anti-thymic stromal lymphopoietin.

In this issue of *Immunology and Allergy Clinics of North America*, coeditors Linda Cox and Anna Nowak-Węgrzyn have done a masterful job of assembling state-of-the-art reviews that span a variety of practical and scientific topics relating to inhalant and/or food allergen immunotherapy. I am confident that this issue will be a valuable resource, whether for the practicing allergist catching up with an "old friend," a clinical scientist seeking a cutting edge review, or a Fellow-in-training who may be learning about immunotherapy for the first time.

Stephen A. Tilles, MD
ASTHMA Inc. Clinical Research Center
Northwest Asthma and Allergy Center
University of Washington
9725–3rd Avenue Northeast, Suite 500
Seattle, WA 98115, USA

E-mail address:
stilles@nwasthma.com

http://dx.doi.org/10.1016/j.iac.2015.09.002
immunology.theclinics.com

Preface

Allergen-specific Immunotherapy—Turning the Tables on the Immune System

CrossMark

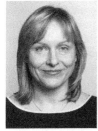 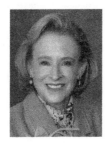

Anna H. Nowak-Węgrzyn, MD   Linda S. Cox, MD
Editors

Allergic disorders have emerged as a major global public health problem.[1] The initial epidemics of asthma, allergic rhinitis, followed by atopic dermatitis, food allergy, and anaphylaxis have predominantly affected the developed counties with a "western lifestyle."[2–4] It is estimated that up to 30% of the general population is affected by at least one allergic condition, posing a significant global socioeconomic burden.[5] In the past decade, allergic disorders have been increasingly recognized in South America, Asia, and Africa. These countries are currently experiencing a rise in the respiratory allergic disorders; it is anticipated that food allergy and anaphylaxis will soon also become more prevalent.[6] Among the various therapeutic options for allergic disorders, allergen-specific immunotherapy (AIT) has the unique potential to induce desensitization and long-lasting tolerance.[7–9] The current issue of the *Immunology and Allergy Clinics of North America* is devoted to the specific immunotherapy with aeroallergens and foods. It provides a comprehensive "bench-to-bedside" review of AIT with 14 articles that explore a number of AIT topics, including mechanisms, current and future approaches, as well as practical considerations and challenges related to adherence, identifying responders, and assessing outcomes.

This issue begins with an overview of the more than 100-year history of AIT written by Passalacqua and Canonica, which also discusses recent regulatory changes and allergy diagnostic testing advances likely to impact future AIT. In 1908, Schofield reported successful oral desensitization to raw egg in a teenage boy with anaphylactic egg allergy.[10] Subcutaneous allergen-specific immunotherapy (SCIT) for the treatment of hay fever was introduced by Leonard Noon in 1911.[11] Epicutaneous immunotherapy (EPIT) as a treatment for allergies was introduced in 1917, and the first case of successful EPIT was reported in 1921 by Vallery-Radot and Hangenau, who found that allergen administration onto scarified skin reduced systemic allergic symptoms in

Immunol Allergy Clin N Am 36 (2016) xv–xxi
http://dx.doi.org/10.1016/j.iac.2015.09.001
0889-8561/16/$ – see front matter © 2016 Published by Elsevier Inc.

patients allergic to horses.[12,13] A decade later, intradermal allergen-specific immunotherapy was shown to be safe and highly efficacious, leading to allergic rhinitis symptom relief after administration of only three doses of pollen.[14,15] Sublingual immunotherapy (SLIT) was introduced in the 1990s. In this issue, Nelson and colleagues compare SLIT with SCIT and conclude that SLIT has a superior safety profile, but available evidence suggests superior short-term efficacy with SCIT.

In 2008, the results of the first clinical trial of intra-inguinal lymhphatic immunotherapy (ILIT) were published by Senti and colleagues,[16] who explore the use of this and other novel delivery routes for aeroallergen allergy in this issue. The safety and efficacy of oral immunotherapy (OIT), SLIT, and EPIT for food allergies are reviewed in two articles in this issue written by Fleisher and colleagues and Vickery and Wood.

The mechanisms of aeroallergen and food AIT are covered in articles by Mübeccel and Cezmi Akdis and Berin and Shreffler, respectively. Comparison among the different routes of AIT is presented in **Table 1**. Probably the most important differences are the antigen uptake and processing and the total dose. Sublingual and epicutaneous routes appear to have specific advantages due to the presence of resident tolerogenic dendritic cell subsets in the sublingual mucosa and in the skin. OIT utilizes the GALT pathways that underlie physiologic responses to food antigens and oral tolerance. ILIT delivers allergens directly to the lymph nodes with minimal likelihood of systemic dissemination.

Regardless of the route of antigen delivery, successful AIT is associated with the induction of Treg cells, modulation of T- and B-cell responses, skewing of allergen specific–antibody isotype from IgE to IgG_4 predominance, early desensitization (increased threshold for activation) of mast cells and basophils, and decreased numbers and activation of eosinophils and mast cells in the tissues.[17–22] Local induction of Treg cells in the nasal mucosa in response to AIT has been observed in allergic rhinitis patients.[23] Allergen-specific Treg cells produce IL-10 and TGF-β cytokines that suppress proliferative and cytokine responses against major allergens and their recognition sites.[24,25] An alternative mechanism of tolerance is deletion of allergen-specific T helper 2 (Th2) cells as a consequence of repeated high-dose allergen exposure.[26] IL-10 promotes a noninflammatory phenotype. Serum levels of IgE decrease gradually, while allergen-specific IgG_4, referred to as blocking antibodies, increase during AIT, which is the result of class-switching of B cells from IgE to IgG_4. IgG_4 competes with Fcϵ receptor-bound IgE for binding allergens, which limits activation and degranulation of mast cells and basophils. IgG_4 has important roles in limiting the activation of $CD4^+$ T cells, by inhibition of CD23-mediated IgE-facilitated antigen presentation.[22,27–35]

In addition to exploring different routes of allergen administration, modifications of native allergens are being actively investigated to enhance safety and efficacy of AIT. Allergenic peptides and various forms of recombinant allergens (hypoallergens, dimers, trimers, and fusion proteins) have been shown to control allergic inflammation by inducing inhibitory antibodies. These novel AIT therapies are discussed in the article by Creticos on AIT vaccine modification.

Efficacy and safety of AIT can be also enhanced by the use of the adjuvants that skew the immune response toward T helper 1, which downregulates the allergic Th2 inflammation. Various adjuvants have been studied, including alum, toll-like receptor agonists, probiotics, and nanoparticles.[36–40] Current and novel AIT adjuvants are reviewed in the article by Schmidt-Weber and Chesné.

Following the AIT studies focusing on the aeroallergens and venom, in the past decade, food allergy has become a prime target for immunomodulation. OIT, SLIT, and EPIT are being currently investigated in clinical trials for milk, egg, and peanut allergy.[41] Pretreatment with anti-IgE antibody (omalizumab) has been shown to

Table 1
Comparison of different routes of allergen-specific immunotherapy

	SCIT	SLIT	OIT	EPIT	ILIT
Allergens	Aeroallergens, venom	Aeroallergens, food, latex	Foods	Aeroallergens: grass pollen, dust mites, cat dander Foods: milk, peanut	Grass pollen, MHC class II-targeting cat dander (MAT-Fel d 1)
Dose	Micrograms	Micrograms (aeroallergens) - miligrams (foods)	Grams	Micrograms	Micrograms (1000-fold less than in SCIT)
Up dosing	Initial dose escalation can be rush or gradual every 1–2 wk	No	Initial rapid dose escalation over 1 day, followed by up-dosing every 2 wk	No	No
Dosing interval	Variable, usually maintenance every 4 wk	Daily	Daily	Daily	3 injections every 4 wk are equivalent to 3 y of SCIT
Allergen uptake	Subcutaneous dendritic cells	Oral mucosal uptake by Langerhans cells	Intestinal mucosal uptake by dendritic cells	Allergens are captured within the superficial layers of intact stratum corneum by Langerhans cells subpopulation of dendritic cells expressing the langerin-specific surface marker cytotoxic T lymphocyte-associated antigen 4	Antigen-presenting cells in the inguinal lymph nodes
Safety/side effects	Most commonly local reactions (induration, erythema) at the site of injection, uncommonly anaphylaxis	Local, mild oropharyngeal	Most commonly mild oropharyngeal and gastrointestinal; systemic reactions may occur in the setting of fever, infection, exercise, or asthma flare	Local skin irritation, eczema, hives, and gastrointestinal (diarrhea)	Infrequent mild urticaria and angioedema

increase safety of the up-dosing during OIT.[42] Multifood OIT has been shown to have a comparable safety profile to a single-food OIT, opening a new venue for patients with multiple food allergies.[41] As an alternative to AIT, diets containing extensively heated (baked) cow's milk and hen's egg are well-tolerated by the majority of the milk and egg-allergic children, and they appear to accelerate development of tolerance to unheated milk and egg, and have already changed the paradigm of strict dietary avoidance for cow milk and hen's egg allergy management.[43] Leonard and Nowak-Węgrzyn discuss this approach.

Practical aspects of AIT are also covered in the issue:

○ Identifying biomarkers to predict and monitor response (Moingeon)
○ Outcome measures for assessing AIT efficacy, the magnitude of improvement that is clinically significant, and unmet needs (Demoly, Bousquet)
○ Use of component-resolved diagnosis to guide AIT prescription (Kleine-Tebbe, Matricardi)
○ Adherence challenges and strategies for improvement (Bender, Lockey)

Considering the unique disease-modifying potential of AIT, it will remain an attractive therapeutic approach to allergic disorders. Currently, SCIT and SLIT are approved for clinical use, whereas OIT, EPIT, and ILIT remain in the sphere of clinical research. The improvements increasing efficacy, safety, and treatment adherence in AIT are needed to take the full advantage of the beneficial immunomodulation afforded by AIT. This issue of *Immunology and Allergy Clinics of North America* provides a wide-ranging review of the "art and science" of current AIT practice and a preview into possible future approaches.

Anna H. Nowak-Węgrzyn, MD
Icahn School of Medicine
at Mount Sinai
Jaffe Family Food Allergy Institute
One Gustave Levy Place, Box 1198
New York, NY 10029, USA

Linda S. Cox, MD
Department of Medicine
Nova Southeastern University Davie Florida
5333 North Dixie Highway
Ft. Lauderdale, FL 33334, USA

E-mail addresses:
anna.nowak-wegrzyn@mssm.edu (A.H. Nowak-Węgrzyn)
lindaswolfcox@msn.com (L.S. Cox)

REFERENCES

1. Lotvall J, Pawankar R, Wallace DV, et al. We call for iCAALL: International Collaboration in Asthma, Allergy and Immunology. J Allergy Clin Immunol 2012;129: 904–5.
2. Pearce N, Ait-Khaled N, Beasley R, et al. Worldwide trends in the prevalence of asthma symptoms: phase III of the International Study of Asthma and Allergies in Childhood (ISAAC). Thorax 2007;62:758–66.

3. Odhiambo JA, Williams HC, Clayton TO, et al. Global variations in prevalence of eczema symptoms in children from ISAAC Phase Three. J Allergy Clin Immunol 2009;124:1251–8.e23.
4. Strachan D, Sibbald B, Weiland S, et al. Worldwide variations in prevalence of symptoms of allergic rhinoconjunctivitis in children: the International Study of Asthma and Allergies in Childhood (ISAAC). Pediatr Allergy Immunol 1997;8: 161–76.
5. Schoenwetter WF, Dupclay L Jr, Appajosyula S, et al. Economic impact and quality-of-life burden of allergic rhinitis. Curr Med Res Opin 2004;20:305–17.
6. Prescott SL, Pawankar R, Allen KJ, et al. A global survey of changing patterns of food allergy burden in children. World Allergy Organ J 2013;6:21.
7. Jutel M, Agache I, Bonini S, et al. International consensus on allergy immunotherapy. J Allergy Clin Immunol 2015;136:556–68.
8. Cox L, Nelson H, Lockey R, et al. Allergen immunotherapy: a practice parameter third update. J Allergy Clin Immunol 2011;127:S1–55.
9. Cox L, Calderon MA. Subcutaneous specific immunotherapy for seasonal allergic rhinitis: a review of treatment practices in the US and Europe. Curr Med Res Opin 2010;26:2723–33.
10. Schofield AT. A case of egg poisoning. Lancet 1908;1:716.
11. Noon L. Prophylactic inoculation against hay fever. Lancet 1911;177:1572–3.
12. Blamoutier P, Blamoutier J, Guibert L. Traitement co-saisonnier de la pollinose par l'application d'extraits de pollens sur des quadrillages cutanés: Résultats obtenus en 1959 et 1961. Rev Fr d'Allerg;1:112–20.
13. Vallery-Radot P, Hangenau J. Asthme d'origine équine. Essai de désensibilisation par des cutiréactions répétées. Bull Soc Méd Hôp Paris 1921;45:1251–60.
14. Hurwitz SH. Medicine: seasonal hay fever-some problems in treatment. Cal West Med 1930;33:520–1.
15. Phillips EW. Relief of hay-fever by intradermal injections of pollen extract. J Am Med Assoc 1926;86:182–4.
16. Senti G, Prinz Vavricka BM, Erdmann I, et al. Intralymphatic allergen administration renders specific immunotherapy faster and safer: a randomized controlled trial. Proc Natl Acad Sci U S A 2008;105:17908–12.
17. Jutel M, Akdis CA. Immunological mechanisms of allergen-specific immunotherapy. Allergy 2011;66:725–32.
18. James LK, Shamji MH, Walker SM, et al. Long-term tolerance after allergen immunotherapy is accompanied by selective persistence of blocking antibodies. J Allergy Clin Immunol 2011;127:509–16.e1-5.
19. Francis JN, James LK, Paraskevopoulos G, et al. Grass pollen immunotherapy: IL-10 induction and suppression of late responses precedes IgG4 inhibitory antibody activity. J Allergy Clin Immunol 2008;121:1120–5.e2.
20. Wachholz PA, Soni NK, Till SJ, et al. Inhibition of allergen-IgE binding to B cells by IgG antibodies after grass pollen immunotherapy. J Allergy Clin Immunol 2003; 112:915–22.
21. Cameron LA, Durham SR, Jacobson MR, et al. Expression of IL-4, Cepsilon RNA, and iepsilon RNA in the nasal mucosa of patients with seasonal rhinitis: effect of topical corticosteroids. J Allergy Clin Immunol 1998;101:330–6.
22. Kucuksezer UC, Ozdemir C, Akdis M, et al. Mechanisms of immune tolerance to allergens in children. Korean J Pediatr 2013;56:505–13.
23. Radulovic S, Jacobson MR, Durham SR, et al. Grass pollen immunotherapy induces Foxp3-expressing CD4+ CD25+ cells in the nasal mucosa. J Allergy Clin Immunol 2008;121:1467–72, 72.e1.

24. Akdis CA, Blesken T, Akdis M, et al. Role of interleukin 10 in specific immunotherapy. J Clin Invest 1998;102:98–106.
25. Jutel M, Akdis M, Budak F, et al. IL-10 and TGF-beta cooperate in the regulatory T cell response to mucosal allergens in normal immunity and specific immunotherapy. Eur J Immunol 2003;33:1205–14.
26. Wambre E, DeLong JH, James EA, et al. Specific immunotherapy modifies allergen-specific CD4(+) T-cell responses in an epitope-dependent manner. J Allergy Clin Immunol 2014;133:872–9.e7.
27. Santos AF, James LK, Bahnson HT, et al. IgG4 inhibits peanut-induced basophil and mast cell activation in peanut-tolerant children sensitized to peanut major allergens. J Allergy Clin Immunol 2015;135:1249–56.
28. Vickery BP, Scurlock AM, Kulis M, et al. Sustained unresponsiveness to peanut in subjects who have completed peanut oral immunotherapy. J Allergy Clin Immunol 2014;133:468–75.
29. Shamji MH, Francis JN, Wurtzen PA, et al. Cell-free detection of allergen-IgE cross-linking with immobilized phase CD23: inhibition by blocking antibody responses after immunotherapy. J Allergy Clin Immunol 2013;132:1003–5.e1-4.
30. Muller U, Akdis CA, Fricker M, et al. Successful immunotherapy with T-cell epitope peptides of bee venom phospholipase A2 induces specific T-cell anergy in patients allergic to bee venom. J Allergy Clin Immunol 1998;101:747–54.
31. Patel D, Couroux P, Hickey P, et al. Fel d 1-derived peptide antigen desensitization shows a persistent treatment effect 1 year after the start of dosing: a randomized, placebo-controlled study. J Allergy Clin Immunol 2013;131:103–9.e1-7.
32. Worm M, Lee HH, Kleine-Tebbe J, et al. Development and preliminary clinical evaluation of a peptide immunotherapy vaccine for cat allergy. J Allergy Clin Immunol 2011;127:89–97. e1-14.
33. Jongejan L, van Ree R. Modified allergens and their potential to treat allergic disease. Curr Allergy Asthma Rep 2014;14:478.
34. Marth K, Focke-Tejkl M, Lupinek C, et al. Allergen peptides, recombinant allergens and hypoallergens for allergen-specific immunotherapy. Curr Treat Options Allergy 2014;1:91–106.
35. Bouchaud G, Braza F, Chesne J, et al. Prevention of allergic asthma through Der p 2 peptide vaccination. J Allergy Clin Immunol 2015;136:197–200.e1.
36. Smarr CB, Bryce PJ, Miller SD. Antigen-specific tolerance in immunotherapy of Th2-associated allergic diseases. Crit Rev Immunol 2013;33:389–414.
37. Creticos PS, Schroeder JT, Hamilton RG, et al. Immunotherapy with a ragweed-toll-like receptor 9 agonist vaccine for allergic rhinitis. N Engl J Med 2006;355:1445–55.
38. DuBuske LM, Frew AJ, Horak F, et al. Ultrashort-specific immunotherapy successfully treats seasonal allergic rhinoconjunctivitis to grass pollen. Allergy Asthma Proc 2011;32:239–47.
39. Mothes N, Heinzkill M, Drachenberg KJ, et al. Allergen-specific immunotherapy with a monophosphoryl lipid A-adjuvanted vaccine: reduced seasonally boosted immunoglobulin E production and inhibition of basophil histamine release by therapy-induced blocking antibodies. Clin Exp Allergy 2003;33:1198–208.
40. Drachenberg KJ, Wheeler AW, Stuebner P, et al. A well-tolerated grass pollen-specific allergy vaccine containing a novel adjuvant, monophosphoryl lipid A, reduces allergic symptoms after only four preseasonal injections. Allergy 2001;56:498–505.
41. Albin S, Nowak-Wegrzyn A. Potential treatments for food allergy. Immunol Allergy Clin North Am 2015;35:77–100.

42. Nadeau KC, Schneider LC, Hoyte L, et al. Rapid oral desensitization in combination with omalizumab therapy in patients with cow's milk allergy. J Allergy Clin Immunol 2011;127:1622–4.
43. Leonard SA, Caubet JC, Kim JS, et al. Baked milk- and egg-containing diet in the management of milk and egg allergy. J Allergy Clin Immunol Pract 2015;3:13–23 [quiz: 4].

Allergen Immunotherapy

History and Future Developments

Giovanni Passalacqua, MD*, Giorgio Walter Canonica, MD

KEYWORDS

- Subcutaneous immunotherapy • Sublingual immunotherapy • Indications
- Allergen immunotherapy • Efficacy • Safety • History • Molecular diagnosis

KEY POINTS

- Allergen immunotherapy (AIT) is a cornerstone in the management of respiratory allergic diseases because it is allergen-specific and immunomodulating and may affect disease progression.
- Sublingual immunotherapy (SLIT) represents a significant advance, offering patients an excellent safety and acceptance profile.
- From a historical viewpoint, in the past three decades there has been an impressive development in this form of treatment, which has lasted more than 100 years.
- The most promising fields are the use of AIT in food allergy, preventative effects, and improvement of routes of administration and standardization of extracts and protocols.

THE HISTORICAL PERSPECTIVE

AIT was introduced into clinical practice more than a century ago by Leonard Noon,[1] with the aim of "vaccinating" against hypothetical "aerogenic toxins". Despite the wrong rationale, the subcutaneous immunotherapy (SCIT) with pollen extracts was effective in reducing hay fever symptoms. Subsequently, the use of SCIT gradually increased and was progressively extended to other allergens. SCIT remained the only mode of administration for more than 70 years, and its use remained totally empirical until 1965 when IgE was discovered (**Fig. 1**).[2] The first randomized controlled study on AIT was published in 1954 by Frankland and Augustin,[3] and a few years later, Johnstone and Dutton[4] suggested that AIT could modify the natural history of respiratory allergy, but this fact was not considered for another 40 years. In 1978, the first randomized, double-blinded, placebo-controlled (RDBPC) trial with AIT for hymenoptera venom allergy appeared,[5] showing the superiority of purified venoms over whole-body

Allergy and Respiratory Diseases, IRCCS San Martino-IST, University of Genoa, Genoa 16132, Italy
* Corresponding author. Allergy and Respiratory Diseases, DIMI, Padiglione Maragliano, Largo Rosanna Benzi 10, Genoa 16132, Italy.
E-mail address: passalacqua@unige.it

Immunol Allergy Clin N Am 36 (2016) 1–12
http://dx.doi.org/10.1016/j.iac.2015.08.001
0889-8561/16/$ – see front matter © 2016 Elsevier Inc. All rights reserved.

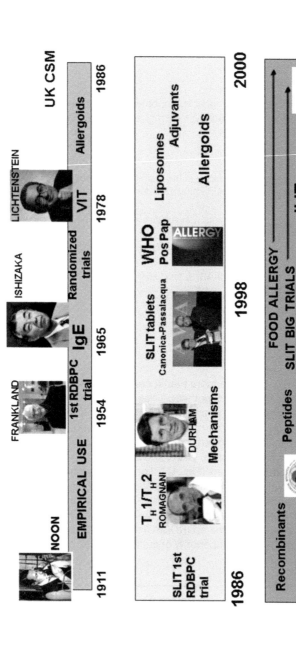

Fig. 1. The history of AIT. ARIA, Allergic Rhinitis and its Impact on Asthma; CSM, Committee on the Safety of Medicines; ITS, immunotherapies; Pos Pap, Position Paper; WAO, World Allergy Organization.

extracts. This was followed by numerous other trials substantially confirming the efficacy and safety of venom immunotherapy (VIT),[6] now widely used and well standardized in procedures.

It became clear that SCIT with respiratory allergens involved a certain risk of severe or even fatal adverse events,[7] as established by the UK Committee on Safety of Medicines in 1986.[8] Many AIT adverse events are due to human errors, but some adverse events are unpredictable and unavoidable.[9,10] This fact prompted the search for safer routes of administration of AIT. Among the proposed routes, SLIT rapidly established scientific credibility and soon remained the most viable alternative to SCIT. Other routes of administration had been proposed: the local bronchial during the 1950s, the local nasal during the 1970s, and the oral at the beginning of the 1980s (for review see Canonica and Passalacqua[11]). The results of clinical trials demonstrated that the efficacy of oral and bronchial routes is unproved and the risk/benefit ratio is unfavorable; thus, these routes of administration were abandoned, although there is currently a renewed interest for the oral route in the desensitization for food allergy. The local nasal immunotherapy proved effective for allergic rhinitis but because of the impractical administration technique, its clinical use rapidly declined.

The first randomized, double-blind, placebo-controlled trial with SLIT appeared in 1986,[12] and it was followed by numerous other trials which, although conducted in small samples, substantially confirmed the efficacy of this route. SLIT was first mentioned as a possible alternative to SCIT in a World Health Organization position paper[13] in 1998, and its role in clinical practice was confirmed in the subsequent official documents.[14,15]

In the meanwhile, other relevant advances about AIT appeared. Among the most important were the discovery of the helper T cell (T_H1/T_H2) system,[16] the re-evaluation of the role of IgG4 as blocking antibodies,[17] and the description of the regulatory T cells.[18,19] The improved knowledge of the mechanisms of action[20] allowed for the introduction of new approaches, such as the use of adjuvants (currently some products are commercialized) and the use of antigenic peptides and the recombinant allergens. In parallel, other specific aspects began to be investigated, namely the preventive effect on the development of asthma, that was demonstrated for both SCIT and SLIT, although in open trials and with relatively small populations.[21–23]

In the past decade, the efficacy of SLIT was clearly confirmed in the so-called big trials, which included hundreds (usually from 250 to more than 800) of patients. Some of those trials involved a dose-ranging design[24–29] and therefore allowed identification of the optimal maintenance dose for each of the tested products, at least for the relevant allergens (grass, mite, and ragweed). There is 1 single dose-ranging large trial performed with SCIT.[30] The introduction of fast-dissolving tablets for SLIT further improved the convenience. The official acceptance of SLIT culminated in 2009 with the publication of a first position paper prepared by the World Allergy Organization,[31] including 60 RDBPC trials, followed by an updated version with 77 trials.[32] During 2014, the Food and Drug Administration (FDA), approved 3 SLIT tablet products to be marketed in the United States.[33]

THE PRESENT SITUATION
Practical Aspects

To date, the practice of AIT is standardized, and numerous official position papers and practice parameters are available worldwide (**Table 1**). In particular, hymenoptera VIT, although there are different extracts available, is well standardized and its practice is uniform.

Table 1
The main position papers and guidelines on allergen immunotherapy

Year	Organization	Type of Allergen Immunotherapy	Reference
1998	World Health Organization	SCIT/SLIT	Ann Allergy Asthma Immunol 1998;81(5 Pt 1):401–5.
1998	European Academy of Allergy and Clinical Immunology	Non injection routes	Allergy 1998;53:933–44.
2001	Allergic Rhinitis and its Impact on Asthma	SCIT/SLIT	J Allergy Clin Immunol 2001;108(5 Suppl):S147–334.
2005	European Academy of Allergy and Clinical Immunology	VIT	Allergy 2005;60:1459–70.
2007	American Academy of Allergy, Asthma & Immunology/ American College of Allergy, Asthma & Immunology	SCIT	J Allergy Clin Immunol 2007;120(Suppl):S25–85, IV.
2008	Allergic Rhinitis and its Impact on Asthma	SCIT/SLIT	Allergy 2008;63(Suppl 86):8–160.
2009	World Allergy Organization	SLIT	Allergy 2009;64(Suppl 91):1–59.
2011	American Academy of Allergy, Asthma & Immunology/ American College of Allergy, Asthma & Immunology	SCIT	J Allergy Clin Immunol 2011;127(1 Suppl):S1–55.
2011	British Society for Allergy and Clinical Immunology	VIT	Clin Exp Allergy 2011;41:1201–20.
2013	World Allergy Organization	SLIT	World Allergy Organ J 2014;7(1):6.

At variance with SCIT, which is standardized in regimens and protocols, SLIT is affected by numerous variables. It can be administered as drops, monodose vials, or tablets and with variable timings and doses. In particular, the maintenance dose is strictly dependent on the method of standardization, which varies from one manufacturer to another. It is also true that all the products that are officially approved (eg, by the FDA or European Medicines Agency) display the content in micrograms of major allergen(s) per dose. At present, tablets that were first introduced in 1998 as monomeric allergoids[34] seem to represent the preferred SLIT formulation because of ease of use. Also, the time interval between each maintenance dose varies from one producer to another (daily, on alternate days, or twice weekly), but the current attitude is to prefer once-a-day administration.[35] For pollen allergies, the pre-coseasonal protocol is the most largely used, because its efficacy does not differ from that of the continuous (all-year-long) administration.[36,37]

Another important and unresolved debate concerns the use of mixtures of allergens. The European view is that AIT is given for no more than 3 allergens in the same patient,[38] and the dose of each allergen is given separately. In the United States, the usual practice is multiple allergens mixed together in a single preparation with attention to not mixing allergens that can degrade other proteins.[39] This dichotomy has cultural and historical reasons and is attributable to different concentrations of allergen solutions, which are usually higher in the United States products.[40] There are few well designed studies that have evaluated and demonstrated the efficacy of allergen mixtures.[41] On the contrary, it is now accepted that AIT with a single allergen is effective in polysensitized patients, provided the allergen chosen is responsible for the disease.[42]

In this regard, the molecular-based diagnosis (molecular allergy) has become a useful tool to refine the prescription of AIT (discussed later).

Other current fields of research in AIT are pharmacoeconomic aspects and adherence. Looking at the published studies, it seems that in the long term both SCIT and SLIT produce economic savings for both patients and health providers.[43] This is a result of a combination of reduced drug consumption and health care utilization (direct costs) as well as improvement of the quality of life (indirect costs). In contrast, adherence is a major problem, particularly for SLIT, which is self-administered: although structured studies provided overall favorable results in terms of adherence,[44] real-life adherence is reported to be poor,[45] although more frequent follow-up of patients seems to increase compliance.[46]

The Role of Molecular Diagnosis

The IgE response is not generically directed toward an allergenic source but rather to specific proteins (or epitopes) that are contained into the raw material. For instance, the IgE response to grasses is directed to a few proteins (Phl p 1, Phl p 5, an Phl p 6), and the IgE response to mite is specific for the proteins Der p 1, Der p 2, Der f 1, Der f 2, and so forth.[47] Such molecules are considered the genuine sensitizers. On the other hand, there are also highly conserved molecules, which are present in different species (eg, profilins, lipid transfer proteins, and storage proteins). They are called pan-allergens or cross-reacting proteins[47] and are often responsible for multiple positivities on the standard diagnostic tests. The relevant implications of pan-allergen sensistization may be particularly pertinent in AIT. The molecular diagnosis allows distinction of genuine sensitizations from the positivities due to cross-reacting proteins, thereby refining the choice of the allergen to be used for AIT.[48] Several studies have shown that molecular diagnosis significantly modifies the prescription of AIT in polysensitized patients.[49,50] Many individual recombinant or purified molecular components for skin testing and immunoassay are available. The multiplexed assay systems allow detecting, in a single analysis, specific IgE toward approximately 130 allergenic molecules.[51]

Regulatory Aspects

Despite the amount of clinical and mechanistic data on AIT and its consolidated use, the regulatory aspects (pharmacologic classification of products, marketing authorization, national and supranational approval, and deputy regulatory authorities) remain vague and largely differ among countries. Although in the United States and in the European Community (EC), there are well-defined regulatory authorities (FDA, European Medicines Agency, and Paul Ehrlich Institute), in other countries, such as those in Latin America, there is no uniform regulation.[52]

In Europe, numerous official regulatory documents have been released (for review, see Kaul and colleagues[53] and Bonini[54]), mainly concerning Good Manufacturing Practice. Those documents impose on all members of the EC specific standards for the production of allergen extracts. Within the EC, apart from a few exceptions, allergen extracts are considered named patient products (NPPs), prepared individually according to a physician's prescription, but almost all extracts are manufactured by industrial procedures. There is a general effort to abolish NPPs, with exceptions of rare allergens or special sensitization profiles, whereas a single preparation should contain in the near future only allergens from homologous groups (trees, grasses, mites, and so forth).[53] In addition, for each new product, a registration dossier (from phase I to III) is required for the marketing authorization.

THE NEAR FUTURE: PERSPECTIVES

After the introduction of SLI and recent mechanistic studies, there was an impressive advancement in the clinical research on AIT, and new opportunities rapidly appeared (**Table 2**).

The current indication for AIT is allergic rhinoconjunctvitis with/without allergic asthma and hymenoptera venom allergy,[13,38,39] but for the SLIT tablets approved in the United States, asthma is not an indication. In recent years, many clinical trials have suggested that the indications of AIT can be expanded. In terms of amount of clinical data, the most promising application is food allergy. As discussed elsewhere, there are many clinical trials proving the efficacy of desensitization for cow's milk, peanut, egg, and some other allergenic foods (for review, see Albin and Nowak-Węgrzyn[55] and Jones and colleagues[56]). Whether administration of gradually increasing amounts of an offending food represents a true AIT or, better, a simple oral induction of tolerance is still not clear. Latex allergy is not an official indication for AIT, although SLIT products are available and commercialized, based on the results of clinical trials.[57] The same is true for atopic dermatitis, for which both SLIT and SCIT were demonstrated partially effective, especially if a sensitization to dust mite is present.[58,59]

According to current knowledge, the goal of AIT is to take the allergen into contact with antigen-presenting cells to develop an immunologic desensitization. This contact can be achieved, in addition to the subcutaneous or sublingual route, by administering an allergen directly into lymph nodes. An innovative clinical trial[60] supports this rationale, showing that the intralymphatic immunotherapy (ILIT) requires much lower doses of allergen and fewer injections than the traditional SCIT modality, while maintaining the same efficacy.[61] Also, skin is a suitable site for presenting antigens. Epicutaneous

Table 2		
The future developments of allergen immunotherapy		
Advancement	**Description**	**Comments**
Route of administration	ILIT Epicutaneous Intradermal	The ILIT allows short courses of administration with lower doses of antigens. EPIT is totally noninvasive and, therefore, particularly suitable for children.
Formulation	Nanoparticles Slow release/mucoadhesive	At early experimental stage, with positive results in animal models
Extract + adjuvants	Bacteria-derived adjuvants DNA-derived adjuvants	Bacterial adjuvants already are commercially available for SCIT. Low number of injections. DNA-adjuvants are under experimental investigation, with a single human trial.
Peptides	Long or short peptides	Under investigation, mainly with Fel d 1 allergen
Molecules	Recombinant/highly purified sensitizing molecules	Some trials available in humans. The single molecules seem not to perform better than the crude extracts.
New indications	Food allergy Atopic dermatitis Latex allergy Nickel allergy?	Despite the existence of numerous trials with positive results, none of these indications is currently approved for clinical practice. Latex SLIT products are commercialized and used.

immunotherapy (EPIT) has been tested with good results for both aeroallergens and food allergens.[62] This route seems particularly suitable in children.

The products commonly used for AIT are crude extracts, derived from allergenic sources (eg, grasses, ragweed, and mite) and, therefore, contain allergenic and nonallergenic proteins and carbohydrates or lipids. They can be improved by adding adjuvants, which provide an additional enhancement of the T_H1 response. An organic adjuvant usually stimulates the Toll-like receptors of the innate immunity, which in turn favor the T_H1-oriented response.[63] Monophosphoryl lipid A, derived from the cell wall of *Salmonella minnesota*, is proved safe, effective, and capable of reducing the number of injections and the dose of allergen and is currently commercialized. Many other trials with adjuvants are ongoing.[64] Also prokaryote-derived oligodenucleotides (CpG sequences) are good adjuvants, because they stimulate the Toll-like receptor 9, with a consequent increase in the T_H1 response. Early trials using this approach provided encouraging results,[65,66] but the clinical research remains at the initial stage. Another possible manipulation is to give only allergenic fragments, instead of the whole allergenic proteins, because antigen-presenting cells recognize linear sequences; this is called peptide-based immunotherapy. There are so far some promising studies with mixtures of peptides from cat and mite allergens.[67]

As discussed previously, it is now possible to synthesize (or highly purify) the most relevant single sensitizer proteins. Thus, if identifying for each subject the allergenic components toward which IgE are directed, it would be possible to vaccinate only with those molecules (tailored immunotherapy). Nonetheless, it seems that the use of single genuine sensitizers does not perform better than the raw extracts.[68] In addition, the sensitization profile, dissected by molecular diagnosis, is largely variable in each subject.[69] Finally, the regulatory authorities require a registration trial for each single allergen product. All those considerations, despite the intriguing immunologic rationale, make this approach so far unfeasible.

UNMET NEEDS AND CONCLUDING REMARKS

The body of evidence for SCIT, SLIT, and VIT is robust, as a result of an abundance of clinical and mechanistic trials. Nonetheless, some points to be clarified, and debated aspects are still present (**Table 3**). For instance, there is a large variability in administration schedules, dosages, and duration of SLIT, which is marketed in numerous countries as NPPs. Only a few products represent exceptions—Oralair (Stallergenes, Antony Cedex, France), Grazax or Grastek (ALK-Abelló, Copenhagen, Denmark), and Ragwitek (Merck, Whitehouse Station, New Jersey)—because they are registered and marketed as pharmaceutical products.[70] Another critical point is the standardization. Almost all AIT vaccines commercialized are standardized either biologically or immunologically, based on in-house references. Thus, extracts are labeled in units that differ from one manufacturer to another, and comparison among trials and products is only rarely possible.

Again, there is no experimental demonstration that the regimens used are the most appropriate and cost effective, that the pre-coseasonal regimen for pollen allergens is better, or that for perennial allergens a continuous treatment is needed. There is no rigorous study on the optimal duration of an AIT treatment; thus, the current suggestions are only empirical or based on sparse clinical data.[71,72] The same is partly true for the preventative effect, demonstration of which is based on only 3 controlled open trials.[73] Finally, there is great heterogeneity in clinical trials, which affects the robustness of meta analyses, and the reporting of trials is unsatisfactory.[74,75]

Table 3
Main unmet needs in allergen immunotherapy

Problem	Comments
Optimal maintenance dose	Currently fixed only for grass, ragweed, and mite (soluble tablets, single products). The optimal maintenance dose remains to be clearly defined for the remaining relevant allergens.
Optimal maintenance regimen	Is it needed to give an all-year treatment of perennial allergens? Is the pre-coseasonal (coseasonal regimen) more convenient than the continuous one?
Use of multiple allergens	Few studies are available. The efficacy of multiple allergens, even mixed, is poorly defined.
Adherence	Data about adherence with AIT differ among controlled and real-life studies.
Standardization of extracts	The use of in-house references and of different units make the clinical studies not comparable. The potency of the extracts is still yet not well defined.
Standardization of studies	Large heterogeneity among clinical trials (design, patients' selection, dose, duration, and analysis). Reporting is still poor.
Duration and long-lasting effect	The optimal duration of an AIT course is not experimentally defined. The demonstration of long-lasting and preventive effects relies on a small number of clinical trials

AIT is a cornerstone in the management of respiratory allergic diseases because it is allergen-specific and immunomodulating and may affect disease progression. SLIT has represented a significant advance, offering patients an excellent safety and acceptance profile. From a historical viewpoint, in the past 3 decades there has been an impressive development of this form of treatment, which has lasted more than 100 years. The most promising fields are the use of AIT in food allergy, the preventative effects, and the improvement of the routes of administration and standardization of extracts and protocols.

REFERENCES

1. Noon L. Prophylactic inoculation against hay fever. Lancet 1911;i:1572–3.
2. Johansson SGO. The History of IgE: from discovery to 2010. Curr Allergy Asthma Rep 2011;11:173–7.
3. Frankland AW, Augustin R. Prophylaxis of summer hay fever and asthma: controlled trial comparing crude grass pollen extracts with isolated main protein component. Lancet 1954;1:1055–7.
4. Johnstone DE, Dutton A. The value of hyposensitization therapy for bronchial asthma in children: a 14-year study. Pediatrics 1968;42:793–802.
5. Hunt KJ, Valentine MD, Sobotka AK, et al. A controlled trial of immunotherapy in insect hypersensitivity. N Engl J Med 1978;299:157–61.
6. Lockey RF, Turkeltaub PC, Olive ES, et al. The Hymenoptera venom study. III: safety of venom immunotherapy. J Allergy Clin Immunol 1990;86:775–80.
7. Lockey RF, Benedict LM, Turkeltaub PC, et al. Fatalities associated with immunotherapy and skin testing. J Allergy Clin Immunol 1987;79:660–4.
8. Committee on the Safety of Medicines. CSM update. Desensitizing vaccines. Br Med J 1986;293:948.

9. Aaronson DW, Gandhi TK. Incorrect allergy injections: allergists' experiences and recommendations for prevention. J Allergy Clin Immunol 2004;113:1117–21.
10. Windom HH, Lockey RF. An update on the safety of specific immunotherapy. Curr Opin Allergy Clin Immunol 2008;8:571–6.
11. Canonica GW, Passalacqua G. Noninjection routes for immunotherapy. J Allergy Clin Immunol 2003;111:437–48.
12. Scadding K, Brostoff J. Low dose sublingual therapy in patients with allergic rhinitis due to dust mite. Clin Allergy 1986;16:483–91.
13. Bousquet J, Lockey R, Malling HJ. World Health Organization Position Paper. Allergen immunotherapy: therapeutical vaccines for allergic diseases. J Allergy Clin Immunol 1998;102(4 Pt 1):558–62.
14. Bousquet J, Van Cauwenberge P. Allergic rhinits and its impact on asthma. J Allergy Clin Immunol 2001;108(5 Supp):S146–50.
15. Bousquet J, Khaltaev N, Cruz AA, et al. Allergic Rhinitis and its Impact on Asthma (ARIA) 2008 update (in collaboration with the World Health Organization, GA2LEN and AllerGen). Allergy 2008;63(Suppl 86):8–160.
16. Romagnani S. Human TH1 and TH2 subsets: doubt no more. Immunol Today 1991;12:256–7.
17. James LK, Shamji MH, Walker SM, et al. Long-term tolerance after allergen immunotherapy is accompanied by selective persistence of blocking antibodies. J Allergy Clin Immunol 2011;127:509–16.
18. Rolland JM, Gardner LM, O'Hehir RE. Functional regulatory T cells and allergen immunotherapy. Curr Opin Allergy Clin Immunol 2010;10(6):559–66.
19. Böhm L, Maxeiner J, Meyer-Martin H, et al. IL-10 and regulatory T cells cooperate in allergen-specific immunotherapy to ameliorate allergic asthma. J Immunol 2015;194(3):887–97.
20. Fujita H, Soyka MB, Akdis M, et al. Mechanisms of allergen-specific immunotherapy. Clin Transl Allergy 2012;2(1):2.
21. Möller C, Dreborg S, Ferdousi HA, et al. Pollen immunotherapy reduces the development of asthma in children with seasonal rhinoconjunctivitis (the PAT-study). J Allergy Clin Immunol 2002;109:251–6.
22. Novembre E, Galli E, Landi F, et al. Coseasonal sublingual immunotherapy reduces the development of asthma in children with allergic rhinoconjunctivitis. J Allergy Clin Immunol 2004;114:851–7.
23. Marogna M, Tomassetti D, Bernasconi A, et al. Preventive effects of sublingual immunotherapy in childhood: an open randomized controlled study. Ann Allergy Asthma Immunol 2008;101:206–11.
24. Durham SR, Yang WH, Pedersen MR, et al. Sublingual immunotherapy with once-daily grass-allergen tablets: a randomised controlled trial in seasonal allergic rhinoconjunctivitis. J Allergy Clin Immunol 2006;117:802.
25. Didier A, Malling HJ, Worm M, et al. Optimal dose, efficacy, and safety of once daily sublingual immunotherapy with a 5-grass pollen tablet for seasonal allergic rhinitis. J Allergy Clin Immunol 2007;120:1338.
26. Creticos PS, Maloney J, Bernstein DI, et al. Randomized controlled trial of a ragweed allergy immunotherapy tablet in North American and European adults. J Allergy Clin Immunol 2013;131:1342–9.
27. Nolte H, Hébert J, Berman G, et al. Randomized controlled trial of ragweed allergy immunotherapy tablet efficacy and safety in North American adults. Ann Allergy Asthma Immunol 2013;110:450–5.
28. Mosbech H, Deckelmann R, de Blay F, et al. Standardized quality (SQ) house dust mite sublingual immunotherapy tablet (ALK) reduces inhaled corticosteroid

use while maintaining asthma control: a randomized, double-blind, placebo-controlled trial. J Allergy Clin Immunol 2014;134:568–75.

29. Bergmann KC, Demoly P, Worm M, et al. Efficacy and safety of sublingual tablets of house dust mite allergen extracts in adults with allergic rhinitis. J Allergy Clin Immunol 2014;133:1608–14.

30. Frew A, Powell JL, Corrigan CJ, et al. Efficacy and safety of specific immuno-therapy with SQ allergen extract in treatment-resistant seasonal allergic rhinocon-junctivitis. J Allergy Clin Immunol 2006;117:319–25.

31. Canonica GW, Bousquet J, Casale T, et al. Sub-lingual immunotherapy World Al-lergy Organization Position Paper 2009. Allergy 2009;64(Supp 91):1–59.

32. Canonica GW, Cox L, Pawankar R, et al. Sublingual immunotherapy: World Allergy Organization position paper 2013 update. World Allergy Organ J 2014;7(1):6.

33. Thompson CA. Sublingual immunotherapy approved for grass pollen allergies. Am J Health Syst Pharm 2014;71:770.

34. Passalacqua G, Albano M, Fregonese L, et al. Randomised controlled trial of local allergoid immunotherapy on allergic inflammation in mite-induced rhinocon-junctivitis. Lancet 1998;351:629–32.

35. Lombardi C, Incorvaia C, Braga M, et al. Administration regimens for sublingual immunotherapy to pollen allergens: what do we know? Allergy 2009;64:849–54.

36. Pajno GB, Caminiti L, Crisafulli G, et al. Direct comparison between continuous and coseasonal regimen for sublingual immunotherapy in children with grass al-lergy: a randomized controlled study. Pediatr Allergy Immunol 2011;22:803–7.

37. Stelmach I, Kaluzińska-Parzyszek I, Jerzynska J, et al. Comparative effect of pre-coseasonal and continuous grass sublingual immunotherapy in children. Allergy 2012;67:312–20.

38. Zuberbier T, Bachert C, Bousquet PJ, et al. GA^2 LEN/EAACI pocket guide for allergen-specific immunotherapy for allergic rhinitis and asthma. Allergy 2010; 65:1525–30.

39. Cox L, Nelson H, Lockey R, et al. Allergen immunotherapy: a practice parameter third update. J Allergy Clin Immunol 2011;127(1 Suppl):S1–55.

40. Cox L, Jacobsen L. Comparison of allergen immunotherapy practice patterns in the United States and Europe. Ann Allergy Asthma Immunol 2009;103: 451–9.

41. Nelson HS. Multiallergen immunotherapy for allergic rhinitis and asthma. J Allergy Clin Immunol 2009;123:763–9.

42. Malling HJ, Montagut A, Melac M, et al. Efficacy and safety of 5-grass pollen sub-lingual immunotherapy tablets in patients with different clinical profiles of allergic rhinoconjunctivitis. Clin Exp Allergy 2009;39:387–93.

43. Hankin CS, Cox L. Allergy immunotherapy: what is the evidence for cost saving? Curr Opin Allergy Clin Immunol 2014;14:363–70.

44. Senna G, Ridolo E, Calderon M, et al. Evidence of adherence to allergen-specific immunotherapy. Curr Opin Allergy Clin Immunol 2009;9:544–8.

45. Senna G, Lombardi C, Canonica GW, et al. How adherent to sublingual immuno-therapy prescriptions are patients? The manufacturers' viewpoint. J Allergy Clin Immunol 2010;126:668–9.

46. Savi E, Peveri S, Senna G, et al. Causes of SLIT discontinuation and strategies to improve the adherence: a pragmatic approach. Allergy 2013;68:1193–5.

47. Sastre J. Molecular diagnosis in allergy. Clin Exp Allergy 2010;40:1442–60.

48. Canonica GW, Ansotegui IJ, Pawankar R, et al. A WAO - ARIA - GA^{2}LEN consensus document on molecular-based allergy diagnostics. World Allergy Or-gan J 2013;6(1):17.

49. Sastre J, Landivar ME, Ruiz-García M, et al. How molecular diagnosis can change allergen-specific immunotherapy prescription in a complex pollen area. Allergy 2012;67(5):709–11.
50. Passalacqua G, Melioli G, Bonifazi F, et al. The additional values of microarray allergen assay in the management of polysensitized patients with respiratory allergy. Allergy 2013;68:1029–33.
51. Melioli G, Passalacqua G, Canonica GW. Novel in silico technology in combination with microarrays: a state-of-the-art technology for allergy diagnosis and management? Expert Rev Clin Immunol 2014;10:1559–61.
52. Baena Cagnani CE, Larenas D, Sisul C, et al. Allergy training and immunotherapy in Latin America: results of a regional overview. Ann Allergy Asthma Immunol 2013;111(5):415–9.
53. Kaul S, May S, Lüttkopf D, et al. Regulatory environment for allergen-specific immunotherapy. Allergy 2011;66:753–64.
54. Bonini S. Regulatory aspects of allergen-specific immunotherapy: europe sets the scene for a global approach. World Allergy Organ J 2012;5:120–3.
55. Albin S, Nowak-Węgrzyn A. Potential treatments for food allergy. Immunol Allergy Clin North Am 2015;35:77–100.
56. Jones SM, Burks AW, Dupont C. State of the art on food allergen immunotherapy: oral, sublingual, and epicutaneous. J Allergy Clin Immunol 2014; 133:318–23.
57. Nettis E, Delle Donne P, Di Leo E, et al. Latex immunotherapy: state of the art. Ann Allergy Asthma Immunol 2012;109:160–5.
58. Gendelman SR, Lang DM. Sublingual immunotherapy in the treatment of atopic dermatitis: a systematic review using the GRADE system. Curr Allergy Asthma Rep 2015;15:498–507.
59. Bae JM, Choi YY, Park CO, et al. Efficacy of allergen-specific immunotherapy for atopic dermatitis: a systematic review and meta-analysis of randomized controlled trials. J Allergy Clin Immunol 2013;132:110–7.
60. Senti G, Prinz Vavricka BM, Erdmann I, et al. Intralymphatic allergen administration renders specific immunotherapy faster and safer: a randomized controlled trial. Proc Natl Acad Sci U S A 2008;105:17908–12.
61. Witten M, Malling HJ, Blom L, et al. Is intralymphatic immunotherapy ready for clinical use in patients with grass pollen allergy? J Allergy Clin Immunol 2013; 132:1248–52.
62. Senti G, von Moos S, Tay F, et al. Determinants of efficacy and safety in epicutaneous allergen immunotherapy: summary of three clinical trials. Allergy 2015. http://dx.doi.org/10.1111/all.12600.
63. Aryan Z, Holgate ST, Radzioch D, et al. A new era of targeting the ancient gatekeepers of the immune system: toll-like agonists in the treatment of allergic rhinitis and asthma. Int Arch Allergy Immunol 2014;164:46–63.
64. Pfaar O, Cazan D, Klimek L, et al. Adjuvants for immunotherapy. Curr Opin Allergy Clin Immunol 2012;12:648–57.
65. Creticos PS, Schroeder JT, Hamilton RG, et al. Immune Tolerance Network Group Immunotherapy with a ragweed-toll-like receptor 9 agonist vaccine for allergic rhinitis. N Engl J Med 2006;355:1445–55.
66. Creticos PS, Chen YH, Schroeder JT. New approaches in immunotherapy: allergen vaccination with immunostimulatory DNA. Immunol Allergy Clin North Am 2004;24:569–81.
67. Créticos PS. Advances in synthetic peptide immuno-regulatory epitopes. World Allergy Organ J 2014;7(1):30.

68. Pauli G, Larsen TH, Rak S, et al. Efficacy of recombinant birch pollen vaccine for the treatment of birch-allergic rhinoconjunctivitis. J Allergy Clin Immunol 2008; 122:951–60.

69. Tripodi S, Frediani T, Lucarelli S, et al. Molecular profiles of IgE to Phleum pratense in children with grass pollen allergy: implications for specific immunotherapy. J Allergy Clin Immunol 2012;129:834–9.

70. Passalacqua G, Canonica GW. Sublingual immunotherapy: focus on tablets. Ann Allergy Asthma Immunol 2015;115(1):4–9.

71. Nakonechna A, Hills J, Moor J, et al. Grazax sublingual immunotherapy in pre-co-seasonal and continuous treatment regimens: is there a difference in clinical efficacy? Ann Allergy Asthma Immunol 2015;114:73–4.

72. Stelmach I, Sobocińska A, Majak P, et al. Comparison of the long-term efficacy of 3- and 5-year house dust mite allergen immunotherapy. Ann Allergy Asthma Immunol 2012;109:274–8.

73. Passalacqua G. Specific immunotherapy: beyond the clinical scores. Ann Allergy Asthma Immunol 2011;107:401–6.

74. Casale TB, Canonica GW, Bousquet J, et al. Recommendations for appropriate sublingual immunotherapy clinical trials. J Allergy Clin Immunol 2009;124: 665–70.

75. Bousquet PJ, Calderon MA, Demoly P, et al. The Consolidated Standards of Reporting Trials (CONSORT) Statement applied to allergen-specific immunotherapy with inhalant allergens: a Global Allergy and Asthma European Network (GA(2)LEN) article. J Allergy Clin Immunol 2011;127:49.

Subcutaneous Immunotherapy and Sublingual Immunotherapy
Comparative Efficacy, Current and Potential Indications, and Warnings—United States Versus Europe

Harold S. Nelson, MD[a],*, Melina Makatsori, MD[b], Moises A. Calderon, MD, PhD[b,c]

KEYWORDS

- SCIT • SLIT • AIT • Immunotherapy • Allergic rhinitis • Allergic asthma

KEY POINTS

- Both SCIT and SLIT are of proven effectiveness in the treatment of allergic rhinitis and allergic asthma with some evidence that both are helpful in selected patients with atopic dermatitis.
- Both SCIT and SLIT modify the underlying immune process resulting in persisting benefits after cessation of treatment.
- The lesser frequency and severity of systemic reactions allows SLIT to be home administered after the first dose.
- SCIT but not SLIT has been demonstrated to be effective using mixtures of multiple, unrelated allergen extracts.
- Although good comparative studies are lacking, available evidence suggests superior short-term efficacy with SCIT.

Disclosure statement: Consultant to Merck and Circassia; grant support from Circassia (H.S. Nelson). Lecture Fees: ALK, Stallergenes, Merck, and Allergopharma, Consultancy Fees: ALK, Stallergenes, Merck, and Hal Allergy (M.A. Calderon).
[a] National Jewish Health and University of Colorado Denver School of Medicine, 1400 Jackson Street, Denver, CO 80206, USA; [b] Section of Allergy and Clinical Immunology, Royal Brompton and Harefield Hospital NHS Trust, National Heart and Lung Institute, Imperial College London, Dovehouse Street, London SW3 6LY, UK; [c] Department of Internal Medicine and Allergy, Faculty of Medicine, University of Costa Rica, San Jose, Costa Rica, USA
* Corresponding author.
E-mail address: nelsonh@njhealth.org

Immunol Allergy Clin N Am 36 (2016) 13–24
http://dx.doi.org/10.1016/j.iac.2015.08.005
0889-8561/16/$ – see front matter © 2016 Elsevier Inc. All rights reserved.

immunology.theclinics.com

INTRODUCTION

Allergy immunotherapy (AIT) was introduced more than a century ago by Leonard Noon as a treatment of allergic rhinitis caused by grass pollen.[1] The subcutaneous injection of increasing and eventually maintenance doses of various seasonal and perennial allergens (subcutaneous immunotherapy [SCIT]) came into widespread use for the treatment of allergic rhinitis, allergic asthma, and allergic sensitization to insect venoms. Although of proved efficacy in allergic rhinitis,[2] allergic bronchial asthma,[3] and Hymenoptera venom sensitivity,[4] the use of SCIT for allergic rhinitis and allergic asthma has been limited by the long course of treatment requiring numerous visits to physicians' offices, by cost, and to some extent by the possibility of local and systemic reactions to the injections. As a result, alternative methods of AIT have been investigated that aim to avoid these SCIT drawbacks by greatly shortening the course of treatment, allowing home administration, or both. Alternatives under active investigation include administering the extract in a limited number of injections intralymphatically, applying the extracts incorporated in a patch (epicutaneously), or treating with modified extracts that are hypoallergenic so that a few large doses are sufficient for a course of treatment.[5] The one alternative approach that has been studied the most and is now an accepted clinical practice is to administer the extract as a liquid or a rapidly dissolving tablet (sublingual immunotherapy [SLIT]).

SCIT and SLIT are directed at modifying immune response to the allergen to which the patient is sensitized and therefore the responses to treatment with these two approaches share many features (**Box 1**). Both have been shown to be effective for allergic rhinitis and allergic asthma and with some support for use in selected patients with atopic dermatitis.[6] There are defined effective doses for most standardized extracts for SCIT, for the SLIT tablets, and liquid ragweed. The sequence of immunologic

---

Box 1
Shared and differing attributes of SCIT and SLIT

Shared

1. Effective treatment of allergic rhinitis and allergic asthma, with some support for use in selected patients with atopic dermatitis.

2. Defined optimal doses for standardized liquid extracts (SCIT) and SLIT tablets.

3. Underlying immunologic response
   a. Early induction of regulatory T cells.
   b. Later immunodeviation from a predominant Th2 to a Th1 response to the administered allergen.
   c. Suppression of Th17 responses.

4. Evidence for disease modification
   a. Reduction of additional sensitization in monosensitized patients.
   b. Reduction in the development of asthma in patients with allergic rhinitis.
   c. Persisting benefit after stopping an effective course of treatment.

Differing

1. Frequency and severity of systemic reactions (favors SLIT).

2. Clinical efficacy with Hymenoptera venom (favors SCIT) and for food allergy (favors SLIT).

3. Lack of defined optimal doses for SLIT liquids (favors SCIT).

4. Proven effectiveness of multiple allergen mixes with SCIT but not SLIT (favors SCIT).

5. Clinical efficacy (currently available studies favor SCIT).

responses is the same, irrespective of the route of administration and not surprising, similar disease modification has been demonstrated with both forms of AIT. However, there are differences between the two approaches. The most important is the greatly reduced likelihood of SLIT producing systemic reactions, a feature that allows home administration and thus overcomes one of the major drawbacks of SCIT. Although there is some evidence of efficacy of SLIT with Hymenoptera venom[7,8] it is not yet clinically recommended. SLIT for food allergy is still under investigation, but studies show some efficacy and good safety,[9] whereas SCIT for food allergy proved too dangerous for clinical application.[10] There are major drawbacks for SLIT in regard to dosing. First is the lack of defined dosing for most liquid extracts,[11] and second is the lack of demonstrated efficacy of SLIT with multiple allergen mixtures.[12] Finally, there is the question of relative clinical efficacy, with the currently available data favoring SCIT.[13,14]

CLINICAL EFFICACY

Meta-analyses (**Table 1**) and more recent systematic reviews[17,18] have confirmed the effectiveness of SCIT and SLIT for treatment of allergic rhinitis and allergic asthma. Meta-analyses using the Cochrane collaboration method demonstrated significant efficacy of SCIT for symptoms of and medication use for allergic rhinitis[2] and allergic asthma.[3] Similar analyses demonstrated significant improvement in symptoms and medication use for allergic rhinitis[15] with SLIT. Trends favored SLIT for the treatment of allergic asthma[16] but the results did not reach statistical significance perhaps because of a smaller number of studies in this category. A more recent systematic review[17] reported high-quality support for the effectiveness of SCIT for reduction of asthma symptoms and medication use and for reduction of rhinoconjunctivitis symptoms and moderate evidence to support reduction in rhinoconjunctivitis medication use. A companion systematic review of SLIT[18] showed high-quality evidence for reduction in asthma symptoms and moderate-quality evidence to support the reduction in symptoms of rhinoconjunctivitis and in the use of rescue medications for rhinitis and asthma.

A meta-analysis of eight randomized, controlled trials provided moderate support of the use of house dust mite (HDM) extracts by SCIT and SLIT for selected patients with atopic dermatitis who are HDM sensitive. Two of the studies coadministered other allergens.[6]

Table 1
Cochrane collaboration and Cochrane method meta-analyses of SCIT and SLIT for allergic rhinitis and allergic asthma

Study	Method	Number of Studies	Allergens	Number of Subjects	Symptoms Scores SMD (95% CI)	Medication Scores SMD (95% CI)
Allergic rhinitis						
Calderon et al,[2] 2007	SCIT	51	S	2871	−0.73 (−0.97 to −0.50)	−0.57 (−0.82 to −0.33)
Radulovic et al,[15] 2011	SLIT	49	S and P	4589	−0.49 (−0.64 to −0.34)	−0.32 (−0.43 to −0.21)
Allergic asthma						
Abramson et al,[3] 2010	SCIT	88	S and P	3459	−0.59 (−0.83 to −0.35)	−0.53 (−0.80 to −0.27)
Calamita et al,[16] 2006	SLIT	25	S and P	1706	−0.38 (−0.79 to 0.03)	−0.91 (−1.94 to 0.12)

Abbreviations: CI, confidence interval; P, perennial; S, seasonal; SMD, standardized mean difference.

SCIT with Hymenoptera venom[4] and whole body extract of imported fire ants[19] is well accepted as effective in treating sensitivity to the stings of these insects. There are limited data for treating Hymenoptera venom sensitivity with SLIT and it is currently not recommended.[7,8]

An attempt was previously made to treat patients with anaphylactic sensitivity to peanuts with injections of peanut extract. Although the level of sensitivity could be reduced, even the maintenance injections resulted in repeated systemic reactions, so the treatment was deemed a failure.[9] Treatment of hazel nut[20] and peanut allergy[10] with SLIT has been reported to increase tolerance with an acceptable rate of systemic reactions. This treatment, although promising, must still be considered experimental.

THE IMMUNOLOGIC RESPONSE

The immunologic response to AIT involves changes in the allergen-specific humoral response, with ultimately a shift from allergen-specific IgE to IgG, and particularly IgG4 responses. These changes in antibody response result from underlying changes in the T-cell responses and it is the latter that are thought to mediate the clinical improvement and ultimate disease modification. The early T-cell response is an increase in allergen-specific regulatory T cells (Tregs) secreting interleukin-10 and sometimes also transforming growth factor-β.[21,22] There is evidence that this initial increase in Tregs is not fully sustained and after one or several years of continuing treatment, the Treg numbers are reduced and the predominant pattern is a shift, again allergen specific, from a T helper (Th) 2 to a Th1 cytokine responses.[22–24] This is known as immune deviation. This same evolving pattern of immunologic changes has been demonstrated with SCIT and SLIT.

Studies with SCIT and SLIT have also demonstrated a suppressive effect of AIT on Th17 cells and their cytokines. After 2 years of SCIT with HDM extract in adults, Th2 and Th17 cells were reduced, Th1 and Tregs were increased, and, strikingly, the decrease in plasma interleukin-17 levels correlated highly with the decrease in symptoms of perennial rhinitis.[25] Sublingual administration of Dermatophagoides farinae extract for 48 weeks to children with allergic asthma also decreased symptoms, increased Tregs, and decreased Th17 cells in the peripheral blood.[26]

DISEASE MODIFICATION

Pharmacotherapy of allergic rhinitis and asthma can to variable degrees control the symptoms but has no effect on the underlying immunologic mechanisms and hence has no persisting benefit after treatment is stopped.

Because SCIT and SLIT have been shown to modify the underlying immunologic process, not unexpectedly both modify the progression of the respiratory allergy and impart persistent benefits after stopping a successful course of treatment. Studies with SCIT[27] and SLIT[28] have shown marked reduction in the development of new sensitivities in monosensitized patients, not only during the period of treatment, but also persisting for several years after its discontinuation. Similarly, when children having only allergic rhinitis were treated with either SCIT[29] or SLIT[30] there was a significant reduction in the number who developed asthma. Again this protection has been shown to persist for years after treatment was discontinued.

The most important effect of modifying the underlying immune process, however, is the persisting remission in symptoms that results from 3 to 5 years of treatment with proved effect doses of allergens. Relapses do occur but some patients may experience long-lasting improvement.[28,31]

DEFINED OPTIMAL DOSES

Ideally, to define optimal doses for AIT a dose-response study should be conducted that includes a low dose that is suboptimal and a high dose that either shows no improvement over a lower dose or is associated with unacceptable side effects. It is surprising how seldom such studies of AIT have been conducted. Nevertheless, there are SCIT studies in which a lower, less-effective dose has been included with standardized extracts of ragweed, timothy grass, HDM, cat, and dog.[32] The effective dose of major allergen was within a fairly narrow range (7–19 µg). This suggests that at least for other pollen and animal dander extracts similar doses are likely to be effective. SCIT with *Alternaria* in this dose range has also proved to be effective.[33]

Studies of rapidly dissolving SLIT tablets for grass, ragweed, and HDM have included dose-ranging studies and higher dose safety studies. Thus optimal doses for safety and efficacy have been identified for these tablets.[34–37] For SLIT with liquid extracts, the same studies have not been conducted. Dose-response studies were conducted with liquid ragweed extract[38] and a birch/hazel nut/alder mix.[39] However, the two doses studied in these studies differed by nearly 10-fold leaving unanswered whether intermediated doses might be equally effective. A two-dose study of HDM liquid SLIT found a daily dose of 1 µg Der f 1 ineffective but a dose of 70 µg per day reduced bronchial allergen sensitivity.[40] Again, the efficacy of intermediate doses was not investigated. Except for these studies, there seems to be little scientific basis for many of the SLIT-liquid doses used, and effective treatment has been reported with a 500-fold range in doses.[11]

MULTIALLERGEN ALLERGY IMMUNOTHERAPY

There is evidence to support the administration of mixtures of unrelated allergens by SCIT. Four double-blind, randomized, controlled studies have shown clinical efficacy, two in patients with allergic rhinitis[41,42] and two in patients with allergic asthma.[43,44] Two studies are often cited in questioning the efficacy of multiallergen SCIT, but both have fatal flaws in their design. One compared the response to AIT in patients monosensitized to grass who received only grass extract with that in patients polysensitized to grass and other pollens who received a mixture of these pollens This was not a randomized study and immunoblotting revealed that the polysensitized subjects were sensitized to more than twice as many proteins in the grass extract as were those monosensitized, thus providing an alternative explanation for their less robust response to AIT.[45] The second, a study of SCIT for polysensitized children with perennial asthma, used largely seasonal allergens for treatment and omitted cat, dog, cockroach, and mouse extracts from the treatment all of which have been shown to be important allergens for perennial asthma in children. Thus the failure of AIT in this study may have been caused by omission of most of the relevant allergens from the treatment extract.[46]

Although there have been many more recent studies of SLIT than SCIT, all but three have used monotherapy. Two studies used two differing extracts that were administered simultaneously from separate dispensers.[47,48] Both demonstrated efficacy for the two components. Only the third examined truly multiallergen immunotherapy.[12] In this study, subjects were randomized to receive SLIT with a timothy grass extract (containing 19 µg at maintenance), the same dose of timothy grass combined with nine other pollen extracts at 1:100 wt/vol, or placebo. After 10 months the subjects receiving timothy grass monotherapy had significant favorable changes compared with those receiving placebo in titrated skin prick tests, titrated nasal challenge, and timothy grass–specific IgG4, whereas those receiving the same dose of timothy grass combined with other pollen extracts differed significantly from placebo only for titrated skin prick tests and then to a lesser degree than those receiving timothy grass mono-therapy. To date, this is the only study conducted of multiallergen SLIT and raises unanswered questions regarding its suitability for clinical use.

SAFETY
Local Reactions

In a systematic review of 61 randomized controlled trials including 3577 subjects local reactions to subcutaneous injections were reported in 5% to 58% of patients and 3% to 10% of injections.[17] Local reactions may be immediate or delayed and vary from small areas of redness and itching to delayed larger swellings. Although patients with frequent large reactions are at increased risk for systemic reactions, individual large local reactions do not predict a systemic reaction and therefore should not be a basis for dose adjustment.[49]

Local or application site reactions are common with SLIT. Among 3314 adults in the timothy grass SLIT tablet studies, 67% receiving active and 24% receiving placebo re-ported treatment-related adverse events.[50] In the active treatment group this included oral pruritus in 27%, throat irritation in 23%, ear pruritus in 13%, and mouth edema in 11%. With the highest dose ragweed SLIT tablet, local reactions were less common than with the timothy grass SLIT tablet: oral pruritus 4%, throat irritation 11%, ear pru-ritus 6%, and mouth edema 7%.[51] Except for localized swelling, which tends to develop only after several days of treatment, the local symptoms occur with the first dose, persist a few minutes, and cease occurring within the first 2 weeks of treatment.

Systemic Reactions

The incidence of systemic reactions to SCIT varies widely with the different doses used in treatment. In the American Academy of Allergy, Asthma and Immunology/American College of Allergy, Asthma and Immunology online surveillance survey, data were submitted by allergists on the outcome from 23.3 million injection visits be-tween 2008 and 2012.[52] Systemic reactions were reported as occurring in 9.4 per 10,000 injection visits and of these 0.4 per 10,000 were severe. There was one fatality reported during these 4 years. Although systemic reactions, even anaphylaxis, can occur with SLIT, there have as yet been no reported fatal or near fatal reactions.[53] A review of studies with the timothy grass SLIT tablet reported eight systemic reactions, all mild or moderate, in 2115 subjects receiving active treatment for a systemic reac-tion rate of 0.38% of patients.[54] In the United States, the Food and Drug Administra-tion's Prescribing Information Guides mandate that recipients of a prescription for SLIT tablets also receive a prescription for and be instructed in the use of autoinject-able epinephrine. The relevance of this mandate was examined in a review of phase III trials conducted with timothy grass SLIT tablets, short ragweed SLIT tablets, and HDM SLIT tablets, which including 8804 subjects treated for 24 to 18 months.[55] Thirteen pa-tients received epinephrine injections for SLIT-tablet related symptoms (8 local and 5 systemic reactions). Four of the systemic reactions occurred with the first dose admin-istered in the physician's office. The fifth occurred on day 6. None of the 5 systemic reactions was considered serious. Patients self-administered epinephrine 8 times, only 3 of which were for SLIT-tablet related symptoms.

COMPARATIVE EFFICACY OF SUBCUTANEOUS IMMUNOTHERAPY AND SUBLINGUAL IMMUNOTHERAPY

In the absence of definitive head-to-head trials, an indirect approach has been used to compare the clinical efficacy of SCIT and SLIT. The reduction in symptoms or medication use with SCIT or SLIT has been compared with that with placebo by meta-analyses and then the standardized mean differences (SMD) from the meta-analyses for SCIT and SLIT have been compared. In the four meta-analyses cited in **Table 2**, the reduction in SMD for symptom scores and medication use in allergic rhinitis was –0.73 and –0.57, respectively, in 51 studies of SCIT and –0.49 and –0.32 in 49 studies for SLIT. This has been interpreted as suggesting a greater efficacy for SCIT. The results for asthma cannot be compared, because the SMD for symptoms and medication with SLIT did not differ significantly from placebo. The studies in these meta-analyses pre-date the large randomized, placebo-controlled trials conducted with SLIT tablets. A meta-analysis, limited to commercially available preparations, that separately assessed the response to SCIT, SLIT tablets, and SLIT drops for grass allergic rhinitis found no significant difference between SCIT and SLIT tablets for symptoms or medication use. The results with SLIT drops were much more variable and for symptom reduction the drops were less effective than the tablets.[56]

Direct head-to-head comparisons between SCIT and SLIT are clearly preferable to indirect comparisons of the response to placebo, but there have been problems with the quality of most of these studies. Eleven direct comparisons, all randomized and four placebo-controlled, were reviewed.[13] Overall, the results with SCIT were superior to those with SLIT when compared with placebo and in some instances when compared with each other (see **Table 2**). The problem with interpretation of these studies is that often the SLIT was low-dose, but more important in 9 of 11 studies SLIT was administered every other day or two or three times a week and daily SLIT has been shown to be more effective than thrice weekly even when the latter delivered a higher cumulative dose.[57] There is one study that seems to overcome the shortcomings of many of the previous studies. Optimal treatment regimens for ALK-Abello' sub-cutaneous (100,000 Standardized Quality units every 2 months) and sublingual timothy grass tablets (75,000 Standardized Quality units daily) were directly compared in a 15-month study, which also included an untreated group.[14] Outcomes included allergen nasal challenges, specific IgG4, and several functional assays of the IgG4 response. The nasal challenge was significantly different from placebo at 3 and

Table 2
Comparative response to SCIT and SLIT in 11 randomized studies

Statistically Significant Differences	Symptoms	Medication	Skin Prick Tests	IgG4	Bronchia/ Nasal Allergen Challenges	Miscellaneous
None reported	3 studies	7 studies	6 studies	4 studies	8 studies	9 studies
SCIT only greater than placebo	3 studies	2 studies	3 studies	6 studies	1 study	1 study
Both greater than placebo	4 studies	2 studies	2 studies	None	1 study	1 study
SLIT only greater than placebo	None	None	None	None	None	None
SCIT greater than SLIT	1 study	None	None	1 study	1 study	None

Adapted from Nelson HS. Subcutaneous immunotherapy versus sublingual immunotherapy: which is more effective? J Allergy Clin Immunol Pract 2014;1:144–9.

15 months in the SCIT-treated group, but not in those receiving SLIT. Both AIT approaches induced significant humoral responses compared with placebo, but those with SCIT were of approximately twice the magnitude of those with SLIT.

WARNINGS

There are still some unanswered questions regarding SCIT and SLIT and their use. These include the optimal length of treatment and clarifications regarding absolute and relative contraindications.

It is also important to consider that clinical efficacy of AIT is greatly affected by patient adherence to the treatment regimen. Several studies have suggested that in clinical practice, adherence to SLIT over the intended 3-year course of treatment is variable.[58] SCIT also suffers from less than optimal adherence; however, because it is administered by allergists nonadherence does not go undetected. Furthermore, adherence to SCIT seems to be better than to SLIT. In a pharmacy data study from the Netherlands, 23% completed a projected 3-year course of SCIT compared with only 7% of those prescribed SLIT. The mean duration of persistence with treatment was 1.7 years for SCIT but only 0.6 years for SLIT.[59] However, more research is required to identify reasons for lack of adherence and develop strategies to improve this.

Different regulatory laws in Europe and the United States currently govern registration and licensing of immunotherapy products.[60] In Europe, regulatory guidance has been published in the form of directives 2001/20/EC and 2003/63/EC, which outlined specifications for allergen products in diagnostics and immunotherapy. The bodies involved in the regulatory process are the European Medicines Agency and national health authorities of the individual member states. A marketing authorization for allergen products is achievable by national or centralized procedures and through mutual recognition.[61] However, there is a need for simplifying and standardizing the process to make immunotherapy more widely available.

In the United States, approval of allergen extracts is the responsibility of the Division of Bacterial, Parasitic and Allergenic Products of the US Food and Drug Administration. Allergenic Products Advisory Committee meetings were held in December 2013 and January 2014 to consider the safety and efficacy of the two grass and one ragweed SLIT tablets.[62] All three products received approval in April 2014. The prescribing information for all three products contains a Black Box warning that the tablets can cause life-threatening allergic reactions; should not be administered to patients with severe, unstable, or uncontrolled asthma; require the patient to be observed for 30 minutes following the initial dose; that patients be provided with and trained in the use of autoinjectable epinephrine; and list patients for whom the treatment may not be appropriate because of underlying medical conditions that reduce their ability to survive and serious allergic reaction or who may be unresponsive to epinephrine or inhaled bronchodilators.[63–65] Additional contraindications listed are a history of any severe systemic allergic reaction or any severe local reaction to SLIT, or a history of eosinophilic esophagitis.

REFERENCES

1. Noon L. Prophylactic inoculation against hay fever. Lancet 1911;i:1572.
2. Calderon MA, Alves B, Jacobson M, et al. Allergy injection immunotherapy for sessional allergic rhinitis. Cochrane Database Syst Rev 2007;(1):CD001936.
3. Abramson MJ, Puy RM, Winer JM. Injection allergen immunotherapy for asthma. Cochrane Database Syst Rev 2010;(8):CD001186.

4. Boyle RJ, Elremelli M, Hockenhull J, et al. Venom immunotherapy for preventing allergic reactions to insect stings. Cochrane Database Syst Rev 2012;(10):CD0008838.
5. Nelson HS. New forms of allergy immunotherapy for rhinitis and asthma. Allergy Asthma Proc 2014;35:271–7.
6. Bae JM, Choi YY, Park CO, et al. Efficacy of allergen-specific immunotherapy for atopic dermatitis: a systematic review and meta-analysis of randomized controlled trials. J Allergy Clin Immunol 2013;132:110–7.
7. Patriarca G, Nucera E, Roncallo C, et al. Sublingual desensitization in patients with wasp venom allergy: preliminary results. Int J Immunopathol Pharmacol 2008;21:669–77.
8. Severino MG, Cortellinii G, Bonadonna P, et al. Sublingual immunotherapy for large local reactions caused by honeybee sting: a double-blind, placebo-controlled trail. J Allergy Clin Immunol 2008;122:4–8.
9. Nelson HS, Lahr J, Rule R, et al. Treatment of anaphylactic sensitivity to peanuts by immunotherapy with injections of aqueous peanut extract. J Allergy Clin Immunol 1997;99:744–51.
10. Burks AW, Wood RA, Jones SM, et al. Sublingual immunotherapy for peanut allergy: long-term follow-up of a randomized multicenter trial. J Allergy Clin Immunol 2015;135(5):1240–8.e1-3.
11. Cox L, Larenas Linnemann D, Nolte H, et al. Sublingual immunotherapy: a comprehensive review. J Allergy Clin Immunol 2006;117:1021–35.
12. Amar SM, Harbeck RJ, Sills M, et al. Response to sublingual immunotherapy with grass pollen extract: monotherapy versus combination in a multiallergen extract. J Allergy Clin Immunol 2009;124:150–6.
13. Nelson HS. Subcutaneous immunotherapy versus sublingual immunotherapy: which is more effective? J Allergy Clin Immunol Pract 2014;1:144–9.
14. Aasbjerg K, Backer V, Lund G, et al. Immunological comparison of allergen immunotherapy tablet treatment and subcutaneous immunotherapy against grass allergy. Clin Exp Allergy 2014;44:417–28.
15. Radulovic S, Wilson D, Calderon M, et al. Systematic reviews of sublingual immunotherapy (SLIT). Allergy 2011;66:740–52.
16. Calamita Z, Saconato H, Pela AB, et al. Efficacy of sublingual immunotherapy in asthma: systematic review of randomize-clinical trials using the Cochrane collaboration method. Allergy 2006;61:1162–72.
17. Erekosima N, Suarez-Cuervo C, Ramanathan M, et al. Effectiveness of subcutaneous immunotherapy for allergic rhinoconjunctivitis and asthma: a systematic review. Laryngoscope 2014;124:616–27.
18. Lin SY, Erekosima N, Kim JM, et al. Sublingual immunotherapy for the treatment of allergic rhinoconjunctivitis and asthma: a systematic review. JAMA 2013;309:1278–88.
19. Tankersley MS. The stinging impact of the imported fire ant. Curr Opin Allergy Clin Immunol 2008;8:354–9.
20. Enrique E, Pineda F, Malek T, et al. Sublingual immunotherapy for hazelnut food allergy: a randomized, double-blind, placebo-controlled study with a standardized hazelnut extract. J Allergy Clin Immunol 2005;116:1073–9.
21. Jutel M, Akdis MN, Budak F, et al. IL-10 and TGF-beta cooperate in the regulatory T cell response to mucosa allergen in normal immunity and specific immunotherapy. Eur J Immunol 2003;33:1205–14.
22. Bohle B, Kinaciyan T, Gerstmayr M, et al. Sublingual immunotherapy induces IL-10-producing T regulator cells, allergen-specific T-cell tolerance, and immune deviation. J Allergy Clin Immunol 2007;120:707–13.

23. Mobs C, Ipsen H, Mayer L, et al. Birch pollen immunotherapy results in long-term loss of Bet v 1-specific Th2 responses, transient TR1 activation, and synthesis of IgE-blocking antibodies. J Allergy Clin Immunol 2012;130:1108–16.

24. Hamid QA, Schotman E, Jacobson MR, et al. Increases in IL-121 messenger RNA+ cells accompany inhibition of allergen-induced late skin responses after successful grass pollen immunotherapy. J Allergy Clin Immunol 1997;99:454–60.

25. Li CW, Lu HG, Chen DH, et al. In vivo and in vitro studies of Th17 response to specific immunotherapy in house dust mite-induced allergic rhinitis patients. PLoS One 2014;9:e91950.

26. Tian M, Wang Y, Lu Y, et al. Effects of sublingual immunotherapy for *Dermatophagoides farina* on Th17 cells and CD4+CD25+ regularity T cells in peripheral blood of children with allergic asthma. Int Forum Allergy Rhinol 2014;4(5):371–5.

27. Pajno G, Barberio G, De Luca F, et al. Prevention of sensitization in asthma children monosensitized to house dust mite by specific immunotherapy. A six-year follow-up study. Clin Exp Allergy 2001;31:1392–7.

28. Marogna M, Spadolini I, Massolo A, et al. Long-lasting effects of sublingual immunotherapy according to its duration: a 15-year prospective study. J Allergy Clin Immunol 2010;126:969–75.

29. Jacobsen L, Niggemann B, Dreborg S, et al. Specific immunotherapy has long-term preventive effect of seasonal and perennial asthma: 10-year follow-8 on the PAT study. Allergy 2007;62:943–8.

30. Marogna M, Tomassetti D, Bernasconi A, et al. Preventive effects of sublingual immunotherapy in childhood: an open randomized controlled study. Ann Allergy Asthma Immunol 2008;101:206–11.

31. Ebner C, Kraft D, Ebner H. Booster Immunotheapy (BIT). Allergy 1994;49:38–42.

32. Nelson HS. Subcutaneous immunotherapy for optimal effectiveness. Immunol Allergy Clin North Am 2011;31:211–26.

33. Kuna P, Kaczmarek J, Kupczyk M. Efficacy and safety of immunotherapy for allergies to *Alternaria alternata* in children. J Allergy Clin Immunol 2011;127:502–8.

34. Didier A, Malling HJ, Worm M, et al. Optimal dose, efficacy, and safety of once-daily sublingual immunotherapy with a 5-grass pollen tablet for seasonal allergic rhinitis. J Allergy Clin Immunol 2007;120:1338–45.

35. Durham SR, Yang WH, Pedersen MR, et al. Sublingual immunotherapy with once-daily grass allergen tablets: a randomized controlled trial in seasonal allergic rhinoconjunctivitis. J Allergy Clin Immunol 2006;117:802–9.

36. Nolte H, Amar N, Bernstein DI, et al. Safety and tolerability of a short ragweed sublingual immunotherapy tablet. Ann Allergy Asthma Immunol 2014;113:93–100.

37. Nolte H, Malone J, Nelson HS, et al. Onset and dose-related efficacy of house dust mite sublingual immunotherapy tablets in an environmental exposure chamber. J Allergy Clin Immunol 2015;135(6):1494–501.

38. Skoner D, Gentile D, Bush R, et al. Sublingual immunotherapy in patients with allergic rhinoconjunctivitis caused by ragweed pollen. J Allergy Clin Immunol 2010;125:660–6.

39. Valovirta E, Jacobsen L, Ljorring C, et al. Clinical efficacy and safety of sublingual immunotherapy with tree pollen extract in children. Allergy 2006;61:117–83.

40. Bush RK, Swenson C, Fahlberg B, et al. House dust mite sublingual immunotherapy results of a US trial. J Allergy Clin Immunol 2011;127:974–81.

41. Lowell FC, Franklin W. A double-blind study of the effectiveness and specificity of injection therapy in ragweed hay fever. N Engl J Med 1965;271:675–9.

42. Franklin W, Lowell FC. Comparison of two dosages of ragweed extract in the treatment of pollenosis. JAMA 1967;201:915–7.

43. Johnstone DE, Dutton A. The value of hyposensitization therapy for bronchial asthma in children: a 14-year study. Pediatrics 1968;42:793–802.
44. Reid MJ, Moss RB, Hsu YP, et al. Seasonal asthma in northern California: allergic causes and efficacy of immunotherapy. J Allergy Clin Immunol 1986; 78:590–600.
45. Bousquet J, Becker WM, Heijjaoui A, et al. Differences in clinical and immunologic reactivity of patients allergic to grass pollen and to multiple pollen species. II. Efficacy of double-blind placebo-controlled specific immunotherapy with standardized extracts. J Allergy Clin Immunol 1991;88:43–53.
46. Adkinson NR Jr, Eggleston PA, Eney D, et al. A controlled trial of immunotherapy for asthma in allergic children. N Engl J Med 1997;336:324–31.
47. Marogna M, Spadolini I, Massolo A, et al. Effects of sublingual immunotherapy for multiple or single allergens in polysensitized patients. Ann Allergy Asthma Immunol 2007;98:274–80.
48. Swamy RS, Reshamwala N, Hunter T, et al. Epigenetic modifications and improved regulatory T-cell function in subjects undergoing dual sublingual immunotherapy. J Allergy Clin Immunol 2012;130:215–24.
49. Lieberman P, Tankersley M. Significance of large local reactions that occur during allergen immunotherapy. J Allergy Clin Immunol Pract 2015;3:310–1.
50. Nelson HS. Oral/sublingual phlegm pretense grass tablet (grazax/grastek) to treat allergic rhinitis in the USA. Expert Rev Clin Immunol 2014;10:1437–51.
51. Creticos PS, Maloney J, Bernstein DI, et al. Randomized controlled trial of a ragweed allergy immunotherapy tablet in North American and European adults. J Allergy Clin Immunol 2013;131:1342–9.
52. Epstein TG, Liss GM, Murphy-Berendts K, et al. AAAAI/ACAAI surveillance study of subcutaneous immunotherapy, years 2008-2012: an update on fatal and nonfatal systemic allergic reactions. J Allergy Clin Immunol Pract 2014;2:161–7.
53. Canonica GW, Cox L, Pawankar R, et al. Sublingual immunotherapy: World Allergy Organization position paper 2013 update. World Allergy Organ J 2014; 7(1):6. Available at: http://www.waojournal.org/content/7/1/6.
54. Maloney J, Durham S, Skoner D, et al. Safety of sublingual immunotherapy timothy grass tablet in subjects with allergic rhinitis with or without conjunctivitis and history of asthma. Allergy 2015;70:302–9.
55. Maloney J, Casale TB, Lockey RF, et al. Epinephrine use in clinical trials of sublingual immunotherapy tablets for treatment of allergic rhinitis with/without conjunctivitis. Abstract presentation, Annual Meeting, American Academy of Allergy, Asthma and Immunology. Houston, Texas, 20–24 February 2015.
56. Nelson H, Carter S, Allen-Ramey F, et al. Network meta-analysis shows commercialized subcutaneous and sublingual grass products have comparable efficacy. J Allergy Clin Immunol Pract 2015;3(2):256–66.e3.
57. Bordignon V, Parmiani S. Variation of the skin endpoint in patients treated with sublingual specific immunotherapy. J Investig Allergol Clin Immunol 2003;13: 170–6.
58. Senna G, Caminati M, Canonica GW. Safety and tolerability of sublingual immunotherapy in clinical trials and real life. Curr Opin Allergy Clin Immunol 2013; 13(6):656–62.
59. Kiel MA, Roder E, van Wijk RG, et al. Real-life compliance and persistence among users of subcutaneous and sublingual allergen immunotherapy. J Allergy Clin Immunol 2013;132:353–60.e2.
60. Bonini S. Regulatory aspects of allergen-specific immunotherapy: Europe sets the scene for a global approach. World Allergy Organ J 2012;5(10):120–3.

61. Kaul S, May S, Lüttkopf D, et al. Regulatory environment for allergen-specific immunotherapy. Allergy 2011;66(6):753–64.
62. Available at: http://www.fda.gov/Advisory. Accessed June 15, 2015.
63. Prescribing information GRASTEK. Whitehouse Station (NJ): Merck Sharp & Dohme Corporation; 2014.
64. Prescribing information RAGWITEK. Whitehouse station (NJ): Merck Sharp & Dohme Corporation; 2014.
65. Prescribing information ORALAIR. Lenoir (NC): Greer Laboratories; 2014.

Novel Delivery Routes for Allergy Immunotherapy

Intralymphatic, Epicutaneous, and Intradermal

Gabriela Senti, MD[a], Thomas M. Kündig, MD[b],*

KEYWORDS

- Epicutaneous allergy immunotherapy • Transcutaneous allergy immunotherapy
- Respiratory allergy • Food allergy

KEY POINTS

- Subcutaneous immunotherapy deposits the allergen in the fat rather than stimulating the immune system. Therefore numerous injections are required to ameliorate symptoms.
- The ideal route for AIT contains dense APCs to enhance effects but few mast cells and blood vessels to reduce local and systemic side effects.
- Lymph nodes contain the highest density of APCs with only few mast cells and blood vessels, making ILIT highly efficient.
- Similar to mucosal epithelium, the epidermis has dense APCs with no mast cells or blood vessels. EPIT should therefore be as safe as SLIT.
- Allergen administered to the epidermis rapidly diffuses to the dermis. We expect diffusion toward blood vessels to be safer than injection into vascularized tissue.

INTRODUCTION

Today, up to 30% of the population in industrialized countries suffers from IgE-mediated allergies, which have therefore become an important socioeconomic burden. Pharmacotherapy with local and oral antihistamines and nasal corticosteroids ameliorates IgE-mediated symptoms efficiently,[1] but cannot stop progression of the causative immunologic imbalance, and therefore progression of rhinoconjunctivitis to asthma and to cross-reactive food allergies. The only disease-modifying treatment that also has a long-term effect is allergy immunotherapy (AIT).[1,2] More than a century ago, Noon[3] introduced subcutaneous allergen-specific immunotherapy (SCIT). However, despite its high efficacy and long-lasting symptom amelioration, less than 4% of allergy patients choose to undergo such AIT, mainly because it has two major

[a] Clinical Trials Center, University Hospital Zurich, Moussonstrasse 2, Zurich 8044, Switzerland;
[b] Department of Dermatology, University Hospital Zurich, Gloriatrasse 31, Zurich 8091, Switzerland
* Corresponding author.
E-mail address: thomas.kuendig@usz.ch

Immunol Allergy Clin N Am 36 (2016) 25–37
http://dx.doi.org/10.1016/j.iac.2015.08.006
0889-8561/16/$ – see front matter © 2016 Elsevier Inc. All rights reserved.

disadvantages. First, AIT is time consuming because it requires 30 to 70 visits to a medical practice. Second, subcutaneous allergen injections are associated with local and systemic allergic side effects.[4–6] Thinking generally, these two drawbacks may be addressed by the following strategies.

Measures to Reduce the Number of Allergen Administrations in Allergy Immunotherapy

To reduce the number of injections, immunogenicity of the allergen administration has to be enhanced, for instance by increasing the allergen dose. AIT has a clear dose effect,[7] but allergic side effects strongly limit the dose that can be given. Making allergens hypoallergenic by chemical modification to allergoids,[8] recombinant modification,[9] or by using non-IgE-binding peptides[10–12] may also permit increased allergen doses, but the modifications often negatively affect allergen immunogenicity. A reduction of injection numbers may also be achieved by replacing the classically used aluminum salts with a more T helper (Th) 1 promoting adjuvant, such as the Toll-like receptor (TLR) ligands CpG oligoeoxynucleotide[13] or monophosphoryl lipid A, a detoxified version of lipopolysaccharide.[14–16] The number of injections may also be reduced by changing to a more efficient route of allergen delivery. Ideally this route would be characterized by a high density of antigen-presenting cells (APCs). The latter are present at highest density in secondary lymphatic organs, such as lymph nodes, and indeed, when allergen is intralymphatically, the number of injections could be reduced to only three.[17–20] Intralymphatic immunotherapy (ILIT) is discussed in detail later.

Measures to Improve Allergy Immunotherapy Safety

To improve safety of AIT, inadvertent allergen delivery to the blood vasculature must be avoided, ideally by delivery of the allergen to nonvascularized tissue. Sublingual immunotherapy (SLIT) fulfills this criterion, because allergen is delivered to the oral mucosa, which is covered by a multilayered epithelium. The allergen diffuses down into deeper mast cell containing layers, and this diffusion is responsible for the frequently observed local oral side effects.[21,22] The layer below the epithelium also contains a high density of blood vessels. However, it seems that when there is no microtrauma to this vasculature, it rarely happens that significant amounts of allergen reach the circulation, for which reason SLIT has proved safe in terms of systemic allergic side effects.[21,22] The same should hold true for epicutaneous allergy immunotherapy (EPIT), where allergen is administered to the nonvascularized epidermis. An advantage of EPIT over SLIT is that keratinocytes can additionally be activated by physical irritation, such as abrasion or adhesive tape stripping, or also by adding adjuvants.[23] Such epithelial irritation increases the expression of proinflammatory cytokines, such as interleukin (IL)-1a, IL-6, and tumor necrosis factor-α, thus skewing the immune response toward Th1,[24] and also activating Langerhans cells (LCs). Therefore, EPIT may not only reduce side effects by minimizing the risk of allergen inadvertently reaching the blood vasculature, but also shorten treatment duration by increasing immunogenicity. We have also observed that epicutaneously administered allergen rapidly and efficiently diffuses down into the dermis.[25] Interestingly, another group has recently demonstrated that intradermal administration of even extremely low doses of allergen was able to induce tolerance.[26]

INTRALYMPHATIC ALLERGEN-SPECIFIC IMMUNOTHERAPY

The concept that antigen localization is a key parameter that determines the strength of the immune response was pioneered in Zurich by the work of Rolf Zinkernagel,

Nobel laureate in Medicine. The concept is simple: because an immune response requires the interaction of three important immune cells (antigen-presenting dendritic cells [DCs], T cells, and B cells), a reaction is more likely to happen at a site where high numbers of these three cell types are present, that is, in lymphoid organs, such as lymph nodes, whereas antigens outside of these organs are largely ignored by the immune system.[27] A great number of preclinical and clinical studies have demonstrated the potency of intralymphatic administration of peptides, proteins, DNA, RNA, bacteria, viruses, or DCs, as comprehensively reviewed.[19,28–31] Studies in mice have demonstrated that ILIT with bee venom allergens, food allergens, such as ovalbumin, and allergen extracts from grass pollen, birch pollen, and cat dander stimulates robust antiallergic and protective B- and T-cell immune responses.[32–36] Compared with SCIT, ILIT enhanced efficiency of immunization, inducing allergen-specific IgG2a antibody responses 10 to 20 times higher with only 0.1% of the allergen dose.[34] Moreover, ILIT enhanced IL-2, interferon-γ, IL-4, and IL-10 secretion when compared with SCIT,[34] suggesting that ILIT did not polarize the response but generated overall stronger responses. The reason seems to be simple: ILIT delivers approximately 100-times more allergen to lymph nodes than any other route, as demonstrated in biodistribution studies after ILIT in mice[34] and humans.[29,30] Because adverse side effects are related to the allergen dose, ILIT would be expected to have a lower incidence of adverse effects.

In a Swiss trial, 165 patients with grass pollen–induced rhinoconjunctivitis were randomized to receive either 54 SCIT injections with pollen extract over 3 years (cumulative allergen dose 4,031,540 subcutaneous units) or three ILIT injections over 2 months (totally 3000 subcutaneous units).[17] Intralymphatic injections were also measured to less painful than venous punctures. Increased nasal tolerance was demonstrated in the ILIT group within 4 months of treatment. Tolerance was long lasting and comparable with SCIT-treated patients who received 3 years of treatment. ILIT ameliorated symptoms, enhanced compliance, reduced skin prick test reactivity, decreased specific serum IgE, and was associated with fewer adverse events than SCIT. Whereas we compared ILIT with SCIT with grass pollen extract, a Swedish study confirmed the positive results of ILIT in a double-blind placebo-controlled trial.[37] By the same token, in a randomized, placebo-controlled, and double-blinded trial, we demonstrated efficacy of ILIT with major histocompatibility complex class II–targeting cat dander allergen (MAT-Fel d 1).[18] Three monthly injections with MAT-Fel d 1 improved nasal allergen tolerance and stimulated significant regulatory T-cell responses and IgG4 without any significant adverse events.

Time Interval Between Injections in Intralymphatic Immunotherapy

In a double-blind placebo-controlled clinical trial, Witten and colleagues[38] found that three or six intralymphatic grass pollen injections induced some desired immunologic changes, such as a regulatory T-cell response and elevated IgG4, but that there was no improvement of clinical parameters, such as symptom or medication scores; if anything, symptoms tended to worsen. The authors concluded that their data were conflicting with ours[17,18] and that of Hylander and colleagues.[20] However, Witten and colleagues[38] used a different protocol. We and Hylander and colleagues[20] used a 4-week time interval between injections, whereas Witten and colleagues[38] used only 2 weeks. It is well known from vaccine immunology[39] that shortening the time interval from 4 to 2 weeks interferes with memory B-cell formation and affinity maturation, which both require phases where only small amounts of antigen are present in lymph follicles. Small amounts enable competition for the antigen, which again positively selects for high-affinity memory B cells. Similar effects are postulated for affinity and functionality of the T-cell response.[40] As a recent example, Patel and colleagues[12] observed that four peptide injections (Cat-PAD) with monthly intervals successfully tolerized patients, whereas eight injections with 2-week intervals did not work. Furthermore, shortening the time interval between injections is known to polarize the immune response toward Th2,[41] which may explain why Witten and colleagues[38] observed symptoms to worsen.

We are meanwhile aware of clinical trials being performed in several centers across the world, such as in Sweden, Norway, Denmark, China, South Korea, and the United States (Cardell LO, Hoffmann HJ, Weinfeld D, Patterson A, personal communication, 2015). In thin-spread societies, such as in Scandinavia, patients have to travel long distances to get immunotherapy, so that a reduction in the number of shots would also have a direct socioeconomic impact, such as less days off from school and work.

Another consideration that speaks for ILIT is that in SCIT and SLIT, nearly half of patients do not finish the whole treatment course.[42] In our trials with ILIT, we observed that everybody who started treatment received all three injections and thus the full treatment course. In conclusion, AIT directly into a subcutaneous lymph node, instead of subcutaneous administration, is (1) practically painless, (2) readily feasible, (3) reduces the required allergen dose and therefore improves safety, (4) reduces the number of allergen injections to three, (5) reduces the treatment duration from 3 years to 2 months, and (6) enhances patient compliance.

ALLERGEN-SPECIFIC EPICUTANEOUS IMMUNOTHERAPY

The epicutaneous route of allergen administration is by no means new. In fact, as a route of vaccination it was used in ancient times, and Edward Jenner applied cow pox virus to scarified human skin. Forgotten for a long time, at the beginning of the twenty-first century epicutaneous vaccination had its second revival, driven by the increasing interest in novel needle-free vaccination routes. Epicutaneous vaccination against *Escherichia coli*–induced traveler's diarrhea made the first step.[43] Animal models have so far shown success against infection with *Helicobacter pylori*,[44] influenza virus,[45] and diphtheria toxin.[46] The protective mechanism in all of these applications relies on induction of humoral immunity dominated by IgG1 and IgA. Studies testing epicutaneous vaccination against human immunodeficiency virus also found induction of mucosal cytotoxic T cells together with secretion of mucosal antibodies.[47] Another field of application is cancer immunotherapy. Several studies revealed promising results with EPIT against skin cancer based on induction of potent CD8[+] T-cell responses.[48,49] Not only has EPIT been demonstrated to induce effector T-cell responses, but also suppressive T-cell responses when EPIT was used to inhibit experimental allergic encephalomyelitis.[50,51]

History of Epicutaneous Immunotherapy in Allergy

EPIT as a treatment of allergies was introduced already in 1917 when Besredka showed that EPIT induced specific antibodies.[52] The first case study on successful EPIT was reported in 1921 by Vallery-Radot and Hangenau,[53] who found that allergen administration onto scarified skin reduced systemic allergic symptoms in patients allergic to horses. A decade later, when the risk of suffering a "pollen shock" during AIT was recognized to be a considerable danger of subcutaneously administering allergen to highly sensitized patients, a method called intradermal allergen specific immunotherapy received much attention.[54,55] Based on the observation that patients with hay fever occasionally experienced symptom amelioration after "intradermal pollen tests," Phillips[55] started to treat highly sensitive patients and patients requesting coseasonal treatment by administration of pollen extract. Strikingly, such intradermal AIT proved to be safe and highly efficacious leading to symptom relief after administration of only three doses.[55] At the same time, Ramirez treated patients allergic to grass pollen with a method he called "cuti-vaccination," which consisted of administration of pollen extract on scarified skin.[52] Based on these results, it was suggested in the 1930s already that the subcutaneous route might not be optimal for AIT.[54]

Between 1950 and 1960, French allergologists revisited EPIT.[52,56,57] Pautrizel and coworkers[57] administered the allergen extract onto slightly rubbed epidermis. Even though the reported results were excellent, a large number of applications were necessary until symptom relief was observed. In contrast, Blamoutier and coworkers[52,56] applied the allergen drops onto heavily scarified skin: "On the proximal volar aspect of the lower arm, in a square area of 4×4 cm, chessboard-like horizontal and vertical scratches are made with a needle [...] These scratches should be superficial and not cause bleeding."[58] Consistently, allergic side effects were observed only rarely when allergen was applied via the skin and they were at all times milder than under conventional SCIT.[52,55,57] These promising results were supported by several studies performed in the subsequent years all over Europe, from Switzerland to Portugal.[58–60] Overall, symptom relief was obtained rapidly and allowed for coseasonal treatment. The reported treatment success rates of 80% exceeded the success rates under conventional SCIT.[58] Despite such successful results with the French *méthode de quadrillage cutané*, reports on this promising administration route disappeared into oblivion for almost half a century.

Epicutaneous Immunotherapy with Aeroallergens

Although there is strong scientific and historical evidence for EPIT in allergy, there existed no double-blind placebo-controlled clinical trials, a fact that led our group to revisit EPIT. Driven by the idea to find a patient-convenient application route of AIT, and based on the good accessibility of the skin and its high density of potent immune cells, our group performed three clinical trials to test efficacy and safety of EPIT. To keep epithelial barrier disruption minimal, we replaced skin scarification by adhesive tape stripping.[61] Besides enhancing the penetration of allergens by removing the stratum corneum,[62] repeated tape stripping also functions as a physical adjuvant through activation of keratinocytes, which then secrete various proinflammatory cytokines (IL-1, IL-6, IL-8, tumor necrosis factor-α, and interferon-γ) favoring maturation and emigration of DCs to the draining lymph nodes.[63,64] The first pilot trial revealed that patients treated with a total of 12 patches containing grass pollen extract experienced significant alleviation of hay fever symptoms compared with placebo-treated patients. In line with the historical study results described previously, no severe systemic allergic reactions were reported. The only adverse events observed were very mild local eczematous reactions under the skin patch.[61] When looking at all 12 patch applications, in 15 out of the 21 verum-treated patients, mild eczema was observed, whereas eczema was seen in only 5 out of the 15 placebo-treated patients. When looking at a single patch application, in roughly half of the verum-treated patients, eczema was observed under the patch, with a severity score between 3 and 6 on a scale ranging from 0 to 18. To exclude that the occurrence of local adverse effects might have partially unblinded the study, we analyzed whether the occurrence of eczema under the patch correlated with symptom amelioration, but could not find such correlation.

Encouraged by these results, a second phase I/IIa trial including a total of 132 patients with grass pollen allergy was initiated to find the optimal treatment dose of EPIT. Enrolled patients were treated with a total of six patches during the pollen season. We found a clear positive correlation between the administered allergen dose and the clinical effect.[65] Also, dose-dependent local adverse effects were observed at the site of patch application. Pruritus was the most frequently reported adverse event, followed by eczema observed after patch removal. Interestingly, with every subsequent patch application, there was a reduction of local adverse events. After the sixth patch application, merely half as many local adverse events were reported. This reduction was not explicable by local depletion of immune cells or degranulation of mast cells, because each of the six patches was applied to a different area of the arm. Therefore, the reduction of local adverse events is likely to be explained by tolerance induction. A third clinical trial investigated the immunologic changes induced during EPIT and found an increase in allergen-specific IgG4.[66] Our results have meanwhile been confirmed by an independent group, demonstrating efficacy and safety of EPIT in children allergic to grass pollen. Hay fever symptoms and the use of antihistamines were significantly reduced in the active treatment group.[67]

So far, there is no head-to-head comparison of EPIT with other routes of administration, except in mouse models. Using the major grass pollen allergen Phl p 5, in the mouse, EPIT was found to be equivalent or better than SLIT.[68] Although EPIT and SLIT induced similar IgG2a levels and also led to a similar reduction in IgE levels in sensitized mice, it was only EPIT that led to a significant reduction of eosinophil counts in the bronchoalveolar lavage in the asthma model. Also in mice, we have compared SCIT with EPIT using ovalbumin as the allergen.[23] Although EPIT without adjuvant was less immunogenic than SCIT, EPIT with an adjuvant was found to be more immunogenic, so that EPIT and SCIT seemed comparable in efficacy.

Epicutaneous Immunotherapy with Food Allergens

A clinical pilot trial to test clinical efficacy and safety of EPIT using the Viaskin EDS (DBV Technologies, Bagneux, France) in children suffering from cow's milk allergy showed a nonsignificant tendency toward increased cumulative tolerance doses after a 3-month treatment period.[69] Treatment was well tolerated with no systemic anaphylactic reactions, but a significant increase of local eczematous skin reactions was observed. Such good safety results are crucial especially when considering the use of EPIT as treatment option for food allergies, for which conventional SCIT is impractical because of an unacceptably high rate of anaphylactic reactions.[70] To substantiate these early findings and aiming to develop a definitive therapeutic option for food allergy patients, an extensive clinical trial program has been initiated with the objective to test treatment efficacy of EPIT with the Viaskin EDS in patients with peanut allergy. A multinational double-blind, placebo-controlled, randomized phase IIb trial has already generated positive clinical results.[71]

Methods for Enhancing Penetration

Methods for enhancing penetration across the skin barrier first include hydration of the stratum corneum, which facilitates diffusion of hydrophilic molecules. Any form of occlusion, such as the allergen patches used by us[61,65,66] and others,[67] hydrates the skin by accumulation of sweat.[68,69] Also, a French group recently developed an alternative form of EPIT based on allergen delivery to the intact skin using an occlusive epidermal delivery system (Viaskin EDS).[68,69,72] Initially developed for diagnostic purposes as an alternative system to the conventional Finn chamber used in atopy patch test,[73] Viaskin relies on the ability to deliver whole protein molecules to the skin.[68,72] Perspiration, generated under an occlusive chamber, dissolves the lyophilized allergen protein loaded on the Viaskin EDS,[68,72] and protein has been demonstrated to accumulate in the stratum corneum, where it efficiently targets immune cells of the superficial skin layer[74] that rapidly migrate to the draining lymph nodes.[68] In murine studies, EPIT with Viaskin EDS has proven efficacy equivalent to SCIT in preventing allergic airway reactions on inhalative allergen challenge.[68] Skin penetration may also be enhanced by adding so-called penetration enhancers, such as salicylic acid,[67] or by packing the antigen into lipid-based colloidal systems.[75] Last but not least, skin penetration can be enhanced by microporation, either using a microneedle patch[45,76] or a laser.[77,78]

Although all of these methods enhance skin penetration of allergens, it remains to be seen to which degree each of these methods also activates keratinocytes, which importantly interact with LCs. It may be speculated that the different outcomes of these methods, such as the relative inefficacy of the Viaskin EDS chamber, may well be explained by the assumption that hydration alone does not activate keratinocytes as much as tape stripping or abrasion. In fact, a heavily disrupted skin barrier has been observed to polarize the immune response toward Th1, whereas slight skin barrier disruption rather induces a noninflammatory Th2/Treg dominated response.[24] The evidence in this area is conflicting. In mouse models of peanut allergy, intact skin and not stripped skin was found to be crucial for efficacy and safety of immunotherapy.[79] In our mouse models with ovalbumin, no therapeutic effect was observed if the skin was not tape stripped before allergen application.[23]

We have recently use microneedle patches and laser microporation of the stratum corneum to enhance allergen penetration into the epidermis (Betschart E, Spina L, Tay F, et al: LASER microporation for epicutaneous allergen immunotherapy. Submitted for publication).[25] In these clinical trials, we found that once the allergen had passed across the stratum corneum and therefore penetrated into the live layers of the epidermis, the basal membrane represented no barrier to diffusion into the dermis. Even when merely the upper 10 μm of the epidermis were perforated, that is, only the stratum corneum, we could observe formation of hives only minutes after application of allergens (unpublished observations).

Adjuvants in Epicutaneous Immunotherapy

Adjuvants in EPIT represent another strategy to enhance efficacy. Aluminum salts, today still the adjuvant used in most marketed vaccines,[80] is not suitable for epicutaneous administration.[81] Thus far, cholera toxin and heat-labile enterotoxin have been successfully used as adjuvants in epicutaneous vaccination against infectious diseases of mice and humans.[43,82,83] However, imidazoquinolines (TLR7 or TLR8 ligands) and CpG (TLR9 ligand) are currently being tested as adjuvants for epicutaneous vaccination against cancer.[49,84] Our group recently tested the immune-enhancing and immune-modulatory potential of diphenylcyclopropenone when used as adjuvant in EPIT.[23]

Outlook for Allergen Epicutaneous Immunotherapy in Humans

With several placebo-controlled double-blind clinical trials confirming the efficacy of EPIT in allergy,[26,61,65–67] there remains little doubt that this method works as a proof of principle. Our clinical trial program has also shown that the allergen dose is an important efficacy parameter,[65,66] but the allergen dose used in skin patches cannot readily be increased beyond a certain concentration. We used 30 μg of major grass pollen allergen Phl p 1 per patch, corresponding to 1 mL of the 10-fold concentration that is used for the skin prick solution. A higher concentration would not only generate considerable material costs, but the application to any accidentally impaired skin barrier would represent a considerate risk for systemic allergic effects. Future research should therefore focus on enhancing penetration of the stratum corneum into the viable layers of the skin where LCs reside, and also on adjuvants suitable for epicutaneous administration.

INTRADERMAL ALLERGEN IMMUNOTHERAPY

In light of the observation that allergen delivery to the epidermis also immediately delivers the allergens by diffusion further down to the dermis, we cannot disentangle whether symptom amelioration in our clinical trials on EPIT actually worked via epidermal delivery to LCs, via dermal delivery to dermal DCs, or by both. In fact, the dermis with its high density of APCs represents an interesting immunotherapy route. Intradermal allergen delivery was shown to reduce hay fever symptoms already in 1926 by Phillips.[55] A recent clinical trial showed that very low allergen doses delivered to the dermis could induce allergen tolerance.[26] Also, intradermal injection of peptides derived from Fel d 1 and other allergens have shown profound clinical symptom amelioration.[12] Also, it should not be forgotten that the higher perfusion rate of the dermis produces per gram of tissue markedly more lymph than is produced in the rather poorly perfused subcutis. This causes intradermally injected substances to be drained into lymph nodes significantly faster than when subcutaneously injected.[85,86] The intradermal route is also gaining attention for other vaccines, such as influenza vaccines.[87,88]

SUMMARY AND FUTURE DIRECTIONS

AIT needs further improvement because the current protocols SCIT and SLIT suffer from long treatment duration and allergic side effects, so that very few patients with allergy choose to undergo these therapies and treatment adherence is low. AIT can be improved by modification of the allergen, by improving the adjuvant, or by changing the route of administration. The ideal route of administration is characterized by a high density of potent APCs and a low density or ideally even the absence of mast cells responsible for local side effects and of vasculature responsible for systemic allergic side effects. The intralymphatic route is interesting in that lymph nodes contain the highest density of DCs found in the human body. We and others demonstrated that as few as three allergen injections into a lymph node are sufficient to ameliorate allergy symptoms.

Also, allergen application to the epidermis is interesting in that epithelia contain a high number of DCs, but neither mast cells nor vasculature. We found, however, that for allergens the basal membrane represents no diffusion barrier toward the dermis, so that epicutaneously applied allergen still reaches the dermis. However, when the epidermis was prepared by adhesive tape stripping, we found EPIT to be safe. Only six patch applications were sufficient to ameliorate allergy symptoms. However, if the epidermis was prepared by abrasion, we observed several systemic allergic reactions. For EPIT we conclude that skin preparation is of key importance. First, the stratum corneum is the main diffusion barrier and must be made permeable for allergens to reach the live epidermis where APCs reside. Second, physical or chemical trauma to the epidermis provides signals and an immunologic milieu for DCs that modulate the efficacy of AIT. For both novel routes of AIT extensive clinical trial programs are under way and are likely to provide for interesting new treatment options in allergy.

REFERENCES

1. Holgate ST, Polosa R. Treatment strategies for allergy and asthma. Nat Rev Immunol 2008;8:218–30.

2. Akdis M, Akdis CA. Therapeutic manipulation of immune tolerance in allergic disease. Nat Rev Drug Discov 2009;8:645–60.
3. Noon L. Prophylactic inoculation against hay fever. Lancet 1911;177:1572–3.
4. Cox L, Calderon MA. Subcutaneous specific immunotherapy for seasonal allergic rhinitis: a review of treatment practices in the US and Europe. Curr Med Res Opin 2010;26(12):2723–33.
5. Cox L, Nelson H, Lockey R, et al. Allergen immunotherapy: a practice parameter third update. J Allergy Clin Immunol 2011;127:S1–55.
6. Bousquet J, Lockey R, Malling HJ. Allergen immunotherapy: therapeutic vaccines for allergic diseases. A WHO position paper. J Allergy Clin Immunol 1998;102:558–62.
7. Frew AJ, Powell RJ, Corrigan CJ, et al. Efficacy and safety of specific immunotherapy with SQ allergen extract in treatment-resistant seasonal allergic rhinoconjunctivitis. J Allergy Clin Immunol 2006;117:319–25.
8. Henmar H, Lund G, Lund L, et al. Allergenicity, immunogenicity and dose-relationship of three intact allergen vaccines and four allergoid vaccines for subcutaneous grass pollen immunotherapy. Clin Exp Immunol 2008;153:316–23.
9. Valenta R, Niespodziana K, Focke-Tejkl M, et al. Recombinant allergens: what does the future hold? J Allergy Clin Immunol 2011;127:860–4.
10. Muller U, Akdis CA, Fricker M, et al. Successful immunotherapy with T-cell epitope peptides of bee venom phospholipase A2 induces specific T-cell anergy in patients allergic to bee venom. J Allergy Clin Immunol 1998;101:747–54.
11. Worm M, Lee HH, Kleine-Tebbe J, et al. Development and preliminary clinical evaluation of a peptide immunotherapy vaccine for cat allergy. J Allergy Clin Immunol 2011;127:89–97. e1–14.
12. Patel D, Couroux P, Hickey P, et al. Fel d 1-derived peptide antigen desensitization shows a persistent treatment effect 1 year after the start of dosing: a randomized, placebo-controlled study. J Allergy Clin Immunol 2013;131:103–9. e1–7.
13. Creticos PS, Schroeder JT, Hamilton RG, et al. Immunotherapy with a ragweed-toll-like receptor 9 agonist vaccine for allergic rhinitis. N Engl J Med 2006;355:1445–55.
14. Dubuske LM, Frew AJ, Horak F, et al. Ultrashort-specific immunotherapy successfully treats seasonal allergic rhinoconjunctivitis to grass pollen. Allergy Asthma Proc 2011;32:239–47.
15. Mothes N, Heinzkill M, Drachenberg KJ, et al. Allergen-specific immunotherapy with a monophosphoryl lipid A-adjuvanted vaccine: reduced seasonally boosted immunoglobulin E production and inhibition of basophil histamine release by therapy-induced blocking antibodies. Clin Exp Allergy 2003;33:1198–208.
16. Drachenberg KJ, Wheeler AW, Stuebner P, et al. A well-tolerated grass pollen-specific allergy vaccine containing a novel adjuvant, monophosphoryl lipid A, reduces allergic symptoms after only four preseasonal injections. Allergy 2001;56:498–505.
17. Senti G, Prinz Vavricka BM, Erdmann I, et al. Intralymphatic allergen administration renders specific immunotherapy faster and safer: a randomized controlled trial. Proc Natl Acad Sci U S A 2008;105:17908–12.
18. Senti G, Crameri R, Kuster D, et al. Intralymphatic immunotherapy for cat allergy induces tolerance after only 3 injections. J Allergy Clin Immunol 2012;129:1290–6.
19. Senti G, Johansen P, Kundig TM. Intralymphatic immunotherapy. Curr Opin Allergy Clin Immunol 2009;9:537–43.

20. Hylander T, Latif L, Petersson-Westin U, et al. Intralymphatic allergen-specific immunotherapy: an effective and safe alternative treatment route for pollen-induced allergic rhinitis. J Allergy Clin Immunol 2013;131:412–20.
21. Cox LS, Larenas Linnemann D, Nolte H, et al. Sublingual immunotherapy: a comprehensive review. J Allergy Clin Immunol 2006;117:1021–35.
22. Canonica GW, Bousquet J, Casale T, et al. Sub-lingual immunotherapy: World Allergy Organization Position Paper. Allergy 2009;64(Suppl 91):1–59.
23. von Moos S, Johansen P, Waeckerle-Men Y, et al. The contact sensitizer diphenyl-cyclopropenone has adjuvant properties in mice and potential application in epicutaneous immunotherapy. Allergy 2012;67:638–46.
24. Swamy M, Jamora C, Havran W, et al. Epithelial decision makers: in search of the "epimmunome". Nat Immunol 2010;11:656–65.
25. Weisskopf M, Spina L, Kündig T, et al. Comparison of microneedles and adhesive tape stripping in skin preparation for epicutaneous allergen delivery. Int Arch Allergy Immunol 2015;167(2):103–9.
26. Rotiroti G, Shamji M, Durham SR, et al. Repeated low-dose intradermal allergen injection suppresses allergen-induced cutaneous late responses. J Allergy Clin Immunol 2012;130:918–924 e1.
27. Zinkernagel RM, Ehl S, Aichele P, et al. Antigen localisation regulates immune responses in a dose- and time-dependent fashion: a geographical view of immune reactivity. Immunol Rev 1997;156:199–209.
28. Johansen P, Mohanan D, Martinez-Gomez JM, et al. Lympho-geographical concepts in vaccine delivery. J Control Release 2010;148:56–62.
29. Kündig TM, Johansen P, Senti G. Intralymphatic vaccination. In: Rapuolli R, Bagnoli F, editors. Vaccine design. Norfolk (United Kingdom): Caister Academic Press; 2011. p. 211–24.
30. Senti G, Johansen P, Kundig TM. Intralymphatic immunotherapy: from the rationale to human applications. Curr Top Microbiol Immunol 2011;352:71–84.
31. von Moos S, Kundig TM, Senti G. Novel administration routes for allergen-specific immunotherapy: a review of intralymphatic and epicutaneous allergen-specific immunotherapy. Immunol Allergy Clin North Am 2011;31:391–406, xi.
32. Johansen P, Senti G, Martinez Gomez JM, et al. Toll-like receptor ligands as adjuvants in allergen-specific immunotherapy. Clin Exp Allergy 2005;35:1591–8.
33. Johansen P, Senti G, Martinez Gomez JM, et al. Heat denaturation, a simple method to improve the immunotherapeutic potential of allergens. Eur J Immunol 2005;35:3591–8.
34. Martinez-Gomez JM, Johansen P, Erdmann I, et al. Intralymphatic injections as a new administration route for allergen-specific immunotherapy. Int Arch Allergy Immunol 2009;150:59–65.
35. Martinez-Gomez JM, Johansen P, Rose H, et al. Targeting the MHC class II pathway of antigen presentation enhances immunogenicity and safety of allergen immunotherapy. Allergy 2009;64:172–8.
36. Mohanan D, Slutter B, Henriksen-Lacey M, et al. Administration routes affect the quality of immune responses: a cross-sectional evaluation of particulate antigen-delivery systems. J Control Release 2010;147:342–9.
37. Cardell LO. Intralymphatic allergen-specific immunotherapy: an effective and safe alternative treatment route for pollen-induced allergic rhinitis. J Allergy Clin Immunol 2012;131(2):412–20.
38. Witten M, Malling HJ, Blom L, et al. Is intralymphatic immunotherapy ready for clinical use in patients with grass pollen allergy? J Allergy Clin Immunol 2013;132:1248–52.e5.

39. Siegrist CA. Vaccine immunology. In: Plotkin SA, editor. Vaccines. 6th edition. Philadelphia: Saunders; 2013. p. 14–32.
40. Kedl RM, Kappler JW, Marrack P. Epitope dominance, competition and T cell affinity maturation. Curr Opin Immunol 2003;15:120–7.
41. Guery JC, Galbiati F, Smiroldo S, et al. Selective development of T helper (Th)2 cells induced by continuous administration of low dose soluble proteins to normal and beta(2)-microglobulin-deficient BALB/c mice. J Exp Med 1996;183:485–97.
42. Makatsori M, Senna G, Pitsios C, et al. Prospective adherence to specific immunotherapy in Europe (PASTE) survey protocol. Clin Transl Allergy 2015;5:17.
43. Frech SA, Dupont HL, Bourgeois AL, et al. Use of a patch containing heat-labile toxin from *Escherichia coli* against travellers' diarrhoea: a phase II, randomised, double-blind, placebo-controlled field trial. Lancet 2008;371:2019–25.
44. Hickey DK, Aldwell FE, Tan ZY, et al. Transcutaneous immunization with novel lipid-based adjuvants induces protection against gastric helicobacter pylori infection. Vaccine 2009;27:6983–90.
45. Sullivan SP, Koutsonanos DG, Del Pilar Martin M, et al. Dissolving polymer microneedle patches for influenza vaccination. Nat Med 2010;16:915–20.
46. Ding Z, Verbaan FJ, Bivas-Benita M, et al. Microneedle arrays for the transcutaneous immunization of diphtheria and influenza in BALB/c mice. J Control Release 2009;136:71–8.
47. Belyakov IM, Hammond SA, Ahlers JD, et al. Transcutaneous immunization induces mucosal CTLs and protective immunity by migration of primed skin dendritic cells. J Clin Invest 2004;113:998–1007.
48. Yagi H, Hashizume H, Horibe T, et al. Induction of therapeutically relevant cytotoxic T lymphocytes in humans by percutaneous peptide immunization. Cancer Res 2006;66:10136–44.
49. Rechtsteiner G, Warger T, Osterloh P, et al. Cutting edge: priming of CTL by transcutaneous peptide immunization with imiquimod. J Immunol 2005;174:2476–80.
50. Bynoe MS, Evans JT, Viret C, et al. Epicutaneous immunization with autoantigenic peptides induces T suppressor cells that prevent experimental allergic encephalomyelitis. Immunity 2003;19:317–28.
51. Bynoe MS, Viret C. Antigen-induced suppressor T cells from the skin point of view: suppressor T cells induced through epicutaneous immunization. J Neuroimmunol 2005;167:4–12.
52. Blamoutier P, Blamoutier J, Guibert L. Traitement co-saisonnier de la pollinose par l'application d'extraits de pollens sur des quadrillages cutanés: Résultats obtenus en 1959 et 1960. Revue Francaise d'Allergie; 1:112–20.
53. Vallery-Radot P, Hangenau J. Asthme d'origine équine. Essai de désensibilisation par des cutiréactions répétées. Bull Soc Méd Hôp Paris 1921;45:1251–60.
54. Hurwitz SH. Medicine: seasonal hay fever-some problems in treatment. Cal West Med 1930;33:520–1.
55. Phillips EW. Relief of hay-fever by intradermal injections of pollen extract. J Am Med Assoc 1926;86:182–4.
56. Blamoutier P, Blamoutier J, Guibert L. Treatment of pollinosis with pollen extracts by the method of cutaneous quadrille ruling. Presse Med 1959;67:2299–301 [in French].
57. Pautrizel R, Cabanieu G, Bricaud H, et al. Allergenic group specificity & therapeutic consequences in asthma; specific desensitization method by epicutaneous route. Sem Hop 1957;33:1394–403 [in French].
58. Eichenberger H, Storck H. Co-seasonal desensitization of pollinosis with the scarification-method of Blamoutier. Acta Allergol 1966;21:261–7.

59. Martin-DuPan RBF, Neyroud M. Treatment of pollen allergy using the cutaneous checker square method of Blamoutier and Guilbert. Schweiz Rundsch Med Prax 1971;60:1469–72.

60. Palma-Carlos AG. Traitement co-saisonnier des pollinoses au Portugal par la méthode des quadrillages cutanés. Revue Francaise d&'apos;Allergie 1967;7: 92–5.

61. Senti G, Graf N, Haug S, et al. Epicutaneous allergen administration as a novel method of allergen-specific immunotherapy. J Allergy Clin Immunol 2009;124: 997–1002.

62. Dickel H, Goulioumis A, Gambichler T, et al. Standardized tape stripping: a practical and reproducible protocol to uniformly reduce the stratum corneum. Skin Pharmacol Physiol 2010;23:259–65.

63. Nickoloff BJ, Naidu Y. Perturbation of epidermal barrier function correlates with initiation of cytokine cascade in human skin. J Am Acad Dermatol 1994;30: 535–46.

64. Dickel H, Gambichler T, Kamphowe J, et al. Standardized tape stripping prior to patch testing induces upregulation of Hsp90, Hsp70, IL-33, TNF-alpha and IL-8/CXCL8 mRNA: new insights into the involvement of "alarmins". Contact Dermatitis 2010;63:215–22.

65. Senti G, von Moos S, Tay F, et al. Epicutaneous allergen-specific immunotherapy ameliorates grass pollen-induced rhinoconjunctivitis: a double-blind, placebo-controlled dose escalation study. J Allergy Clin Immunol 2012;129:128–35.

66. Senti G, von Moos S, Tay F, et al. Determinants of efficacy and safety in epicutaneous allergen immunotherapy: summary of three clinical trials. Allergy 2015;70: 707–10.

67. Agostinis F, Forti S, Di Berardino F. Grass transcutaneous immunotherapy in children with seasonal rhinoconjunctivitis. Allergy 2010;65:410–1.

68. Mondoulet L, Dioszeghy V, Larcher T, et al. Epicutaneous immunotherapy (EPIT) blocks the allergic esophago-gastro-enteropathy induced by sustained oral exposure to peanuts in sensitized mice. PLoS One 2012;7:e31967.

69. Dupont C, Kalach N, Soulaines P, et al. Cow's milk epicutaneous immunotherapy in children: a pilot trial of safety, acceptability, and impact on allergic reactivity. J Allergy Clin Immunol 2010;125:1165–7.

70. Scurlock AM, Jones SM. An update on immunotherapy for food allergy. Curr Opin Allergy Clin Immunol 2010;10:587–93.

71. Sampson HA, Agbotounou W, Thébault C, et al. Epicutaneous immunotherapy (EPIT) is effective and safe to treat peanut allergy: a multi-national double-blind placebo-controlled randomized phase IIb trial. J Allergy Clin Immunol 2015; 1135:AB390.

72. Mondoulet L, Dioszeghy V, Vanoirbeek JA, et al. Epicutaneous immunotherapy using a new epicutaneous delivery system in mice sensitized to peanuts. Int Arch Allergy Immunol 2010;154:299–309.

73. Kalach N, Soulaines P, de Boissieu D, et al. A pilot study of the usefulness and safety of a ready-to-use atopy patch test (Diallertest) versus a comparator (Finn Chamber) during cow's milk allergy in children. J Allergy Clin Immunol 2005;116:1321–6.

74. Soury D, Barratt G, Ah-Leung S, et al. Skin localization of cow's milk proteins delivered by a new ready-to-use atopy patch test. Pharm Res 2005;22: 1530–6.

75. Rattanapak T, Birchall J, Young K, et al. Transcutaneous immunization using microneedles and cubosomes: mechanistic investigations using optical

coherence tomography and two-photon microscopy. J Control Release 2013; 172:894–903.
76. Bal SM, Ding Z, van Riet E, et al. Advances in transcutaneous vaccine delivery: do all ways lead to Rome? J Control Release 2010;148(3):266–82.
77. Weiss R, Hessenberger M, Kitzmuller S, et al. Transcutaneous vaccination via laser microporation. J Control Release 2012;162:391–9.
78. Scheiblhofer S, Thalhamer J, Weiss R. Laser microporation of the skin: prospects for painless application of protective and therapeutic vaccines. Expert Opin Drug Deliv 2013;10:761–73.
79. Mondoulet L, Dioszeghy V, Puteaux E, et al. Intact skin and not stripped skin is crucial for the safety and efficacy of peanut epicutaneous immunotherapy (EPIT) in mice. Clin Transl Allergy 2012;2:22.
80. Marrack P, McKee AS, Munks MW. Towards an understanding of the adjuvant action of aluminum. Nat Rev Immunol 2009;9:287–93.
81. Scharton-Kersten T, Yu J, Vassell R, et al. Transcutaneous immunization with bacterial ADP-ribosylating exotoxins, subunits, and unrelated adjuvants. Infect Immun 2000;68:5306–13.
82. Yu XL, Cheng YM, Shi BS, et al. Measles virus infection in adults induces production of IL-10 and is associated with increased CD4+ CD25+ regulatory T cells. J Immunol 2008;181:7356–66.
83. Glenn GM, Rao M, Matyas GR, et al. Skin immunization made possible by cholera toxin. Nature 1998;391:851.
84. Stoitzner P, Sparber F, Tripp CH. Langerhans cells as targets for immunotherapy against skin cancer. Immunol Cell Biol 2010;88:431–7.
85. Kersey TW, Van Eyk J, Lannin DR, et al. Comparison of intradermal and subcutaneous injections in lymphatic mapping. J Surg Res 2001;96:255–9.
86. O'Mahony S, Solanki CK, Barber RW, et al. Imaging of lymphatic vessels in breast cancer-related lymphedema: intradermal versus subcutaneous injection of 99mTc-immunoglobulin. AJR Am J Roentgenol 2006;186:1349–55.
87. Belshe RB, Newman FK, Cannon J, et al. Serum antibody responses after intradermal vaccination against influenza. N Engl J Med 2004;351:2286–94.
88. Kenney RT, Frech SA, Muenz LR, et al. Dose sparing with intradermal injection of influenza vaccine. N Engl J Med 2004;351:2295–301.

Advances in the Treatment of Food Allergy

Sublingual and Epicutaneous Immunotherapy

Sayantani Sindher, MD[a], David M. Fleischer, MD[b],
Jonathan M. Spergel, MD, PhD[a],*

KEYWORDS

- Allergen immunotherapy (AIT) • Sublingual immunotherapy (SLIT)
- Epicutaneous immunotherapy (EPIT) • Food allergy • Desensitization
- Oral tolerance • Sustained unresponsiveness

KEY POINTS

- Food allergies have continued to increase in prevalence in the past decade and have become a significant health issue.
- In the search for efficacious, yet well-tolerated therapies, sublingual immunotherapy (SLIT) and epicutaneous immunotherapy (EPIT) are being explored for the treatment of food allergy.
- SLIT and EPIT can increase threshold doses, which may provide at least partial protection against accidental exposures without suffering severe symptoms.
- More research is needed to define the optimal doses and administration protocol before these therapies can be offered to patients in clinical practice.

INTRODUCTION

Food allergies have continued to increase in prevalence in the past decade and have emerged as a significant health issue.[1] Three percent to 6% of the population in the United States suffers from food allergy (FA),[2] and its prevalence in children has increased by 18% in the past decade.[3] Although 85% of patients may outgrow

Disclosure of Potential Conflict of Interest: Dr J.M. Spergel is on the Scientific Advisory Board for DBV. S. Sindher has no commercial conflicts of interest to disclose.
[a] Division of Allergy and Immunology, Department of Pediatrics, The Children's Hospital of Philadelphia, Perelman School of Medicine at University of Pennsylvania, 34th Street and Civic Center Boulevard, Philadelphia, PA 19104-4399, USA; [b] Section of Allergy, Department of Pediatrics, Children's Hospital Colorado, University of Colorado Denver School of Medicine, 13123 East 16th Avenue, B518, Aurora, CO 80045, USA
* Corresponding author.
E-mail address: spergel@email.chop.edu

cow's milk and egg allergies, only approximately 20% of peanut-allergic and 10% of tree nut-allergic patients outgrow their allergies.[4,5]

The current standard of care in treating FA is a strict elimination diet and being prepared to treat allergic reactions owing to accidental exposures of trigger foods with medications such as antihistamines and self-injectable epinephrine. Despite careful avoidance, life-threatening reactions can still occur secondary to accidental exposures,[6] and the unpredictability of these acute reactions can significantly decrease the quality of life of individuals with FA.[7] A strict elimination diet can also lead to severe malnutrition in infancy and early childhood[8] when there is a higher nutritional demand for adequate growth and development.[9,10] For these reasons, safe and effective therapies for FA are necessary.

Allergen-specific immunotherapy (AIT) has the most potential for treating FA.[11] It relies on administering incremental doses of allergen by various routes, such as the subcutaneous, oral, sublingual, or epicutaneous.[11] The goal of AIT is to reorient the immune system; however, the precise mechanisms through which AIT affects this change are incompletely understood.[11] Evidence from studies suggest that AIT is involved in suppressing mast cell and basophil reactivity, reducing allergen-specific immunoglobulin (Ig)E while increasing allergen-specific IgG4 antibodies, skewing T-helper (Th)2 responses toward a Th1 phenotype, and stimulating the production of regulatory T cells (Tregs) that seem to be fundamental in inducing long-term tolerance.[12,13]

Food immunotherapy relies on the concept of desensitization and sustained unresponsiveness. The goal of early clinical trials in food immunotherapy was to desensitize patients to a maintenance dose, thus increasing the antigen threshold that can lead to an allergic reaction.[11] Studies being performed now are aimed at achieving a more sustained protective effect, termed sustained unresponsiveness, where patients have the ability to consume a large amount of an allergenic food without adverse reactions after discontinuing immunotherapy.[14,15] Permanent tolerance, in the context of FA immunotherapy, remains to be demonstrated.

Trials investigating immunotherapy to treat FA using subcutaneous administration of peanut extract were first conducted in the early 1990s.[16,17] However, subcutaneous immunotherapy (SCIT) was largely abandoned owing to the high level of anaphylactic reactions.[17,18] Since then, research in food immunotherapy has surged in the past 10 years.[18] Many studies have investigated oral immunotherapy (OIT), and the technique seems to be efficacious; however, a high rate of adverse reactions leading to patient withdrawal continues to drive the search for safer therapeutic options such as sublingual immunotherapy (SLIT) and epicutaneous immunotherapy (EPIT).[11] In this article, we review the advances in SLIT and EPIT for the treatment of food allergies.

SUBLINGUAL IMMUNOTHERAPY

SLIT uses the tolerogenic environment of the oral mucosa and is a well-established method of modulating the aberrant immune responses in individuals with allergic rhinitis.[19] Allergens in the form of drops or tablets are held under the tongue, using the immunogenic properties of the oral mucosa, thus promoting tolerance to the allergen.[19] The sublingual route of administering AIT was first studied in 1986 for the treatment of dust mite allergy.[20] Since then, numerous randomized, controlled trials have confirmed the safety and efficacy of SLIT in both adults and children for the treatment of environmental allergies.[21–23] Although the primary indication for SLIT remains allergic rhinoconjunctivitis, it is currently being explored for the treatment of FA.[19,24]

Since the first reported use of SLIT in FA in 2003,[25] several clinical trials have shown promising results. Studies examining SLIT for specific foods are described herein and listed in **Table 1**.

Kiwi

SLIT was first used for the treatment of FA in a 29-year-old woman with a severe kiwi allergy.[25] During the 5-week buildup phase, the patient kept incremental doses of kiwi extract under her tongue for 1 minute and then swallowed. The patient reached a 3 times daily maintenance treatment regimen and tolerated consuming 1 cm^3 of fresh kiwi after sublingual application of the food for 1 minute. After 5 years, owing to other health concerns, the patient discontinued daily kiwi intake. She was able to resume kiwi consumption without any adverse effects 4 months later.[25,26]

Hazelnut

In 2005, Enrique and colleagues[27] performed the first double-blind, placebo-controlled (DBPC) SLIT trial. The study included 23 adults with hazelnut allergy, who were randomized to receive either hazelnut extract (n = 12) or placebo (n = 11). Although all subjects were positive on initial DBPC food challenge (DBPCFC) to hazelnut, 54.5% had oral allergy syndrome (OAS). The subjects held the extract under their tongue for 3 minutes and then spit it out. During the 4-day buildup phase, 11 of the 12 individuals (92%) from the active group were able to reach the target dose of 188.15 µg of major hazelnut allergen Cor a1 and 121.9 µg of Cor a8. They continued maintenance dosing at home for 8 to 12 weeks, and 5 of 11 individuals (45%) were able to ingest 20 g of hazelnut (about 15–20 hazelnuts) in a posttreatment DBPCFC without any symptoms. The mean tolerated dose in the treated individuals increased from 2.29 to 11.56 g.[27] Consistent with the desensitization, actively treated subjects had significantly increased levels of interleukin (IL)-10 in the peripheral blood compared with the placebo treated subjects. During a 1-year follow-up study, a subsequent DBPCFC was performed, and the mean tolerated dose further increased to 14.57 g and 5 of the 7 reached the highest planned dose of 20 g. Although SLIT seemed to be an effective tool in this study for desensitization, the high rate of OAS in the subjects (54.5%) makes it difficult to interpret the success in patients with hazelnut-induced anaphylaxis.[27,28]

Milk

In 2006, de Boissieu and colleagues[29] included 8 children (age 6–17 years) with cow's milk allergy in an open-label, pilot study. After reacting to an initial milk challenge, the subjects underwent milk SLIT to a goal dose of 1 mL/d of cow's milk over 6 months. The milk extract was kept under the tongue for 2 minutes and then spit out. Although 6 of the 8 children (75%) completed the protocol, only 3 (38%) were able to consume 200 mL of milk without symptoms during a posttreatment DBPCFC. The children did, however, have a higher posttreatment mean challenge threshold that increased from 39 to 143 mL.[29]

Peach

In 2008, Fernandez-Rivas and coworkers[30] conducted a DBPC trial for treatment of peach allergy with SLIT. Fifty-six adult subjects were randomized to receive active treatment (n = 37) or placebo (n = 19). A large number of the patients (63%) had only OAS to peach. The individuals underwent a 5-day inpatient buildup, which was followed by a maintenance dosing schedule of 3 times a week administration of 10 µg of the peach lipid protein Pru p 3 for 6 months. The doses were placed under

Table 1
Studies examining SLIT and EPIT for the treatment of food allergy

Study (Year)	Food	Modality	Design	No. of Patients (Age Range)	Withdrawals/ Active Group	Maintenance Dose	Challenge Dose	Duration	Clinical Outcome	Adverse Events
SLIT										
Enrique et al,[27] 2005	Hazelnut	SLIT	DBPC RCT	23 (19–53)	1/12	13.25 mg/d	20 g	8–12 wk	5/11 completed OFC; ↑ threshold	Systemic reactions 0.2% of total doses (1466); local reactions 7.4% of total doses (1466)
Fernandez-Rivas et al,[30] 2009	Peach	SLIT	DBPC RCT	56 (18–65)	4/37	0.01 mg 3×/wk	3249 μg	6 mo	↑ threshold	Systemic reactions 0.4% and local reactions 39% of total doses (3378)
De Boissieu & Dupont[29] 2006	Milk	SLIT	Prospective case series	8 (6–17)	1/8	1 mL/d	200 mL	6 mo	3/8 completed OFC; ↑ threshold	No systemic reactions; 75% of patients reported subjective local symptoms
Keet et al,[34] 2012	Milk	SLIT/OIT	Open RCT	30 (6–17)	2/10	7 mg (SLIT) 1000 mg/d (OITA) 2000 mg/d (OITB)	8 g	60 wk (off 6 wk)	1/10 SLIT vs 14/20 OIT completed OFC; 9/15 (OIT) sustained unresponsive	Systemic reactions 0.10% (buildup) and 0.02% (maintenance); OP reactions 26.82% (buildup) and 27.99% (maintenance)
Kim et al,[31] 2011	Peanut	SLIT	DBPC RCT	18 (1–11)	0/11	2000 μg/d	2.5 g	12 mo	↑ threshold	Reactions 11.5% and OP itching 9.3% of total doses (4182)

Study	Allergen	Treatment	Design	Age (range)	Reactions	Maintenance dose	Dose	Duration	Results	Outcomes
Chin et al,[35] 2013	Peanut	SLIT/OIT	DBPC RCT	27 (2–11) / 23 (3–10)	0/27 / 5/23	2 mg/d (SLIT), 4000 mg/d (OIT)	2.5 g / 5 g	12 mo	8/27 SLIT vs 16/18 OIT completed OFC	No serious events (SLIT), No epi used (SLIT)
Fleischer et al,[32] 2013	Peanut	SLIT	DBPC RCT	40 (12–37)	3/20 / 5/17	1386 µg / 3696 µg	5 g	68 wk / 44 wk	5/15 SLIT (low dose, 68 wk) vs 0/17 (high dose, 44 wk); ↑ threshold	No severe symptoms; OP reactions 37.3% of initial total SLIT doses (5825); 31.4% in
Nariisety et al,[38] 2015	Peanut	SLIT/OIT	DBPC RCT	21 (7–13)	3/10 / 4/11	3.7 mg/d (SLIT), 2000 mg/d (OIT)	10 g	12 mo (off 4 wk)	5/10 SLIT vs 4/6 OIT completed OFC; 1/10 SLIT and 3/11 (OIT) sustained unresponsiveness; ↑ threshold	No severe symptoms; reactions in 9% of total doses (4578); No epi used (SLIT)
EPIT										
Dupont et al,[47] 2010	Milk	EPIT	DBPC RCT	18 (0.3–15)	0/10	1 mg 3 × 48 h/wk	20 mL	3 mo	12-fold increase in dose (20 mL)	Reactions 25% and OP itching 20% of total doses (470)
MILES (2014) [NCT02223182]	Milk	EPIT	DBPC RCT	150 (2–17)	NA	150, 300 µg, or 500 µg/d	1444 mg cumulative reactive dose	24 mo	Ongoing study	Ongoing study
ARACHILD-2010 [NCT01197053]	Peanut	EPIT	DBPC RCT	54 (5–18)	NA/28	100 µg/d	1 g	18 mo reported	↑ threshold	Ongoing study
CoFAR6 (2013) [NCT01904604]	Peanut	EPIT	DBPC RCT	75 (4–25)	NA	100 µg/d, 250 µg/d	5044 mg	30 mo	Ongoing study	Ongoing study

(continued on next page)

Table 1 (*continued*)

Study (Year)	Food	Modality	Design	No. of Patients (Age Range)	Withdrawals/ Active Group	Maintenance Dose	Challenge Dose	Duration	Clinical Outcome	Adverse Events
VIPES (2012) [NCT01675882]	Peanut	EPIT	DBPC RCT	221 (6–65)	NA/55	50, 100, or 250 µg/d	1 g	12 mo	Response rate (10-fold increase or tolerate 1 g): placebo-, 25%; 50 µg, 45.3%; 100 µg, 41.1%; 250 µg, 50%	No serious events in active groups reported
OLFUS-VIPES (2013) [NCT01675882]	Peanut	EPIT	DBPC RCT	170 (6–65)	NA	250 µg/d	1 g	36 mo	Ongoing study	Ongoing study

Abbreviations: ↑, increased; DBPC, double-blind placebo-controlled; epi, epinephrine; EPIT, epicutaneous immunotherapy; NA, not applicable; OFC, open food challenge; OIT, oral immunotherapy; OITA, oral immunotherapy group A (goal dose 2 g/d), OITB, oral immunotherapy group B (goal dose 1 g/d); OP, oropharyngeal; RCT, randomized, controlled trial; SLIT, sublingual immunotherapy.

the tongue and then swallowed. After 6 months of therapy, 33 active subjects (89%) were rechallenged and demonstrated up to a 9-fold higher threshold to elicit local symptoms compared with baseline. No changes were observed within the placebo group. Because a large portion of the patients had only OAS (63%), the success of SLIT in desensitizing patients with peach-induced anaphylaxis is unclear.[30]

Peanut

Two randomized, DBPC trials for peanut SLIT have been published in the past several years.[31,32] The first study, conducted by Kim and colleagues,[31] enrolled 18 children (ages 1–11 years) randomized to SLIT (n = 11) or placebo (n = 7) groups. Each dose was kept under the tongue for 2 minutes and then swallowed. Over a 6-month period, all subjects in the active group achieved a goal daily dose of 2500 μg in the dose escalation phase and continued for an additional 6 months in the maintenance phase. After completing the maintenance phase, the subjects underwent a DBPCFC. Although baseline thresholds were not established with a pretreatment oral food challenge, the treatment group safely ingested 20 times more peanut protein (1710 mg) than the placebo group (85 mg).[31]

Two years later, Fleischer and colleagues[32] reported the results of the first multicenter, randomized, DBPC clinical trial of peanut SLIT. The group randomized 40 individuals (age 12–37 years) equally to either active treatment with peanut SLIT or placebo after a study initial 2 g peanut DBPCFC, during which subjects had to react to qualify for study entry. In the first blinded phase of the trial, after 44 weeks on a goal dose of 1386 μg/d, the subjects underwent a 5 g DBPCFC to peanut. During this challenge, 14 of 20 individuals (70%) were considered to be "responders," which was defined as the ability to tolerate either 5 g of peanut or a 10-fold higher amount than their baseline DBPCFC. The median tolerated dose in the active group increased from 3.5 to 496 mg. During the second unblinded phase of the trial, the original active group continued an additional 24 weeks months of maintenance therapy, and the placebo-treated subjects crossed over to a higher active peanut SLIT dose of 3696 μg daily. After completing 68 weeks of therapy, the median tolerated peanut dose increased further to 996 mg for the original active group. For the placebo-treated subjects who crossed over to higher dose SLIT, after 44 weeks of active therapy, 7 of 20 subjects (35%) were "responders," with the median dose increasing from 71 mg at the baseline challenge to 603 mg. The authors concluded that the longer duration of treatment was more efficacious than the higher dose based on the results of the DBPCFCs.[32] The study continued with a 3-year open-label period of active peanut SLIT with annual DBPCFCs, after which time analyses were performed to further evaluate long-term safety and efficacy outcomes.[33] For subjects who passed any 10-g DBPCFC during the study, SLIT therapy was discontinued, and the subjects were rechallenged 8 weeks later with a 10-g DBPCFC, followed by an open serving of peanut if challenge negative. Only 4 of the original 40 subjects (10%) demonstrated what has been termed sustained unresponsiveness, the ability to consume without symptoms a predetermined amount of protein after a period of abstinence from immunotherapy. The authors did not find outcome differences between the groups on 1386 versus 3696 μg of daily peanut protein.[33]

SUBLINGUAL IMMUNOTHERAPY VERSUS ORAL IMMUNOTHERAPY

Three studies to date have directly compared OIT and SLIT. In 2012, in a randomized, open-label protocol, Keet and colleagues[34] compared OIT versus SLIT in children with milk allergy. Thirty children (ages 6–17 years), who reacted at initial DBPCFC, underwent at least 6 weeks of initial SLIT to a goal dose of 3.7 mg of milk protein daily, held under the tongue for 2 minutes and then swallowed. The group was then randomized equally into 3 groups: SLIT (goal dose 7 mg/d), OITA (goal dose 2 g/d), and OITB (goal dose 1 g/d). The children continued on the maintenance dose, and after 12 and 60 weeks, underwent DBPCFCs to 8 g of cow's milk protein. Children who passed this challenge were then instructed to stop therapy and were challenged 1 and 6 weeks later. The results showed that after SLIT therapy the challenge threshold increased in all 3 groups from baseline, but therapy with SLIT followed by OIT was much more effective at desensitization than SLIT alone. After the full 60 weeks of maintenance therapy, the median fold increase in threshold increased 40-fold for SLIT (10 subjects), 54-fold for OITA (9 subjects), and 159-fold for OITB (9 subjects). One patient from the SLIT group tolerated the full challenge dose, compared with 8 in OITA and 6 in OITB. After discontinuing therapy for 1 week, 2 subjects from OITB group failed rechallenge. After discontinuing therapy for 6 weeks, 1 subject from the SLIT (10%), 5 from OITA (50%), and 3 from OITB (30%) demonstrated sustained unresponsiveness.[34]

In a second study published the following year, Chin and colleagues[35] performed a retrospective comparison of peanut SLIT versus OIT using data from 2 previously published SLIT and OIT protocols for peanut allergy.[36,37] Twenty-seven children underwent peanut SLIT to a goal dose of 2 mg/d, and 23 children were treated with peanut OIT to a goal dose of 4000 mg/d. After 12 months of therapy, the children underwent a DBPCFC to 2500 mg (SLIT) and 5000 mg (OIT). Among the children who underwent OIT, 70% passed the DBPCFC, in contrast with the SLIT group where only 30% passed the 1-year DBPCFC.[35] Similar to Keet and colleagues,[34] the authors found that OIT was more efficacious than SLIT for inducing desensitization to peanut protein.[35]

A third DBPC trial comparing peanut OIT and SLIT performed by Narisety and colleagues[38] was published recently. In this study, 21 children (ages 7–13 years) with peanut allergy were randomized to receive active SLIT versus placebo OIT or active OIT versus placebo SLIT. Doses were escalated to 3.7 mg/d (SLIT) or 2000 mg/d (OIT), and the patients were rechallenged after 6 and 12 months of maintenance. At this point, the subjects were unblinded, and patients received an additional 6 months of therapy. The patients who passed challenges at 12 or 18 months were taken off therapy for 4 weeks and rechallenged. The results showed that 16 of the 21 subjects (76%) had a greater than 10-fold increase in challenge threshold after 12 months, which was significantly greater in the active OIT group compared with the SLIT group (141-fold vs 22-fold, respectively). At study completion, 1 subject in the SLIT group and 3 from the OIT group demonstrated sustained unresponsiveness. The authors concluded that OIT seemed far more effective than SLIT for the treatment of peanut allergy.[38]

Safety

In the studies described herein, the superior safety of SLIT compared with OIT has been proven repeatedly, which is largely owing to the site of immunotherapy administration. Human oral tissues have low numbers of mast cells, eosinophils, and basophils, making them an ideal site for AIT. This results in decreased release of proinflammatory mediators and fewer adverse reactions.[18,19]

The adverse reactions that occur in 7.4% to 29% of SLIT doses tend to be local, mild, and transient,[29] and observed at a similar frequency in both SLIT and placebo groups.[30] Almost 99% of the reported reactions are local, and of these, the majority of reactions (≤95%) are restricted to the oral cavity, presenting as oropharyngeal itching.[27,30] When oropharyngeal symptoms were excluded, Fleischer and colleagues[32] found that 94% of the received doses were symptom free.

Systemic symptoms in SLIT are very rare, and most adverse reactions occur during the initial buildup phase.[27,31,32] In their study, Enrique and colleagues[27,28] reported only 0.2% systemic reactions, whereas Fernandez-Rivas and associates[30] reported 13.5%, but in both studies the reactions were mild and resolved either spontaneously or with antihistamines, antacids and sometimes omeprazole.[27,28,30]

The studies that compared OIT with SLIT for FA found that OIT caused nearly 4 times more multisystem symptoms.[34,38] Symptoms with OIT also were more likely to require more β-agonist, antihistamine, and injectable epinephrine for treatment.[34,35,38] A greater number of treatment withdrawals owing to intolerable symptoms were also noted in the OIT groups (10%–40%)[34,38] compared with SLIT groups (0%–30%).[34,38]

Immune Mechanisms

The underlying immune mechanisms involved in SLIT have been investigated in several studies.[19] SLIT uses the unique tolerogenic property of the oral mucosa.[19] Regulatory myeloid dendritic cells, which are predominantly oral mucosal Langerhans cells, seem to be the primary target cells of SLIT.[19] It has been proposed that oral mucosal Langerhans cells remain immature after SLIT and do not rapidly migrate to the lymph node, but present to T cells directly in the mucosa instead,[19] thus promoting sustained unresponsiveness. Oral mucosal Langerhans cells further contribute to a tolerogenic environment by producing the regulatory cytokines IL-10 and transforming growth factor-β1 once they have taken up the allergen.[19] Peripheral myeloid dendritic cells can also be involved in cytokine production by allergen-specific T cells and promote a tolerogenic environment after SLIT.[19]

After therapy with SLIT, the myeloid dendritic cells drive the polarization from the proallergic Th2 to the Th1 response.[19] A late phase of the immune response to SLIT shows significantly decreased IL-4 production but increased interferon-γ production, indicating a shift toward a Th1 phenotype.[39] In their peanut study, Kim and colleagues[31] noted decreased IL-4 production but did not find any significant differences in interferon-γ production. Additionally, induction of Tregs is an important aspect of AIT,[40] because through transforming growth factor-β and IL-10 production, Tregs suppress effector immune responses.[41] IL-10 was found to be significantly increased in some FA SLIT studies,[27,28] but not all.[31]

AIT is also proposed to function through inhibiting allergen-specific IgE production and enhancing allergen-specific IgG4 production, both of which are mediated by IL-10 and can be markers of clinical efficacy after SLIT.[19,42] Decreased allergen-specific IgE levels after SLIT for FA have been seen in several studies[25,26,31,34,35,38]; however, clinical improvement was not always associated with this decrease.[32] Increased IgG4 levels have also been observed in multiple studies,[25,27,28,30,31,35,38] but they did not always correlate with clinical outcome.[32,34]

EPICUTANEOUS IMMUNOTHERAPY

EPIT is another method that is being explored currently for the treatment of FA.[11] The allergen delivery through EPIT is limited to active immune cells of the epidermis.[43] In this process, the allergen is contained within a skin patch in soluble form. After the patch's application, the allergen is absorbed into the stratum corneum.[11] The first case study on successful EPIT was reported in 1921 by Vallery-Radot.[44] He was able to successfully reduce systemic allergic symptoms in patients allergic to horses after allergen administration on scarified skin.[44] Several studies have since been performed in Europe that show successful results and fewer side effects compared with SCIT.[45] Nonetheless, the method fell out of favor owing to the uncomfortable process of skin scarification.[46]

Recently, EPIT has experienced a revival in the treatment of FA. Viaskin (DBV Technologies SA, Paris, France) is a new epicutaneous delivery system (EDS) that allows the application of allergens on intact skin and facilitates diffusion of allergens into the stratum corneum.[46] Mondoulet and colleagues[46] initially used EPIT with Viaskin for FA on intact skin in a pilot study with mice sensitized to egg and peanut. They concluded that EPIT was as efficacious as SCIT,[46] and also provided a reassuring safety profile. To date, 1 DBPC pilot study investigating EPIT in children has been published.[47] There are several other EPIT trials in milk and peanut sensitized subjects that are currently ongoing or waiting to be published, having been presented as abstracts at the American Academy of Allergy, Asthma and Immunology (AAAAI) as well as the European Academy of Allergy and Clinical Immunology (ECAAI) meetings.[48,49] Studies examining EPIT for specific foods are described elsewhere in this article and in **Table 1**.

Milk

In 2010, Dupont and colleagues[47] conducted a 3-month-long bicenter, DBPC study to assess the efficacy and safety of EPIT administered using Viaskin EDS after its initial success in animal models.[46] The study enrolled 18 children with cow's milk allergy who were randomized to either active treatment with EPIT (n = 10) or placebo (n = 8). The treatment included three 48-h applications of the EDS per week for 3 months. Active EDS contained 1 mg of cow's milk powder that was applied onto intact skin in the interscapular area. An oral food challenge was performed after 3 months of therapy, which showed an increase in the threshold dose from 1.77 mL to 23.61 mL, a 12-fold increase in the active group. The mean cumulative dose did not vary in the placebo group.[47]

In 2014, the currently ongoing MILES trial, a multicenter, DBPC, randomized phase I/II trial to evaluate the efficacy and safety of Viaskin Milk, was initiated. The study has enrolled 150 children (ages 2–17 years) with cow's milk allergy. Part A of the MILES trial involves daily administration of 3 doses of Viaskin Milk (150, 300, and 500 μg of cow's milk protein) versus placebo for 3 weeks to assess safety and determine dosing for Part B. Part B will evaluate the safety and efficacy of 3 selected doses of Viaskin Milk compared with placebo. After 12 months of therapy, all subjects will be unblinded and will continue therapy for another 12 months at the highest tolerated dose [NCT02223182].

Peanut

The Epicutaneous Immunotherapy in Peanut Allergy in Children (ARACHILD) trial was a multicenter, DBPC, randomized, pilot trial conducted in France in 2010. Fifty-four patients (ages 5–18 years) were enrolled and randomized into 2 treatment arms to assess 100 μg of Viaskin peanut (n = 28) compared with placebo (n = 26). After 6 months of therapy, patients in the placebo arm crossed over to Viaskin peanut without unblinding, followed by an open-label period of 30 months. DBPCFCs were performed at 6, 12, and 18 months after onset of therapy. Successful therapy was defined as the ability to tolerate at least 1 g of peanut protein (4 peanuts) or a 10-fold higher dose than the baseline reactive dose. In the active group, 7.4%, 20% and 40% of subjects were able to consume at least 10 times more peanut protein compared with the beginning of the trial at 6, 12 ,and 18 months, respectively

[NCT01197053]. In children, there was a higher response rate of 12.5%, 33.3%, and 66.7% at the same time points.

In 2010, another multicenter, DBPC, phase Ib, randomized, clinical trial was initiated with Viaskin peanut in the United States to access safety. The trial recruited 100 peanut-allergic subjects (ages 6–50 years) that were randomized to receive treatment for 2 weeks with 250 μg or 500 μg of Viaskin peanut or with placebo. The study found that adolescents and adults tolerated 500 μg of Viaskin peanut well, whereas children tolerated the 250 μg better [NCT01170286]. There were no serious adverse events in the trial owing to Viaskin patch.

The Efficacy and Safety of Several Doses of Viaskin Peanut in Adults and Children With Peanut Allergy (VIPES) study, a multicenter, DBPC, phase IIb, clinical trial of Viaskin peanut was initiated in 2012 in North America and Europe to study efficacy of the therapy. The largest clinical trial in peanut allergy desensitization ever completed, the VIPES trial enrolled 221 peanut-allergic individuals (ages 6–55 years) who were randomized into 4 treatment arms (n = 55 per treatment group) to assess 3 doses of Viaskin Peanut (50, 100, and 250 μg peanut protein) compared with placebo. Successful therapy, defined after 12 months of therapy as the ability to tolerate at least 1 g of peanut protein or a 10-fold higher dose needed to elicit a reaction, was seen in all 3 groups (45.3%, 41.1%, and 50%, respectively). If the criteria were changed to stricter endpoint of 10-fold and minimum of 1000 mg, the study was successful with response rate of 6.5% in the placebo, 28.6% (50 μg), 30.8% (100 μg), and 32.1% (250 μg) [NCT01675882]. The change in cumulative reactive dose of peanut that elicited a reaction at 12 months of therapy was +62.8 mg in placebo, +471.2 mg at 50 μg, +617.5 mg at 100 μg, and +1121 mg at 500 μg dose in the children less 12 years of age. In comparison, the adolescent and adults had less effect but with a trend toward better response with higher dose of EPIT with cumulative reactive dose of 528, 619, 842, and 837 mg for placebo and increasing doses of peanut EPIT.[48,49] These data suggest a significant response to EPIT therapy for peanut.

The VIPES Open-Label Follow-up Study (OLFUS), a phase IIb clinical trial, was initiated in 2013 to assess the safety and efficacy of Viaskin peanut after 36 months of therapy. It included 170 (82%) of the patients who completed 12 months of therapy in the VIPES trial. Patients who show desensitization after 36 months discontinue therapy to evaluate for sustained unresponsiveness [NCT01955109]. The data from this study have not been presented at the current time.

In 2013, another randomized, DBPC trial was initiated by the Consortium of Food Allergy Research to evaluate Viaskin peanut. The trial enrolled 75 patients who were randomized to 2 doses of Viaskin (100 and 250 μg) or placebo. After 52 weeks of therapy, oral food challenges are to be performed. Patients who successfully complete the desensitization protocol with undergo another DBPCFC after 30 months of therapy. Those who pass the challenge will discontinue therapy for up to 20 weeks to assess for sustained unresponsiveness. The placebo group will crossover to active therapy after 52 weeks and a DBPCFC will be performed after 30 months. The anticipated duration of the study is 4 years and has not been presented at the current time [NCT01904604].

Safety

Studies evaluating EPIT for FA have displayed an excellent safety profile.[46–48] The epidermis does not contain blood vessels; therefore, allergen delivery to the epidermis does not cause a large release of allergens into the blood stream,[43] leading to a low risk of systemic reactions. From the only fully published trial, the pilot milk EPIT study by Dupont and colleagues[47] the authors concluded that EPIT is well tolerated and local reactions did not require treatment with epinephrine. Based on data presented in abstracts at the AAAAI and ECAAI on the VIPES and ARACHILD studies, there are no systemic reactions owing to Viaskin patch and only well-tolerated localized reactions to EPIT with 2 patients withdrawing owing to localized dermatitis.[48,49]

Immune Mechanisms

The goal of EPIT is to safely and effectively administer allergen to the epidermis.[11] Several mouse studies have elucidated the mechanism by which EPIT modulates the immune system.[46,50,51] Application of EDS on intact skin enhances the skin hydration through sweat and promotes allergen diffusion through the superficial layers of the skin. Subsequently, dermal dendritic cells uptake the allergen, which becomes concentrated inside the stratum corneum, without free passage through the skin.[43,46,50] Dermal dendritic cells and Langerhans cells are involved in transporting antigen from the epidermis to afferent lymph nodes to activate immune responses.[43] Repeated applications down-regulate local eosinophil recruitment and decrease systemic allergen-specific immune responses while increasing Tregs.[43]

Previous studies show an association between AIT and Tregs.[13,52] CD4$^+$ Tregs include inducible Tregs and naturally occurring Tregs.[13] Inducible Tregs consist of different subsets and they each suppress the immune response differently.[13] These include IL-10–producing Tr1 cells (Tr1), transforming growth factor-β–inducing Th3 cells, and CD4$^+$ CD25$^+$ Foxp3$^+$ Tregs (Foxp3$^+$).[13,53] Different immunotherapy routes may induce different Tregs.[13] SCIT and SLIT induces a transient increase in Tr1, followed by an immune deviation toward the Th1 response.[13,39] EPIT increased peripheral Foxp3$^+$ CD4$^+$ T cells and expression of Foxp3, which leads to a decrease in the allergen-specific cytokine production.[13,43,51]

Dioszeghy and colleagues[43] showed that EPIT-induced Tregs play an important role in developing tolerance. EPIT induces both effector and naïve Foxp3$^+$ Tregs, but not IL-10$^+$ Tr1 cells (which differs from SCIT and SLIT).[50] Foxp3 is critical for the stability of Tregs and allows CD4$^+$ CD25$^+$ Foxp3$^+$ Tregs to persist potentially for a longer period of time. The suppressive activity of Tregs is maintained even after the cessation of EPIT.[13]

In their research involving mouse models, Mondoulet and colleagues[46] found that in sensitive treated animals, EPIT decreased Th2-related cytokines (IL-4 and IL-5) and eotaxin, in addition to decreasing eosinophil infiltration in serum and Bronchoalveolar lavage (BAL). EPIT also strongly influences specific antibody levels.[46] Mouse IgG2a, which is the human equivalent of IgG4, was increased after treatment with food allergens.[46] Although SLIT also increases IgG2a after therapy, it is significantly higher with EPIT.[50] These changes reflect the switch of the immune response from a Th2 to a Th1 profile.[50] Compared with SLIT, EPIT induces a stronger reduction of the Th2 response with a greater decrease in IL-4, IL-5, IL-10, and IL-13.[50]

SUMMARY

Over the past several years, there has been an increase in studies investigating the best modality to treat food allergies. Although SCIT is known to be the most efficacious route for the treatment of environmental allergies, it has not been adopted into practice for FA treatment owing to the high rate of systemic side effects. OIT has shown promising results and is able to induce desensitization, but it too is accompanied by an increased risk of systemic reactions compared with SLIT and EPIT. In the search for efficacious, yet well-tolerated therapies, both SLIT and EPIT have great potential.

SLIT improves the safety of the therapy, but its efficacy remains uncertain and seems lower compared with OIT. As it presently stands, SLIT may be useful as a bridging technique before initiating OIT, or it may need to be optimized with adjuvants to make it more efficacious when used alone. EPIT seems to be more promising owing to a potentially better safety profile, but there are limited data at this time with respect to this and its efficacy, because the data have only been presented as abstracts and have not been peer reviewed. Both SLIT and EPIT show that patients can theoretically increase their threshold doses to a food allergen, thus providing at least partial protection against accidental exposures without suffering severe symptoms. Additionally, several strategies are currently being investigated to improve the immunologic properties of both SLIT and EPIT.[24,45]

More research is needed to define the optimal doses and administration protocol for both SLIT and EPIT. Little is known about the long-term efficacy of these therapies, which can potentially expose treated patients to a high risk of subsequent reactions even with brief lapses in exposure.[34] Although emerging evidence suggests that SLIT and EPIT may be effective in the treatment of FA, further studies are needed before these therapies can be offered to patients in clinical practice.

REFERENCES

1. Savage J, Johns CB. Food allergy: epidemiology and natural history. Immunol Allergy Clin N Am 2015;35:45–59.
2. Sicherer SH, Sampson HA. Food allergy: recent advances in pathophysiology and treatment. Annu Rev Med 2009;60:261–77.
3. Branum AM, Lukacs SL. Food allergy among children in the United States. Pediatrics 2009;124:1549–55.
4. Lee LA, Burks AW. Food allergies: prevalence, molecular characterizations, and treatment/prevention strategies. Annu Rev Nutr 2006;26:539–65.
5. Skolnick HS, Conover-Walker MK, Koerner CB, et al. The natural history of peanut allergy. J Allergy Clin Immunol 2001;107:367–74.
6. Yu JW, Kogan R, Verreault N, et al. Accidental ingestions in children with peanut allergy. J Allergy Clin Immunol 2006;118:466–72.
7. Flokstra-de Blok BM, Dubois AE, Vlieg-Boerstra BJ, et al. Health-related quality of life of food allergic patients: comparison with the general population and other diseases. Allergy 2010;65:238–44.
8. Diamanti A, Pedicelli D, D'Argenio P, et al. Iatrogenic Kwashiorkor in three infants on a diet of rice beverages. Pediatr Allergy Immunol 2011;22:878–9.
9. Flammarion S, Santos C, Guimber D, et al. Diet and nutritional status of children with food allergies. Pediatr Allergy Immunol 2011;22:161–5.
10. Groetch M, Nowak-Wegrzyn A. Practical approach to nutrition and dietary intervention in pediatric food allergy. Pediatr Allergy Immunol 2013;24:212–21.
11. Kostadinova A, Willemsen LEM, Knippels LMJ, et al. Immunotherapy – risk/benefit in food allergy. Pediatr Allergy Immunol 2013;24:633–44.
12. Akdis M, Akdis CA. Mechanisms of allergen-specific immunotherapy: multiple suppressor factors at work in immune tolerance to allergens. J Allergy Clin Immunol 2014;133:621–31.
13. Dioszeghy V, Mondoulet L, Dheift V, et al. The regulatory T cells induction by epicutaneous immunotherapy is sustained and mediates long-term protection from eosinophilic disorders in peanut-sensitized mice. Clin Exp Allergy 2014;44:867–81.

14. Nowak-Wegrzyn A, Fiocchi A. Is oral immunotherapy the cure for food allergies? Curr Opin Allergy Clin Immunol 2010;10:214–9.
15. Rolinck-Werninghaus C, Staden U, Mehl A, et al. Specific oral tolerance induction with food in children: transient or persistent effect on food allergy? Allergy 2005; 60:1320–2.
16. Oppenheimer JJ, Nelson HS, Bock SA, et al. Treatment of peanut allergy with rush immunotherapy. J Allergy Clin Immunol 1992;90:256–62.
17. Nelson HS, Lahr J, Rule R, et al. Treatment of anaphylactic sensitivity to peanuts by immunotherapy with injections of aqueous peanut extract. J Allergy Clin Immunol 1997;99:744–51.
18. McGowan EC, Wood RA. Sublingual (SLIT) versus oral immunotherapy (OIT) for food allergy. Curr Allergy Asthma Rep 2014;14:486.
19. Jay DC, Nadeau KC. Immune mechanisms of sublingual immunotherapy. Curr Allergy Asthma Rep 2014;14:473.
20. Scadding K, Brostoff J. Low dose sublingual therapy in patients with allergic rhinitis due to dust mite. Clin Allergy 1986;16:483–91.
21. Bousquet J, Lockey R, Malling HJ. WHO position paper. Allergen immunotherapy: therapeutic vaccines for allergic diseases. Allergy 1998;53(Suppl S44):1–42.
22. Bousquet J, VanCauwenberge P, Khaltaev N. Aria workshop group: WHO. Allergic rhinitis and its impact on asthma. J Allergy Clin Immunol 2001; 108(Suppl 5):S147–334.
23. Canonica GW, Bousquet J, Casale T, et al. Sublingual immunotherapy: world allergy organization position paper 2009. Allergy 2009;64(Suppl 91):1–59.
24. Compalati E, Braido F, Canonica GW. Sublingual immunotherapy: recent advances. Allergol Int 2010;62:415–23.
25. Mempel M, Rakoski J, Ring J, et al. Severe anaphylaxis to kiwi fruit: immunologic changes related to successful sublingual allergen immunotherapy. J Allergy Clin Immunol 2003;111:1406–9.
26. Kerzl R, Simonowa A, Ring J, et al. Life-threatening anaphylaxis to kiwi fruit: protective sublingual allergen immunotherapy effect persists even after discontinuation. J Allergy Clin Immunol 2006;119:507–8.
27. Enrique E, Pineda F, Malek T, et al. Sublingual immunotherapy for hazelnut food allergy: A randomized, double-blind, placebo-controlled study with a standardized hazelnut extract. J Allergy Clin Immunol 2005;116:1073–9.
28. Enrique E, Malek T, Pineda F, et al. Sublingual immunotherapy for hazelnut food allergy: A follow-up study. Ann Allergy Asthma Immunol 2008;100:283–4.
29. de Boissieu D, Dupont C. Sublingual immunotherapy for cow's milk protein allergy: a preliminary report. Allergy 2006;61:1238–9.
30. Fernandez-Rivas M, Garrido Fernancez S, Nadal JA, et al. Randomized double-blind, placebo-controlled trial of sublingual immunotherapy with a Pru p 3 quantified peach extract. Allergy 2009;64:876–83.
31. Kim EH, Bird JA, Kulis M, et al. Sublingual immunotherapy for peanut allergy: clinical and immunologic evidence of desensitization. J Allergy Clin Immunol 2011; 127:640–6.e1.
32. Fleischer DM, Burks AW, Vickery BP, et al. Sublingual immunotherapy for peanut allergy: a randomized, double-blind, placebo-controlled multicenter trial. J Allergy Clin Immunol 2013;131:119–27.e1-7.
33. Burks AW, Wood RA, Jones SM, et al. Sublingual immunotherapy for peanut allergy: Long-term follow- up of a randomized multicenter trial. J Allergy Clin Immunol 2015;135:1240–8.e3.

34. Keet CA, Frischmeyer-Guerrerio PA, Thyagarajan A, et al. The safety and efficacy of sublingual and oral immunotherapy for milk. J Allergy Clin Immunol 2012;129:448–55.
35. Chin SJ, Vickery BP, Julis MD, et al. Sublingual versus oral immunotherapy for peanut-allergic children: a retrospective comparison. J Allergy Clin Immunol 2013;132:476–8.
36. Varshney P, Jones SM, Scurlock AM, et al. A randomized controlled study of peanut oral immunotherapy: clinical desensitization and modulation of the allergic response. J Allergy Clin Immunol 2014;132(2):476–8.
37. Skripak JM, Nash SD, Rowley H. A randomized, double-blind, placebo-controlled study of milk oral immunotherapy for cow's milk allergy. J Allergy Clin Immunol 2008;122(6):1154–60.
38. Narisety S, Frischmeyer-Guerrerio PA, Keet CA, et al. A randomized, double-blind, placebo-controlled pilot study of sublingual versus oral immunotherapy for the treatment of peanut allergy. J Allergy Clin Immunol 2015;135:1275–82.
39. Bohle B, Kinaciyan T, Gerstmayr M, et al. Sublingual immunotherapy induces IL-10-producing T regulatory cells, allergen-specific T-cell tolerance, and immune deviation. J Allergy Clin Immunol 2007;120:707–13.
40. Jones SM, Burks AW, Dupont C. State of the art on food allergen immunotherapy: oral, sublingual, and epicutaneous. J Allergy Clin Immunol 2014;133:318–23.
41. Pellerin L, Jenks J, Begin P, et al. Regulatory T cells and their roles in immune dysregulation and allergy. Immunol Res 2014;133:318–23.
42. Suarez-Fueyo A, Ramos T, Galan A, et al. Grass tablet sublingual immunotherapy downregulates the TH2 cytokine response followed by regulatory T-cell generation. J Allergy Clin Immunol 2014;133:130–8.
43. Dioszeghy V, Mondoulet L, Dhelft V, et al. Epicutaneous immunotherapy results in rapid allergen uptake by dendritic cells through intact skin and downregulates the allergen-specific response in sensitized mice. J Immunol 2011;186:5629–37.
44. Vallery-Radot P, Hangenau J. Asthme d'origine equine. Essai de desensibilisation par des cutireactions repetees. Bull Soc Med Hop Paris 1921;45:1251–60.
45. Senti G, von Moos S, Kundig TM. Epicutaneous immunotherapy for aeroallergen and food allergy. Curr Treat Options Allergy 2013;1:68–78.
46. Mondoulet L, Dioszeghy V, Ligouis M, et al. Epicutaneous immunotherapy on intact skin using a new delivery system in a murine model of allergy. Clin Exp Allergy 2010;40:659–67.
47. Dupont C, Kalach N, Soulaines P, et al. Cow's milk epicutaneous immunotherapy in children: a pilot trial of safety, acceptability, and impact on allergic reactivity. J Allergy Clin Immunol 2010;125:1165–7.
48. DBV Technologies, European Academy of Allergy and Clinical Immunology Annual Meeting. Barcelona, Spain, June 7, 2015. Available at: http://media.dbv-technologies.com/a6bf4/ressources/_pdf/2/2057,DBV-EAACI-symposium-full-presentati.pdf. Accessed July 9, 2015.
49. Sampson HA, Agbotounou W, Thébault C, et al. Epicutaneous Immunotherapy (EPIT) is effective and safe to treat peanut allergy: a multi-national double-blind placebo-controlled randomized phase IIb trial. J Allergy Clinic Immunol 2015;135:SAB390.
50. Mondoulet L, Dioszeghy V, Ligouis M, et al. Epicutaneous immunotherapy compared with sublingual immunotherapy in mice sensitized to pollen (Phleum pretense). ISRN Allergy 2012;2012:375735.
51. Mondoulet L, Dioszeghy V, Puteaux E, et al. Intact skin and not stripped skin is crucial for the safety and efficacy of peanut epicutaneous immunotherapy (EPIT) in mice. Clin Transl Allergy 2012;2:22.

52. Jutel M, Akdis M, Budak F, et al. IL-10 and TGF-beta cooperate in the regulatory T cell response to mucosal allergens in normal immunity and specific immunotherapy. Eur J Immunol 2003;33:1205–14.

53. Akdis CA, Akdis M. Mechanisms and treatment of allergic disease in the big picture of regulatory T cells. J Allergy Clin Immunol 2009;123:735–46.

Oral Immunotherapy for Food Allergy

Allison J. Burbank, MD[a], Puja Sood, MD[c], Brian P. Vickery, MD[a],*,
Robert A. Wood, MD[b]

KEYWORDS

- Food allergy • Oral immunotherapy (OIT) • Desensitization • Tolerance
- Sustained unresponsiveness • Skin prick test (SPT) • Immunoglobulin E (IgE)
- Omalizumab

KEY POINTS

- There are no approved interventional treatments for food allergy.
- Multiple studies have demonstrated the ability of oral immunotherapy (OIT) to induce desensitization to cow's milk, hen's egg, and peanut.
- There are limited data available to support a disease-modifying effect of OIT.
- Adverse reactions are common in patients receiving OIT and can be life threatening.

INTRODUCTION

Food allergy is a potentially life-threatening condition and is now estimated to affect up to 8% of children and up to 2% to 3% of adults in the United States.[1,2] Cow's milk (CM), hen's egg, peanut, tree nut, wheat, soy, fish, and shellfish are the foods most often associated with food allergy in the United States.[2] Avoidance is currently the only approved therapy for food allergy. Strict avoidance diets can be difficult, especially because most of these foods are commonly used in food preparation. Avoidance diets may also put children at risk of nutritional deficiencies and impaired growth.[3,4] Although approximately 85% of milk- and egg-allergic children are expected to achieve natural tolerance to these foods by adulthood, only 15% to 20% of peanut or tree nut allergic individuals "outgrow" their allergies.[5]

Peanut is a particularly important food allergen in Westernized countries, affecting up to 1% of children in the United States.[6,7] Peanut is implicated in more than one-half of all fatal food allergy–related deaths in the United States, and a disproportionate number of patients experiencing fatal reactions are teenagers and young adults.[8,9] One case series of 32 fatal reactions reported 69% were between the ages of 13 and 21 years.[10,11]

[a] Department of Rheumatology, Allergy, and Immunology, University of North Carolina, CB #7231, Chapel Hill, NC 27599, USA; [b] Johns Hopkins University School of Medicine, Baltimore, MD 21218, USA; [c] Department of Pediatrics, University of Maryland Children's Hospital, Baltimore, MD 21201, USA
* Corresponding author.
E-mail address: bvickery@email.unc.edu

Immunol Allergy Clin N Am 36 (2016) 55–69
http://dx.doi.org/10.1016/j.iac.2015.08.007
0889-8561/16/$ – see front matter © 2016 Elsevier Inc. All rights reserved.

immunology.theclinics.com

Accidental exposures affect an estimated 12.5% of children with peanut allergy annually.[12] Food allergy has a negative impact on quality of life owing to food-related anxiety, fear of accidental exposures, and social and dietary limitations.[7,13] Currently there is no known cure or disease-modifying treatment for food allergy.

WHAT IS ORAL IMMUNOTHERAPY?

Oral immunotherapy (OIT) involves mixing an allergenic food into a vehicle and consuming it in gradually increasing doses. Protocols vary in the type of food and vehicle substance used for OIT, with some using commercially available foods in their natural forms (eg, liquid milk, ground peanuts) whereas others use prepared products such as defatted peanut flour or dehydrated egg white. Currently, virtually all OIT research studies ongoing at US academic centers require Investigational New Drug status, and these US Food and Drug Administration–regulated forms of therapy require additional standards and safeguards. For example, allergenic proteins must be identified and quantified and the product must be shown to be free of common microbial contaminants.

Most OIT protocols include an initial escalation phase, followed by dose buildup phase and maintenance phases with considerable variability depending on the study (**Fig. 1**).[14] The initial escalation phase is often done over a single day and involves rapid updosing starting from a very small dose that is rapidly increased.[14] The purpose of this initial dose escalation is to safely begin OIT in a subthreshold starting dose and identify a safe starting daily dose for home administration. Generally, the initial doses are in microgram quantities of allergenic protein, often requiring liquid preparation/dilution, and can be advanced to the solid OIT product in the range of several milligrams by the end of this phase. If well-tolerated, the dose is escalated incrementally (usually biweekly or weekly) until a target maintenance dose is reached or the subject reaches dose-limiting toxicity. There is considerable variation between studies regarding the target maintenance dose, in large part because formal pharmacokinetic and pharmacodynamic studies of OIT are lacking. In addition, there has been no attempt to harmonize the approaches toward demonstrating clinical efficacy. Maintenance therapy continues with daily administration in the home, and the duration of maintenance therapy varies and can continue for months to years.[15]

EFFICACY OF ORAL IMMUNOTHERAPY

The efficacy of an OIT trial depends on the defined endpoints, namely whether the goal is to induce desensitization alone or to induce a more durable state of clinical

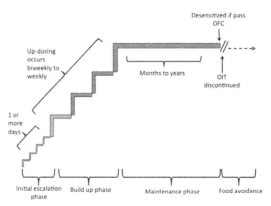

Fig. 1. Typical oral immunotherapy (OIT) protocol. OFC, open food challenge.

tolerance, which is often referred to as "sustained unresponsiveness."[16,17] Desensitization is defined as a temporary increase in the threshold for reactivity, and maintenance of the desensitized state requires continued consumption of the allergenic protein to prevent the reappearance of reactivity. Most of the studies described in this review include an end-of-study, double-blind, placebo-controlled food challenge (DBPCFC) to determine which subjects were desensitized successfully. In some trials, subjects who are desensitized successfully are then required by the protocol to restrict the allergenic food from their diet. After some defined period of time, which is not universally established but conventionally 4 to 8 weeks, the participant again undergoes a DBPCFC to determine whether or not they have achieved sustained unresponsiveness to the food. In this context, sustained unresponsiveness is defined as the consumption of all of the challenge material without dose-limiting symptoms. Most studies then follow this blinded challenge with an open feeding of a serving size portion. If a subject is able to consume all of these exposures successfully, then the individual is encouraged to incorporate the previously allergenic food regularly into the diet. Although a number of studies have demonstrated that the majority of allergic subjects treated with OIT can be desensitized successfully to a particular food, sustained unresponsiveness is achieved less commonly.

The implications of these observed changes remain poorly understood. This is owing largely to the majority of studies lacking (1) rigorously designed control groups designed to clearly show the effect of OIT and (2) long-term follow-up after OIT. However, taken together several lines of evidence from published studies described in detail herein suggest that the clinical effects after OIT are transient.[16–22] This lack of sustained protection against allergic symptoms has important implications for the future of OIT and reinforces the experimental nature of this treatment.

SUMMARY OF CLINICAL TRIALS
Peanut Oral Immunotherapy

Desensitization with injection peanut immunotherapy was first described in 1992 with an unacceptable systemic reaction rate of 13.3%.[23] After 2 case reports of successful peanut OIT in 2006,[24,25] the first open-label trial of peanut OIT was published in 2009 in a prospective cohort study.[14,26] This study showed successful induction of desensitization, an overall reassuring safety profile, as well as humoral and cellular changes demonstrating immune modulation. Using a maintenance dose of 1800 mg of peanut protein, at 36 months 27 of 29 patients (93%) who completed the protocol were able to tolerate an oral challenge with a cumulative dose of 3.9 g of peanut protein.[26] In 2010, Blumchen and colleagues[19] reported that 23 children with significant risk factors (history of high sensitivity and comorbidities such as asthma) were able to be maintained at 500 mg peanut protein daily over a 9-week period, although the success rate for passing oral food challenges was less than in the Jones study.

With regard to randomized clinical trials, in 2011 Varshney and colleagues[27] reported the first multicenter, randomized, double-blind, placebo-controlled study of peanut OIT. The study included 28 subjects, ages 1 through 16, who underwent oral sensitization with peanut flour or placebo to a daily maintenance dose of 4 g, and were followed for about 1 year. In a DBPCFC, 16 subjects who completed OIT in the active treatment arm were able to ingest a maximum cumulative dose of 5 g of peanut (~20 peanuts) compared with the placebo group of 9 subjects who tolerated a median of 280 mg of peanut. Three patients withdrew early owing to adverse reactions. The study also showed a significant decrease in skin test wheal size as well as serum interleukin (IL)-5 and IL-13 levels in the active group compared with the placebo, as well as an increase in the proportion of CD4$^+$ CD25$^+$ FoxP3$^+$ T-regulatory cells.

In 2011, Anagnostou and colleagues[28] published a prospective cohort study of peanut OIT, in which 22 children received daily maintenance dosing of 800 mg of peanut protein for 32 weeks. This study showed a significant increase in peanut tolerance with immunotherapy, with 86% of subjects tolerating updosing and 14 of 22 (64%) tolerating 6.6 g protein at completion of treatment. In 2014, the same group completed the largest peanut OIT randomized, controlled trial using a maintenance dosing of 800 mg.[29] The trial was split into 2 phases. In the first phase, each arm underwent 26 weeks of peanut OIT versus standard of care, peanut avoidance, after which subjects underwent a food challenge to 1400 mg of peanut protein. In the active OIT group, 24 of 39 participants (62%) had no reaction compared with no participants in the control group. The second phase allowed participants in the control group to receive active peanut OIT. Eighty-four percent Of the active group at the end of the first phase and 91% of the control group at the end of the second phase were able to tolerate daily ingestion of 800 mg protein for 26 weeks.

In 2014, Vickery and colleagues[17] published the first study of sustained unresponsiveness after peanut OIT. Twenty-four subjects ages 1 to 16 completed OIT with maintenance dosing of 4000 mg of peanut protein for up to 5 years. One month after stopping OIT, 50% of the subjects demonstrated sustained unresponsiveness to a 5000 mg DBPCFC. They also showed patients passing the challenge had other evidence of sustained immunomodulatory effects with smaller skin test results, lower peanut immunoglobulin (Ig)E levels (especially Ara h 1 and Ara h 2), and lower ratios of peanut-specific IgE/total IgE. With sublingual immunotherapy (SLIT) therapy also emerging, Narisety and colleagues[30] conducted a randomized, double-blind, placebo-controlled pilot study comparing peanut SLIT and OIT, demonstrating a significant increased challenge threshold at 12 months for OIT, but with a greater rate of adverse reactions and early study withdrawal. Only 4 of 20 subjects were shown to have sustained unresponsiveness. A summary of the findings of several landmark trials of peanut OIT can be found in **Table 1**.

Egg Oral Immunotherapy

In 2 early studies, Patriarca and colleagues[31,32] reported on a small series of patients treated with egg OIT. In one, desensitization was successful in 5 of 5 patients and in the other it was successful in 11 of 15 patients. In one of the first studies in the United States, Buchanan and colleagues[33] treated 7 children aged 14 months to 7 years with 24 months of maintenance OIT at a dose of 300 mg/d, with 57% passing an oral food challenge at treatment completion. In a follow-up study at the same center, patients were treated with a higher, individualized dose (median, 2400 mg) for a longer duration (median, 33 months) with a goal of reducing the egg IgE level below 2 kU$_A$/L.[34] Six of the 6 patients, including 3 patients whose egg white IgE remained more than 4 kU$_A$/L, passed a DBPCFC 1 month after stopping treatment and were considered "tolerant," with the study reporting a 75% "tolerance" rate from the original 8 participants.

In the first randomized trial of egg OIT, Staden and colleagues[18] reported on 45 children who were randomized to receive either egg or milk OIT, with maintenance dosing of 1.6 or 3.5 g/d, respectively, or an elimination diet as a control. Eleven of the patients were egg allergic. Although the milk and egg results were not separated, after a median of 21 months of therapy, 16 of the 25 (64%) were able to introduce the previously allergenic food into their diet, 9 with complete tolerance and 7 with partial tolerance, compared with 7 of 20 children (35%) in the control group. In the same year, Morisset and colleagues[35] published a randomized study of 60 children with milk allergy (13

Table 1
Peanut OIT studies

Reference, Year	Design	Samples Size (n)	Subject Age	Maintenance Dose (mg)	Duration	Conclusions
Jones et al,[26] 2009	Open label	29	1–16	1800 mg	36 mo	93% passed 3.9 g peanut OFC
Blumchen et al,[19] 2010	Randomized, open label	23	3–14	500	7-day rush escalation, 8 wk maintenance	64% reached their maintenance dose of 500 mg peanut
Varshney et al,[27] 2011	Randomized, placebo controlled	19	3–11	2000	48 wk	84% passed 5000 mg peanut OFC
Anagnostou et al,[28] 2011	Open label	22	4–18	800	32 wk	64% tolerated 6.6 g OFC
Anagnostou et al,[29] 2014	Randomized, placebo controlled	39	7–16	800	26 wk	62% tolerated 1400 mg challenge
Vickery et al,[17] 2014	Open label	24	1–16	≤4000	≤5 y	1 mo after OIT stopped, 50% achieved sustained unresponsiveness to 5000 mg OFC
Narisety et al,[30] 2014	Randomized, placebo controlled	16	7–13	2000	12 mo	Significantly greater increase in OFC threshold in OIT vs SLIT, low rate of sustained unresponsiveness

Abbreviations: OFC, open food challenge; OIT, oral immunotherapy; SLIT, sublingual immunotherapy.

months-6.5 years), and 90 children with egg allergy (12 months-8 years). Patients were randomized to OIT or allergen avoidance, and after 6 months of treatment 69% of those receiving egg OIT showed successful induction of desensitization.

In 2012, Burks and colleagues[16] published results of a multicenter, double-blind, randomized, placebo-controlled trial of egg OIT in 55 subjects, ages 5 to 11 years, with persistent egg allergy. The maintenance phase of the study consisted of 2 g of egg protein daily with egg DBPCFCs performed at 10 and 22 months. For those without reaction at the 22-month challenge, OIT was discontinued for 6 to 8 weeks with repeat food challenge to test for sustained unresponsiveness. At the 10-month DBPCFC, none of the placebo patients (n = 15) were desensitized compared with 55% of those treated with active OIT. After 22 months of OIT, 30 of 40 subjects (75%) were effectively desensitized, but only 11 (28%) demonstrated sustained unresponsiveness on rechallenge 6 to 8 weeks later. Participants who had smaller egg skin tests and higher egg-specific IgG4 were more likely to have sustained unresponsiveness.

Caminiti and colleagues[22] conducted a randomized, placebo-controlled trial of egg OIT in which egg-allergic children were treated with OIT or placebo for 4 months. Sixteen of the 17 subjects enrolled in the OIT group were desensitized and added egg to their diet. After 6 months of OIT, they avoided egg for a 3-month period followed by DBPCFC. In the OIT group, 5 patients (31%) remained tolerant to egg, whereas only 1 patient in the placebo group was tolerant to egg during the final oral challenge. Some of the discrepancy in desensitization rates between Burks and colleagues[16] and Caminiti and colleagues[22] could be owing to differences in trial design and subject selection. For example, the study by Burks and colleagues excluded patients with egg-specific IgE of less than 5 kU/L in children aged 6 years and older and less than 12 kU/L in children 5 years and younger in an attempt to exclude subjects who were likely to achieve natural tolerance to egg during the study period. Additionally, Caminiti and colleagues used a similar target dose of egg for their OIT protocol as for the DBPCFC dose used to confirm desensitization (about 4 g). In contrast, Burks and colleagues used a maintenance dose of 2 g of egg with a DBPCFC dose of 5 g at 10 months or 10 g at 22 months.

Other studies of egg OIT have included small randomized, controlled trials by Dello Iacono and colleagues[36] and Meglio and colleagues[37] with desensitization rates of 80% to 90%, including children with severe egg allergy, and 2 studies using rush protocols with desensitization induced in as few as 5 days.[38,39] **Table 2** contains a summary of the findings of key studies of egg OIT.

Milk Oral Immunotherapy

As with egg, Patriarca and colleagues[31,32] reported the first studies of milk OIT, with desensitization rates of 65.5% and 100% in 2 small trials. Meglio and colleagues[40] reported a pilot study in 2004 of 21 children at least 6 years of age with a 6-month oral desensitization protocol that resulted in a 72% success rate in achieving the target dose of 200 mL of CM daily, with an additional 14% of subjects achieving partial desensitization with 40 to 80 mL of CM per day. Of note, at a 4-year follow-up of 20 of the original participants, 65% and 5% showed total and partial tolerance, respectively, with a significant reduction in serum-specific CM IgE and negative skin prick testing for all tolerant subjects.[41] A number of other nonrandomized studies have also demonstrated overall success in desensitization with milk OIT.[42–44]

As noted for egg OIT, the first randomized, controlled trial of milk OIT was reported by Staden and colleagues.[18] In 2008, Longo and colleagues[45] reported a randomized, controlled trial of 60 children aged 5 or older with a history of severe CM allergy and

Table 2 Egg OIT studies						
Reference, Year	Design	Samples Size (n)	Subject Age	Maintenance Dose	Duration	Conclusions
Buchanan et al,[33] 2007	Open label	7	1–16	0.3 g	24 mo	57% passed 8 g OFC. 29% passed OFC after 3–4 mo period of egg avoidance
Vickery et al,[34] 2010	Open label	8	3–13	0.3–3.6 g	18– 50 mo	75% passed a 10 g OFC 1 mo after stopping OIT
Burks et al,[16] 2012	Randomized, placebo controlled	40	5–11	1.6 g	22 mo	75% passed 10 g OFC, but only 28% demonstrated sustained unresponsiveness on re-challenge 6–8 wk later

very high CM-specific IgE levels, randomized to milk OIT or avoidance. All 30 of the participants in the control group failed a DBPCFC at the 1-year mark, compared with 11 treated subjects (36%) who were completely tolerant and 16 (54%) who were partially tolerant. The first placebo-controlled OIT trial for any food in a study of milk OIT by Skripak and colleagues,[46] was undertaken in 2008, in which 21 subjects ages 6 to 17 were treated for 3 to 4 months with 500 mg of milk protein or placebo. In those on active therapy, the median milk challenge threshold increased from 40 mg at baseline to 5140 mg after treatment, with no change in the placebo group. A follow-up open-label study using individualized, ongoing milk intake demonstrated the ability to tolerate from 1000 to 16,000 mg (median of 7000, with 33% tolerating 16,000 mg) of CM protein in 13 subjects over 3 to 17 months.[47]

Pajno and colleagues[48] conducted a randomized, controlled trial of CM OIT in 2010, and their findings are summarized in **Table 3**. In 2013, the same group published data from a randomized, controlled trial suggesting that maintenance dosing after desensitization with milk OIT can be done with equal success daily or twice weekly.[49] Martorell and colleagues[50] completed a randomized, controlled trial in 2011 of 60 children ages 24 to 36 months that showed complete desensitization in 90% at 1 year. In 2012, Salmivesi and colleagues[51] published a randomized, controlled trial in school-age children showing similar effectiveness of milk OIT at the 1-year follow-up.

Also in 2012, Keet and colleagues[52] published an open-label randomized, controlled trial comparing milk OIT with SLIT in 30 children ages 6 to 17. Initial dose escalation was conducted with SLIT in all subjects followed by OIT in two-thirds of the patients. The study showed that the efficacy for desensitization was greater in patients undergoing OIT compared with SLIT, but that OIT was associated with more adverse effects. Only 40% of subjects receiving milk OIT passed an OFC when treatment was discontinued for 6 weeks, and 2 lost protection in the first week off therapy. A follow-up study of 32 patients from the 2 prior Johns Hopkins' milk OIT studies 3 to 5 years after completing therapy showed full milk tolerance in only 31% of patients, suggesting that protection is more difficult to maintain than previously described.[20]

Table 3
Milk OIT studies

Reference, Year	Design	Samples Size (n)	Subject Age	Maintenance Dose	Duration	Conclusions
Meglio et al,[40] 2004	Open label	21	6–10	200 mL	6 mo	72% achieved desensitization to 200 mL of cow's milk daily
Longo et al,[45] 2008	Randomized open label	30	5–17	150 mL	10-day rush escalation, 1 y maintenance	36% completely tolerant ($\geq$150 mL) and 54% partially tolerant (5–150 mL)
Skripak et al,[46] 2008	Randomized, placebo controlled	13	6–17	500 mg milk protein	23 wk	Median milk challenge threshold increased from 40 mg at baseline to 5140 mg after OIT
Narisety et al,[47] 2009	Open label (follow-up)	13	6–16	500–4000 mg milk protein	3–17 mo	Ongoing milk intake demonstrated tolerance from 1000 to 16,000 mg (median, 7000) with 33% tolerating 16,000 mg on OFC
Pajno et al,[48] 2010	Randomized, placebo controlled	15	4–10	200 mL	18 wk	67% tolerant to 200 mL cow's milk
Martorell et al,[50] 2011	Randomized, placebo controlled	30	2–3	200 mL	1 y	90% showing complete desensitization
Keet et al,[52] 2012	Randomized, placebo controlled	20 for OIT	6–17	1000–2000 mg	60 wk	70% of patients receiving OIT passed an 8 g OFC; only 40% passed OFC when treatment was discontinued for 6 wk

Abbreviations: OFC, open food challenge; OIT, oral immunotherapy.

MULTIPLE FOODS

Begin and colleagues[53] conducted a phase I single-center study of OIT in patients with multiple food allergies to determine the safety of multifood OIT compared with single food OIT. Of the 40 subjects who underwent DBPCFC to peanut as well as other allergenic foods, 25 were reactive to peanut plus at least 1 other food during challenge. The remaining 15 were reactive only to peanut. Patients were started on OIT containing either peanut only or peanut plus up to 4 additional foods. The frequency of adverse reactions was similar between the peanut OIT group and the multiple food OIT group. However, dose escalation occurred more rapidly in the peanut OIT group than in the multiple food OIT group.

IMMUNOLOGIC CHANGES WITH ORAL IMMUNOTHERAPY

The mechanisms of OIT are still under investigation. Active suppression of immune responses seems to occur with an increase in food-specific IgG4 during OIT, which is thought to have an antigen-neutralizing effect, and decreased basophil and mast cell responsiveness.[16,17,21,26] Some studies have shown that OIT alters the binding pattern of antigen to antigen-specific IgE, either by a decrease in the amount of specific IgE, a decrease in the diversity of epitope recognition, or altered affinity of IgE for antigen.[54] Studies of OIT have demonstrated decreased allergen-induced SPT and basophil activation in the first few months of immunotherapy.[21,26] After 6 to 12 months of OIT, there seems to be a shift away from T-helper 2 cytokine production toward a proinflammatory profile characterized by increased production of IL-1β and tumor necrosis factor-α.[26] Immune suppression by T-regulatory cells and clonal anergy are thought to occur later in the course of OIT. Syed and colleagues[55] demonstrated increased function of antigen-specific CD4$^+$ CD25$^+$ FoxP3$^+$ T-regulatory cells after OIT supporting the theory of active suppression of immune responses to food allergens.[21] Oral antigen-induced deletion of food-specific T cells in Peyer's patches has been demonstrated in mouse models.[56] In a recent publication by Begin and colleagues,[57] T-cell receptors of peanut-proliferative CD4 T cells were sequenced. They found an initially highly diverse polyclonal response to incubation with peanut, but only a small number of clones were consistent over time. When these clones were followed over time in peanut-allergic patients receiving peanut OIT and omalizumab compared with patients on avoidance diets, the authors noted a change in clonal frequency among these consistent clones was demonstrated only in subjects receiving peanut OIT, suggesting possible deletion and/or anergy of peanut-proliferative T cells.

SAFETY OF ORAL IMMUNOTHERAPY

Adverse reactions are common with OIT, with similar rates reported for milk, egg, and peanut. Local symptoms such as oral itching are most common and reactions are generally mild, requiring either no treatment or antihistamines. Abdominal pain is the most common symptom leading to withdrawal from treatment, and moderate reactions, such as rhinoconjunctivitis, wheezing, vomiting, and urticaria, occur in a small percent of all doses. However, given that doses are given daily, the risk for each patient over an extended course of treatment is substantial. For example, in a study of milk OIT in young children, 47% of subjects developed moderate reactions over the course of treatment.[50] More severe reactions requiring treatment with epinephrine and β-agonists are most common during dose escalation, but can also occur during maintenance therapy.[30,45,46,48,50] Wasserman and colleagues[58] reported that 95 reactions requiring epinephrine occurred during peanut OIT for 352 patients. It is especially concerning that most severe reactions occur unpredictably, with a dose that has been previously tolerated, possibly triggered by cofactors such as infection, exercise, anxiety, or allergen coexposure.[14,29,46,47]

A particular obstacle to moving these treatments to clinical practice is the high percent of patients who cannot tolerate OIT. Overall, 10% to 20% of subjects have dropped out of OIT trials, with rates as high as 36% in some studies. Although some participants have withdrawn owing to anaphylaxis or other acute reactions, the vast majority of withdrawals are owing to chronic abdominal pain. Eosinophilic esophagitis has been documented in some of these cases and it is not clear how frequently undiagnosed disease may complicate OIT.[59,60] A recent metaanalysis of these reports revealed that eosinophilic esophagitis occurred in as many as 2.7% of patients undergoing OIT to milk, peanut, egg, or wheat.[61] However, using funnel plot analysis, the authors found a significant degree of publication bias and indicated that the actual prevalence of eosinophilic esophagitis after OIT is much less. Further studies directed at minimizing adverse reaction are therefore critically important to move these treatments forward.

ADJUNCTIVE THERAPIES

Several potential adjunctive therapies to OIT have been studied, with the goal of improving both safety and efficacy. Two studies have examined the use omalizumab in combination with OIT. In 2011, Nadeau and colleagues[62] treated 11 children with omalizumab for 9 weeks, at which time they underwent rapid desensitization to milk (0.1 to 1000 mg). For the next 8 weeks, they increased their milk dose to a goal of 2000 mg. At week 16, omalizumab was discontinued and milk consumption was maintained at 2000 mg/d for another 8 weeks. Nine of the 10 patients reached the daily maintenance dose of 2000 mg/d, and all 9 children passed the DBPCFC to 7250 mg at week 24. This study suggested that OIT can be escalated more rapidly when combined with omalizumab, although adverse reactions were still relatively common.

In another study, the combination of OIT and omalizumab was examined in peanut allergy in a pilot study of 13 children.[63] The children were treated with omalizumab for 12 weeks, at which time they underwent rapid desensitization to peanut (from 0.1 to 500 mg) over 6 hours. For the next 8 weeks, they underwent weekly updosing to a goal of 4000 mg peanut flour daily (2000 mg protein). Omalizumab was discontinued at week 20, and the children underwent an 8000-mg peanut flour DBPCFC at week 32. Twelve of the 13 children reached the goal dose, and 1 patient withdrew because of persistent nausea and vomiting. All 12 patients passed the DBPCFC at week 32 and continued to eat 10 to 20 peanuts daily until the end of the study.

Case reports and small open trials have been conducted with a number of other adjunctive therapies, including probiotics, interferon gamma, premedication with ketotifen, and more recently leukotriene receptor antagonists.[64–68] A recent placebo-controlled, randomized trial with probiotic and peanut OIT was published by Tang and colleagues[64] that suggested that the coadministration of *Lactobacillus rhamnosus* with peanut OIT facilitates sustained unresponsiveness and induces immunologic changes that can modulate food allergic responses. Unfortunately, it is not clear what, if any, were the specific effects of the probiotics because there was no OIT-only control group. In 2013, a randomized single-blind placebo-controlled study of 6 subjects undergoing peanut OIT showed that ketotifen premedication at 2 mg twice daily might decrease the incidence of gastrointestinal symptoms during active OIT.[66] Finally, Takahashi and colleagues[67] proposed the possibility of leukotriene receptor antagonists such as montelukast as an aid in OIT for the prevention of adverse allergic reactions in a retrospective study of 5 children, where leukotriene receptor antagonist intervention seemed to help patients reach their target dose. Each of these possible adjunctive therapies requires further study.

LIMITATIONS

OIT protocols are both time and labor intensive, requiring close monitoring and involvement of ancillary staff, physicians, and family members. Compliance is essential, because regular dosing is required to minimize risk and, as noted, the risk is substantial even in the clinical trial setting. Most important, the risk does not disappear once treatment is complete, because reactivity will almost certainly return without regular exposure.

FUTURE CONSIDERATIONS/SUMMARY

Food allergy is a potentially life-threatening disease affecting up to 8% of children and 3% of adults in Westernized countries. Despite the significant impact of food allergy on patients and health care systems, there are currently no approved therapies for food allergy apart from strict avoidance. Milk, egg, and peanut OIT studies have shown consistently successful desensitization to allergenic foods, although whether or not treatment is capable of inducing lasting tolerance remains to be seen. Further mechanistic studies are needed to improve understanding of the immunologic changes induced by OIT, and to identify biomarkers of response. Safety is a significant concern, and adverse events are common during OIT. Investigational therapies including coadministration of anti-IgE antibody are being studied with the hopes of making OIT safer and better tolerated. There are limited data on the ability of OIT to induce lasting tolerance to foods and warrants further study. Incorporation of novel therapies such as modified food allergens, probiotics, and other immunomodulator therapies in conjunction with OIT are underway with the goals of improving both safety and efficacy. Larger, well-designed, randomized, placebo-controlled trials are needed to determine the efficacy and acute and long-term safety of OIT before it can be implemented in general clinical practice.

REFERENCES

1. Gupta RS, Springston EE, Warrier MR, et al. The prevalence, severity, and distribution of childhood food allergy in the United States. Pediatrics 2011;128(1): e9–17.
2. Chafen JJ, Newberry SJ, Riedl MA, et al. Diagnosing and managing common food allergies: a systematic review. JAMA 2010;303(18):1848–56.
3. Kim J, Kwon J, Noh G, et al. The effects of elimination diet on nutritional status in subjects with atopic dermatitis. Nutr Res Pract 2013;7(6):488–94.
4. Hobbs CB, Skinner AC, Burks AW, et al. Food allergies affect growth in children. J Allergy Clin Immunol Pract 2015;3(1):133–4.e1.
5. Nowak-Wegrzyn A, Sampson HA. Future therapies for food allergies. J Allergy Clin Immunol 2011;127(3):558–73 [quiz 574-5].
6. Nurmatov U, Venderbosch I, Devereux G, et al. Allergen-specific oral immunotherapy for peanut allergy. Cochrane Database Syst Rev 2012;(9):CD009014.
7. Sicherer SH, Sampson HA. Food allergy. J Allergy Clin Immunol 2010;125(2 Suppl 2):S116–25.

8. Bock SA, Munoz-Furlong A, Sampson HA. Further fatalities caused by anaphylactic reactions to food, 2001-2006. J Allergy Clin Immunol 2007;119(4):1016–8.

9. Wensing M, Penninks AH, Hefle SL, et al. The range of minimum provoking doses in hazelnut-allergic patients as determined by double-blind, placebo-controlled food challenges. Clin Exp Allergy 2002;32(12):1757–62.

10. Sampson MA, Munoz-Furlong A, Sicherer SH. Risk-taking and coping strategies of adolescents and young adults with food allergy. J Allergy Clin Immunol 2006; 117(6):1440–5.

11. Bock SA, Munoz-Furlong A, Sampson HA. Fatalities due to anaphylactic reactions to foods. J Allergy Clin Immunol 2001;107(1):191–3.

12. Nguyen-Luu NU, Ben-Shoshan M, Alizadehfar R, et al. Inadvertent exposures in children with peanut allergy. Pediatr Allergy Immunol 2012;23(2):133–9.

13. Lieberman JA, Sicherer SH. Quality of life in food allergy. Curr Opin Allergy Clin Immunol 2011;11(3):236–42.

14. Hofmann A, Scurlock AM, Jones SM, et al. Safety of a peanut oral immunotherapy protocol in children with peanut allergy. J Allergy Clin Immunol 2009;124(2): 286–91, 291.e1-6.

15. Kulis M, Wright BL, Jones SM, et al. Diagnosis, management, and investigational therapies for food allergies. Gastroenterology 2015;148(6):1132–42.

16. Burks AW, Jones SM, Wood RA, et al. Oral immunotherapy for treatment of egg allergy in children. N Engl J Med 2012;367(3):233–43.

17. Vickery BP, Scurlock AM, Kulis M, et al. Sustained unresponsiveness to peanut in subjects who have completed peanut oral immunotherapy. J Allergy Clin Immunol 2014;133(2):468–75.

18. Staden U, Rolinck-Werninghaus C, Brewe F, et al. Specific oral tolerance induction in food allergy in children: efficacy and clinical patterns of reaction. Allergy 2007;62(11):1261–9.

19. Blumchen K, Ulbricht H, Staden U, et al. Oral peanut immunotherapy in children with peanut anaphylaxis. J Allergy Clin Immunol 2010;126(1):83–91.e1.

20. Keet CA, Seopaul S, Knorr S, et al. Long-term follow-up of oral immunotherapy for cow's milk allergy. J Allergy Clin Immunol 2013;132(3):737–9.e6.

21. Gorelik M, Narisety SD, Guerrerio AL, et al. Suppression of the immunologic response to peanut during immunotherapy is often transient. J Allergy Clin Immunol 2015;135(5):1283–92.

22. Caminiti L, Pajno GB, Crisafulli G, et al. oral immunotherapy for egg allergy: a double-blind placebo-controlled study, with postdesensitization follow-up. J Allergy Clin Immunol Pract 2015;3(4):532–9.

23. Oppenheimer JJ, Nelson HS, Bock SA, et al. Treatment of peanut allergy with rush immunotherapy. J Allergy Clin Immunol 1992;90(2):256–62.

24. Patriarca G, Nucera E, Pollastrini E, et al. Oral rush desensitization in peanut allergy: a case report. Dig Dis Sci 2006;51(3):471–3.

25. Mansfield L. Successful oral desensitization for systemic peanut allergy. Ann Allergy Asthma Immunol 2006;97(2):266–7.

26. Jones SM, Pons L, Roberts JL, et al. Clinical efficacy and immune regulation with peanut oral immunotherapy. J Allergy Clin Immunol 2009;124(2):292–300, 300.e1-97.

27. Varshney P, Jones SM, Scurlock AM, et al. A randomized controlled study of peanut oral immunotherapy: clinical desensitization and modulation of the allergic response. J Allergy Clin Immunol 2011;127(3):654–60.

28. Anagnostou K, Jones SM, Scurlock AM, et al. Efficacy and safety of high-dose peanut oral immunotherapy with factors predicting outcome. Clin Exp Allergy 2011;41(9):1273–81.

29. Anagnostou K, Islam S, King Y, et al. Assessing the efficacy of oral immuno-therapy for the desensitisation of peanut allergy in children (STOP II): a phase 2 randomised controlled trial. Lancet 2014;383(9925):1297–304.
30. Narisety SD, Frischmeyer-Guerrerio PA, Keet CA, et al. A randomized, double-blind, placebo-controlled pilot study of sublingual versus oral immunotherapy for the treatment of peanut allergy. J Allergy Clin Immunol 2014;135(5):1275–82.e1-6.
31. Patriarca G, Nucera E, Roncallo C, et al. Oral desensitizing treatment in food al-lergy: clinical and immunological results. Aliment Pharmacol Ther 2003;17(3): 459–65.
32. Patriarca G, Nucera E, Roncallo C, et al. Food allergy in children: results of a stan-dardized protocol for oral desensitization. Hepatogastroenterology 1998;45(19): 52–8.
33. Buchanan AD, Green TD, Jones SM, et al. Egg oral immunotherapy in nonana-phylactic children with egg allergy. J Allergy Clin Immunol 2007;119(1):199–205.
34. Vickery BP, Pons L, Kulis M, et al. Individualized IgE-based dosing of egg oral immunotherapy and the development of tolerance. Ann Allergy Asthma Immunol 2010;105(6):444–50.
35. Morisset M, Moneret-Vautrin DA, Guenard L, et al. Oral desensitization in children with milk and egg allergies obtains recovery in a significant proportion of cases. A randomized study in 60 children with cow's milk allergy and 90 children with egg allergy. Eur Ann Allergy Clin Immunol 2007;39(1):12–9.
36. Dello Iacono I, Tripodi S, Calvani M, et al. Specific oral tolerance induction with raw hen's egg in children with very severe egg allergy: a randomized controlled trial. Pediatr Allergy Immunol 2013;24(1):66–74.
37. Meglio P, Giampietro PG, Carello R, et al. Oral food desensitization in children with IgE-mediated hen's egg allergy: a new protocol with raw hen's egg. Pediatr Allergy Immunol 2013;24(1):75–83.
38. Itoh N, Itagaki Y, Kurihara K. Rush specific oral tolerance induction in school-age children with severe egg allergy: one year follow up. Allergol Int 2010;59(1): 43–51.
39. Garcia Rodriguez R, Urra JM, Feo-Brito F, et al. Oral rush desensitization to egg: efficacy and safety. Clin Exp Allergy 2011;41(9):1289–96.
40. Meglio P, Bartone E, Plantamura M, et al. A protocol for oral desensitization in chil-dren with IgE-mediated cow's milk allergy. Allergy 2004;59(9):980–7.
41. Meglio P, Giampietro PG, Gianni S, et al. Oral desensitization in children with immunoglobulin E-mediated cow's milk allergy–follow-up at 4 yr and 8 months. Pediatr Allergy Immunol 2008;19(5):412–9.
42. Zapatero L, Alonso E, Fuentes V, et al. Oral desensitization in children with cow's milk allergy. J Investig Allergol Clin Immunol 2008;18(5):389–96.
43. Alvaro M, Giner MT, Vázquez M, et al. Specific oral desensitization in children with IgE-mediated cow's milk allergy. Evolution in one year. Eur J Pediatr 2012;171(9): 1389–95.
44. Sanchez-Garcia S, Rodríguez del Río P, Escudero C, et al. Efficacy of oral immu-notherapy protocol for specific oral tolerance induction in children with cow's milk allergy. Isr Med Assoc J 2012;14(1):43–7.
45. Longo G, Barbi E, Berti I, et al. Specific oral tolerance induction in children with very severe cow's milk-induced reactions. J Allergy Clin Immunol 2008;121(2): 343–7.
46. Skripak JM, Nash SD, Rowley H, et al. A randomized, double-blind, placebo-controlled study of milk oral immunotherapy for cow's milk allergy. J Allergy Clin Immunol 2008;122(6):1154–60.

47. Narisety SD, Skripak JM, Steele P, et al. Open-label maintenance after milk oral immunotherapy for IgE-mediated cow's milk allergy. J Allergy Clin Immunol 2009;124(3):610–2.

48. Pajno GB, Caminiti L, Ruggeri P, et al. Oral immunotherapy for cow's milk allergy with a weekly up-dosing regimen: a randomized single-blind controlled study. Ann Allergy Asthma Immunol 2010;105(5):376–81.

49. Pajno GB, Caminiti L, Salzano G, et al. Comparison between two maintenance feeding regimens after successful cow's milk oral desensitization. Pediatr Allergy Immunol 2013;24(4):376–81.

50. Martorell A, De la Hoz B, Ibáñez MD, et al. Oral desensitization as a useful treatment in 2-year-old children with cow's milk allergy. Clin Exp Allergy 2011;41(9): 1297–304.

51. Salmivesi S, Korppi M, Mäkelä MJ, et al. Milk oral immunotherapy is effective in school-aged children. Acta Paediatr 2013;102(2):172–6.

52. Keet CA, Frischmeyer-Guerrerio PA, Thyagarajan A, et al. The safety and efficacy of sublingual and oral immunotherapy for milk allergy. J Allergy Clin Immunol 2012;129(2):448–55, 455.e1-5.

53. Begin P, Winterroth LC, Dominguez T, et al. Safety and feasibility of oral immunotherapy to multiple allergens for food allergy. Allergy Asthma Clin Immunol 2014; 10(1):1.

54. Vickery BP, Lin J, Kulis M, et al. Peanut oral immunotherapy modifies IgE and IgG4 responses to major peanut allergens. J Allergy Clin Immunol 2013;131(1): 128–34.e1-3.

55. Syed A, Garcia MA, Lyu SC, et al. Peanut oral immunotherapy results in increased antigen-induced regulatory T-cell function and hypomethylation of forkhead box protein 3 (FOXP3). J Allergy Clin Immunol 2014;133(2):500–10.

56. Chen Y, Inobe J, Marks R, et al. Peripheral deletion of antigen-reactive T cells in oral tolerance. Nature 1995;376(6536):177–80.

57. Begin P, Nadeau KC. Changes in peanut-specific T-cell clonotype with oral immunotherapy. J Allergy Clin Immunol 2015;135(6):1636–8.e3.

58. Wasserman RL, Factor JM, Baker JW, et al. Oral immunotherapy for peanut allergy: multipractice experience with epinephrine-treated reactions. J Allergy Clin Immunol Pract 2014;2(1):91–6.

59. Sanchez-Garcia S, Rodríguez Del Río P, Escudero C, et al. Possible eosinophilic esophagitis induced by milk oral immunotherapy. J Allergy Clin Immunol 2012; 129(4):1155–7.

60. Ridolo E, De Angelis GL, Dall'aglio P. Eosinophilic esophagitis after specific oral tolerance induction for egg protein. Ann Allergy Asthma Immunol 2011;106(1): 73–4.

61. Lucendo AJ, Arias A, Tenias JM. Relation between eosinophilic esophagitis and oral immunotherapy for food allergy: a systematic review with meta-analysis. Ann Allergy Asthma Immunol 2014;113(6):624–9.

62. Nadeau KC, Schneider LC, Hoyte L, et al. Rapid oral desensitization in combination with omalizumab therapy in patients with cow's milk allergy. J Allergy Clin Immunol 2011;127(6):1622–4.

63. Schneider LC, Rachid R, LeBovidge J, et al. A pilot study of omalizumab to facilitate rapid oral desensitization in high-risk peanut-allergic patients. J Allergy Clin Immunol 2013;132(6):1368–74.

64. Tang ML, Ponsonby AL, Orsini F, et al. Administration of a probiotic with peanut oral immunotherapy: a randomized trial. J Allergy Clin Immunol 2015;135(3): 737–44.e8.

65. Noh G, Lee SS. A pilot study of interferon-gamma-induced specific oral tolerance induction (ISOTI) for immunoglobulin E-mediated anaphylactic food allergy. J Interferon Cytokine Res 2009;29(10):667–75.
66. Jagdis A, Berlin N, Barron C, et al. Effect of ketotifen premedication on adverse reactions during peanut oral immunotherapy. Allergy Asthma Clin Immunol 2014; 10(1):36.
67. Takahashi M, Taniuchi S, Soejima K, et al. New efficacy of LTRAs (montelukast sodium): it possibly prevents food-induced abdominal symptoms during oral immunotherapy. Allergy Asthma Clin Immunol 2014;10(1):3.
68. Lee SJ, Noh G, Lee JH. In vitro induction of allergen-specific interleukin-10-producing regulatory b cell responses by interferon-gamma in non-immunoglobulin e-mediated milk allergy. Allergy Asthma Immunol Res 2013;5(1):48–54.

Mechanisms of Aeroallergen Immunotherapy

Subcutaneous Immunotherapy and Sublingual Immunotherapy

Cevdet Ozdemir, MD[a,1], Umut Can Kucuksezer, PhD[b,1],
Mübeccel Akdis, PD, MD, PhD[c], Cezmi A. Akdis, MD[c],*

KEYWORDS

- Allergy • Allergens • Immunotherapy • T regulatory cells • Tolerance

KEY POINTS

- SCIT and SLIT use similar immune mechanisms to induce tolerance development to allergens.
- Role of oral mucosa and tonsil immunity is noteworthy during SLIT, where allergens before reaching mast cells are mostly captured by tolerogenic dendritic cells.
- The very early desensitization effect and marked allergen-specific IgG4 responses are the outstanding features of SCIT.

Conflict of Interest: C.Ozdemir and U.C. Kuzuksezer declare no conflict of interest. M. Akdis has received research support from the Swiss National Science Foundation and the European Commission's Seventh Framework Programmes MeDALL and PREDICTA. C.A. Akdis has consultant arrangements with Actellion, Aventis, Stallergenes, Allergopharma, and Circacia; is employed by the Swiss Institute of Allergy and Asthma Research, University of Zurich; and has received research support from Novartis, PREDICTA: European Commission's Seventh Framework, the Swiss National Science Foundation, MeDALL: European Commission's Seventh Framework, and the Christine Kühne-Center for Allergy Research and Education. The authors' laboratories are supported by the Swiss National Science Foundation No. 310030_156823, 320030-159870, and Christine Kühne-Center for Allergy Research and Education (CK-CARE).
 a Department of Pediatric Allergy, Memorial Atasehir Hospital, Memorial Health Group, Vedat Gunyol Cad. 28-30, Istanbul 34758, Turkey; b Department of Immunology, Institute of Experimental Medicine (DETAE), Vakif Gureba Cad, Istanbul University, Istanbul 34093, Turkey; c Swiss Institute of Allergy and Asthma Research (SIAF), University of Zurich, Obere Strasse, CH-7270, Davos, Switzerland
1 These authors contributed equally to this work.
* Corresponding author. Swiss Institute of Allergy and Asthma Research (SIAF), University of Zurich, Obere Strasse 22, Davos Platz CH-7270, Switzerland.
E-mail address: akdisac@siaf.uzh.ch

Immunol Allergy Clin N Am 36 (2016) 71–86
http://dx.doi.org/10.1016/j.iac.2015.08.003
0889-8561/16/$ – see front matter © 2016 Elsevier Inc. All rights reserved.

INTRODUCTION

As the frequency of allergic disorders has increased in recent decades, concerns have been focused on how to develop preventive approaches and implement novel treatment strategies to control allergic disorders. Conventionally used pharmacotherapy regimens in various combinations with different routes of corticosteroids, antihistamines, and antileukotrienes and specific monoclonal antibodies can successfully control the symptoms in most cases during regular usage. However, on cessation of pharmacotherapy, relapse of symptoms and signs of allergic disorders emerge. Allergen immunotherapy (AIT) remains as the modality of choice and the most effective treatment of allergic disorders by targeting the underlying mechanisms and possibly altering the disease course by inducing a long-lasting tolerance to allergens.[1–3]

Allergen-specific subcutaneous immunotherapy (SCIT) has served as an active tool in the management of allergic rhinitis and allergic asthma and also for venom allergy. Sublingual immunotherapy (SLIT) has provided an alternative to SCIT in patients with allergic rhinitis and asthma in whom fear of adverse reactions and discomfort from injections limit the treatment chance. Both of these AIT routes provide a causal therapeutic approach in the management of allergic disorders, but more studies are needed to clarify certain clinical aspects.[4,5] Generation of allergen-specific peripheral tolerance is the principal event during AIT. T and B cells, mainly naturally occurring $Foxp3^+CD4^+CD25^+$ regulatory T cells (Treg) and inducible type 1 Treg cells, play key roles in tolerance development. Suppression of allergen-specific IgE production and induction of allergen-specific IgG4 antibody generation, in addition to other multiple suppressor roles on dendritic cells (DCs), T cell subsets, mast cells, basophils, and eosinophils, lead to improvement in tissue inflammation and attenuate early and late-phase inflammatory responses.[2,6,7] Hence, it is essential to describe the underlying mechanism of allergic disorders to generate more rationale and effective AIT regimens.

ALLERGIC IMMUNE RESPONSE

Aeroallergens (mainly house dust mites, pollens, molds, animal dander), certain foods, and insect venoms constitute the most common allergens responsible for clinical symptoms of allergic disorders. Individual allergic immune response depends on various factors including the presence of atopy-genetic tendency to develop allergy. In addition to dose, type, and route of allergen exposure and presentation to the immune system, the status of the surrounding microenvironment with the dominant type of effector cells and their products, microbiota, and other small molecules with costimulatory and inhibitory activity may play a role.[6,8] Naive $CD4^+$ T cells can differentiate into T helper cell (Th) 1, Th2, Th9, Th17, or Th22 type effector and memory cells, depending on microenvironmental conditions.[6,9,10] Peripheral Th2 response is dominant and interleukin (IL)-4, IL-5, and IL-13 are the leading cytokines enrolled in Th2-type immune response of allergy.[11] It has been proposed that allergic immune response is an IgE antibody-mediated disorder caused by a dysregulation in T-cell immunity.[12] The concept of allergen-specific tolerance induction and the role of immune regulatory mechanisms over Th1 and Th2 imbalance have greatly increased understanding of the mechanisms of allergic disorders.[6]

ANTIGEN PRESENTATION, CELLULAR INTERACTIONS, AND ANTIBODY RESPONSES IN ALLERGIC IMMUNE RESPONSE

Skin and mucosal surfaces (airway mucosa and gastrointestinal mucosa) are a huge area of contact with external antigens or allergens.[13–15] Presentation of the antigen or allergen is one of the pivotal steps, where a decision is made for development of immune response toward allergy. The highly specialized antigen-presenting cells, mainly DCs, reside as sentinels in an immature form at these entry surfaces. On activation, DCs migrate to local lymph nodes, where they lose their phagocytic properties with an improved antigen-presenting capacity and interact with T and B cells.[7,16] DCs can recognize the antigenic epitopes, process, and present them by coupling to major histocompatibility complex-II molecules to Th cells.

In allergic immune response, activated naive Th cells markedly differentiate into Th2-type cells in the presence of IL-4. They produce IL-4 and IL-13, which induces IgE class switch of B cells and development to allergen-specific IgE-producing plasma cells. IgE binds to its high affinity Fcε receptors on mast cells and basophils. On re-exposure with the relevant allergen, sensitized mast cells and basophils release their preformed mediators located within the intracellular granules and also synthesize new biogenic mediators, such as histamine, proteases, and newly generated lipid-derived mediators, such as leukotrienes and cytokines, causing the symptoms and signs of allergic acute-phase type-1 hypersensitivity reactions **(Fig. 1)**.[17] IL-5 is another key cytokine in allergic inflammatory immune response, which exerts its function on eosinophils by recruiting, activating, and prolonging their survival and also has stimulatory effect on B-cell growth.[18]

Cytokines released from these effector cells increase vascular permeability, angiogenesis, and fibrosis, and prosecute infiltration by eosinophils, basophils, neutrophils, macrophages, and T cells, which augment the late-phase response that is thought to

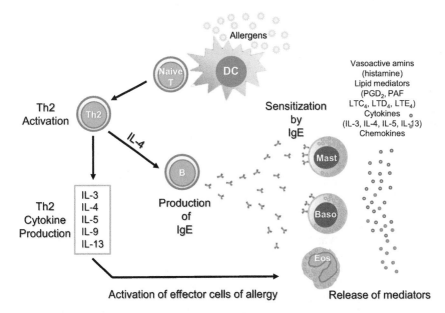

Fig. 1. Initiation of allergic response. Th2 cells are induced when allergen peptides are presented to naive CD4[+] T cells by DC, together with presence of IL-4. Th2 cells produce cytokines IL-3, IL-4, IL-5, IL-9, and IL-13, which are named as Th2-type cytokines. B cells class-switch to produce IgE, which binds to specific Fcε receptors on mast cells (Mast) and basophils (Baso) in sensitization phase. On encountering the same allergen for a second time, degranulation of mast cells and basophils leads to immediate hypersensitivity. Th2-type cytokines are important survival signals for mast cells, basophils, and eosinophils (Eos).

be responsible for the persistent, chronic signs and symptoms of allergy.[19] Moreover, IL-13 has essential roles on epithelial cell maturation and mucus production, airway smooth muscle contractility, and extracellular matrix protein production.[20] Th2 cell differentiation has been shown to be reprogrammed by transforming growth factor (TGF)-β with coexistence of IL-4, which leads to development of Th9 cells with capacity to produce IL-9 and IL-10.[21,22] IL-9 plays an essential role in the growth and survival of mast cells.[23,24]

Furthermore, IL-25, IL-31, and IL-33 are other cytokines mainly secreted by epithelial cells and DCs, which also contribute to Th2 responses.[25–27] However, Th22 cells have been shown to produce IL-22 together with low levels of IL-4, and their contribution to atopic diseases especially in atopic dermatitis has been revealed.[28] Additionally, Th17 cells express IL-17A, IL-17F, IL-6, IL-8, tumor necrosis factor-α, IL-22, and IL-26 and are shown to contribute to some autoimmune pathologies, whereas neutralization of IL-17- and Th17-related functions has been related to limitation of neutrophil infiltration in experimental models of asthma.[29]

Innate lymphoid cells (ILCs) are newly discovered subsets of the immune network, which may have possible contributions to inflammatory diseases. Type 2 ILCs have been found to have possible roles in asthma and upper respiratory inflammation and AIT to grass pollen has been shown to inhibit seasonal increases of peripheral population of type 2 ILCs.[6,30]

IMMUNE TOLERANCE TO ALLERGENS IN HEALTHY IMMUNE RESPONSE

The immune system has the capacity to tolerate self-antigens and non-self-antigens, such as allergens caused by central and peripheral tolerance, as essential mechanisms of immune homeostasis. Excessive immune tolerance may lead to loss of defense against microorganisms and cancer. In contrast, exaggerated immune response to external antigens or allergens may lead to hypersensitivity reactions that may present as allergic rhinitis, asthma, atopic dermatitis, food allergy, and anaphylaxis. During developmental stages of T cells in the thymus and B cells in bone marrow, cells with tendency to autoreactivity are deleted via apoptosis before complete differentiation. Whereas B cells become unresponsive through receptor editing, some T cells can escape from thymic deletion and reach periphery.[31,32] Peripheral tolerance mechanisms regulate this condition through T-cell anergy, apoptosis, and action of Treg cells.[33] Because allergen-specific Th2 and Treg cell repertoire specific to same allergen are reported to be present in those with allergy and healthy individuals, their ratio is claimed to determine the outcome (**Fig. 2**).[19]

It has been shown that certain innate immune response signals including proinflammatory cytokines, such as IL-1β and IL-6, and danger signals, such as Toll-like receptor (TLR) 4 and TLR8 ligands, have the capacity to break allergen-specific T-cell tolerance in healthy subjects.[34] Several viral upper respiratory tract infections as triggers of innate inflammation are known to exacerbate asthma attacks. Human rhinovirus infection has been shown to induce proinflammatory cytokine profiles with elevated IL-1β, IL-2, IL-7, and IL-8 levels, whereas bocavirus infection cannot do so, or induce a Th1 or a Th2 cytokine profile. A simultaneous infection with both viruses has induced a non-Th2 but a modified cytokine response. Immunologic responses in acute wheezing are shown to depend on host (atopy-related inflammation) and virus-specific factors, and interaction of two different virus strains may modulate immune responses.[35] In addition, the development of a healthy immune response during high-dose allergen exposure in beekeepers and cat owners has been intensively

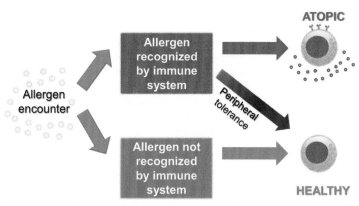

Fig. 2. Allergy versus tolerance. Allergic and nonallergic phenotypes are defined by genetic factors, which define the T-cell receptor specificity of an individual, and also by establishment and maintenance of specific tolerance to allergens. T cells with capacity to recognize allergens are present in healthy individuals and in individuals with allergy.

studied to understand mechanisms of allergen tolerance in humans. IL-10-secreting Treg cells and IgG4 production dominate the mechanisms in both models.[36-38]

REGULATORY CELLS OF THE IMMUNE SYSTEM

In the course of normal immune responses, regulation is a sine qua non. This important role is maintained by several cells with suppressor capacity. Treg cells orchestrate cells and several cellular interactions. Naturally occurring thymus-derived Forkhead box P3 (Foxp3)$^+$ CD4$^+$CD25$^+$ Treg cells and inducible type 1 Treg (Tr1) cells are the major subsets of Treg cells that have regulatory roles on other effector cells of the immune system. Foxp3 is the lineage-specific transcription factor for Treg cells, which regulates Treg cell development.[39] Gut-associated lymphoid tissue serves as a primary area of peripheral conversion of CD4$^+$ cells to Treg cells, where numerous dietary antigens are tolerated as a requisite for healthy immune response.[40] Although FoxP3 is the transcription factor for Treg cells, GATA3 drives Th2 cell differentiation. Both of these transcription factors have been upregulated simultaneously in CD4$^+$ T cells of sensitized subjects, which may suggest that Treg cells and effector T cells have the capacity to be converted to each other.[41]

It has been reported that CD4$^+$CD25$^+$ Treg cells from nonsensitized healthy donors have the capacity to suppress allergen-specific proliferative responses compared with cells obtained from sensitized individuals.[42] In addition to naturally occurring thymus-derived Treg cells in the presence of TGF-β, CD4$^+$CD25$^-$FOXP3$^-$ cells can be induced into Treg cells in the periphery.[43] Tr1 cells regulate immune homeostasis by coordinating peripheral T-cell tolerance. Treg cells have distinct cytokine profiles other than Th1 and Th2 cells, are characterized by IL-10 and TGF-β secretion capacity, and express suppressor molecules, such as cytotoxic T-lymphocyte-associated protein 4 and programmed cell death protein 1. IL-10 is the leading cytokine, which in Treg cell–B cell interaction suppresses specific IgE production. In addition, IL-10 induces specific IgG4 production. IgG4 and probably IgG1 compete with IgE on the surface of mast cells and basophils for allergen binding.[44] Novel techniques are expected to enlighten mechanisms at the single cell level. It has been recently demonstrated that clonal distribution of the peanut Ag-specific T cells changes with peanut oral immunotherapy, supporting the T-cell "replacement" hypothesis as a mechanism of food oral immunotherapy.[45]

Other immune cells have been shown to suppress allergen-specific responses. Inducible IL-10-secreting B regulatory cells have recently been demonstrated, which contribute to allergen tolerance through suppression of effector T cells and induction of IgG4 antibodies.[2,46,47] Although not studied as aeroallergen immunotherapy so far, it was demonstrated that early peanut oral immunotherapy induced an oligoclonal and somatically hypermutated allergen-specific B-cell receptor repertoire.[48] Natural killer cells are important key players of immunity to viral infections and tumors, and they also contribute to immune regulation by their cytokine secretions. A subset of natural killer cells with capacity to produce IL-10 and suppress allergen-specific T-cell responses has also been described.[49,50] Strategies to modulate natural killer cell functions may contribute to treatment of allergy.[51]

MECHANISMS OF ALLERGEN-SPECIFIC IMMUNOTHERAPY

Allergen-specific immunotherapy is an efficient disease-modifying treatment option in the management of allergic disorders with apparent immune regulatory functions. The major aim of a successful AIT is to induce a long-lasting clinically tolerant state to allergens by using peripheral immune tolerance mechanisms. Disease modification in AIT leads to decreased severity of disease together with decreased need for medications, and prevention of further IgE sensitizations to other allergens, all of which may end up with a long-term curative effect.[6,52]

Mechanisms of action of AIT are claimed to be the induction of Treg cells, modulation of T- and B-cell responses, skewing of specific-antibody isotype to IgG4 predominance from IgE, early desensitization of mast cells and basophils, and decreases in numbers and activity of eosinophils and mast cells in the tissues.[53–57] After AIT, allergen-specific Treg cells are generated, which produce IL-10 and TGF-β cytokines that suppress proliferative and cytokine responses against major allergens and their recognition sites.[58,59] Suppressive role of IL-10 on T cells is marked by CD2, CD28, and inducible costimulator costimulatory signal blockage via use of Src-homology-2 domain-containing protein tyrosine phosphatase 1 that dephosphorylates CD2 and inducible costimulator in the rapid signal transduction cascade.[60] Local induction of Treg cells in the nasal mucosa in response to AIT has been observed in patients with allergic rhinitis.[61] Recent studies suggested a role for Treg cells with novel surface molecules, which can be used as a biomarker.[62] Deletion of allergen-specific Th2 cells as a consequence of repeated high-dose allergen stimulation may possibly be an independent mechanism to restore allergen-specific tolerance during immunotherapy.[63] Induction of allergen-specific IgG4 antibodies and reduction of mast cell and eosinophil numbers with increased thresholds for mediator release are also marked after successful AIT.[64,65] Peripheral tolerance induction as a consequence of AIT influences antibody isotypes. Serum levels of IgE decrease gradually whereas allergen-specific IgG4, namely blocking antibodies, increase during AIT, which is the result of class-switching of B cells from IgE to IgG4. This switching effect is the result of IL-10, which promotes a noninflammatory phenotype. IgG4 competes with Fcε receptor-bound IgE for binding allergens, which limits activation and degranulation of mast cells and basophils (**Fig. 3**). IgG4 has important roles in limiting the activation of CD4$^+$ T cells, by inhibition of CD23-mediated IgE-facilitated antigen presentation.[44,57,66,67] Presence of IgG4-isotype antibodies has importance in defining the therapy-responsive phenotype in sensitized individuals, whether this individual will show clinical reactivity. IgG4 has been demonstrated to inhibit peanut-induced

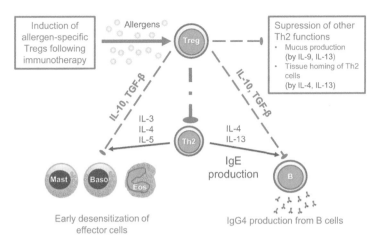

Fig. 3. Development of allergen tolerance. Allergen-specific immunotherapy and natural encounter with high-dose allergens induce Treg cells. As a consequence, peripheral tolerance is induced, which in turn regulates the effector cells of allergy in various ways. Treg cells suppress Th2 cells and their cytokine production (IL-3, IL-4, IL-5, IL-9, and IL-13), which are indispensable for the differentiation, survival, and activity of mast cells, basophils, eosinophils, and mucus-producing cells and for tissue homing of Th2 cells. IL-10 and TGF-β suppress IgE production, while inducing IgG4, a noninflammatory immunoglobulin isotype.

basophil and mast cell activation in peanut-tolerant children sensitized to peanut major allergens.[44] These findings in human cell cultures and tissues have been recently supported in a study in mouse model of AIT. It has been demonstrated that peripherally induced Ag-specific Foxp3[+] Treg cells and thymic Foxp3[+] Treg cells play essential roles in mouse model of AIT. Thymic Treg cells by promoting IL-10 production in Foxp3[−] T cells also crucially contribute to the effectiveness of allergen-specific immunotherapy.[68]

INNATE IMMUNE RESPONSES IN SUBLINGUAL IMMUNOTHERAPY AND SUBCUTANEOUS IMMUNOTHERAPY

SCIT and SLIT are the two globally accepted routes of AIT with worldwide clinical usage.[5,69] SLIT is also used for food allergy with promising results,[70] but in a recent head-to-head study oral immunotherapy was more efficient compared with SLIT.[71] Many other immunotherapies have been suggested or are under development with efficient results[72,73]; however, their mechanisms of action were demonstrated in single studies so confirmation is needed in further studies. Although routes and doses of allergen administration in SLIT and SCIT regimens differ, mechanisms of action of both routes show similarities on an immunologic basis in many aspects.[74] The oral mucosal area is an important entry site for commensal microbes and numerous daily dietary antigens, where peripheral tolerance is induced in a quick manner to maintain immune homeostasis. The sublingual area stands as a quick tolerance induction area by inducing Th1/Treg cells in the absence of danger signals.[75] The oral cavity hosts several subsets of tolerogenic DCs, which induce Treg cell responses. Subsets of DCs include CD11b[+]CD11c[−] and CD11b[+]CD11c[+] myeloid DCs at the mucosal/submucosal interface, plasmacytoid DCs found in submucosal tissues, and a minor subset of CD207[+] Langerhans cells located in the mucosa itself. Both myeloid and plasmacytoid oral DCs have been shown to capture and process the antigen efficiently and can elicit interferon-γ and/or IL-10 production in naive CD4$^+$ T cells.[76] Plasmacytoid DCs have capacity to secrete interferon-α in response to TLR7 and TLR9 stimulation, and may have roles in tolerance induction following AIT.[77] IgE receptor bearing antigen-specific DCs take up allergens that activate IgE and IgG receptors simultaneously. Both of these stimulatory and inhibitory signals in costimulation of pattern recognition molecules TLR4 and CD14 induce tolerogenic mechanisms. Activated DCs migrate to local lymphoid tissue where they induce Th1 and Treg cells.[78] Lower numbers of mast cells and eosinophils in the upper layers of the oral cavity arise as proposed mechanisms about the safety concern of sublingual allergen administration.[79] During SLIT allergens are mostly captured by tolerogenic DCs, before reaching mast cells, which gains advantage over SCIT with virtually no risk of severe systemic reactions.[78,80]

Detailed mapping of the oral cavity has gained interest. Recently, in comparison of sublingual and vestibular regions, higher numbers of DCs have been observed in the vestibular region, which may result with faster induction of IgE-blocking factors. Taken together, these differences between the regions led to discovery of a novel route: oral vestibule immunotherapy. However, study investigating the differences of conventional SLIT and oral vestibule immunotherapy has revealed similar results of IgE-blocking factor and no significant differences between adverse effects of the two different routes. Further studies are needed before application of the vestibular route in clinical settings.[81]

As an alternative mechanism for allergen-presentation and induction of local Treg cells tonsils are strategically located in the gateway of the alimentary and respiratory tracts representing the first contact point of food and aeroallergens with the immune system. Lingual tonsil is anatomically big and remains intact lifelong. Only palatine tonsils and sometimes adenoids are removed by tonsillectomy. High numbers of allergen-specific CD4$^+$Foxp3$^+$ Treg cells are identified in human tonsils.[82] A positive correlation between the percentages of Foxp3$^+$ Treg cells and pDCs is observed in tonsils from individuals with no atopy. Tonsiller plasmocytoid DC can induce Treg cells.

ILCs play an essential role in many inflammatory diseases including allergic diseases and asthma.[83–85] Recent data suggest roles for them for persistence and chronicity of these diseases.[86,87] Lung type 2 ILCs play a critical role in priming the adaptive type 2 immune response to inhaled allergens, including serum IgE levels, recruitment of eosinophils, and Th2 cytokine production. They respond to IL-33 from epithelial cells and initiate inflammation.[88] The effect of grass pollen SCIT on type 2 ILCs in patients with seasonal allergic rhinitis has been recently demonstrated, and their seasonal increase was to be inhibited by subcutaneous grass pollen immunotherapy.[30]

INFLUENCE OF SUBLINGUAL IMMUNOTHERAPY AND SUBCUTANEOUS IMMUNOTHERAPY ON T-CELL RESPONSES

In SCIT, allergen-specific T-cell proliferation has been reduced because of peripheral tolerance mechanisms. Treg cells are induced in SCIT and their immunoregulatory activity has been claimed to be the main mechanism for clinical efficacy of SCIT. Production of IL-10 and TGF-β from and expression of cytotoxic T-lymphocyte-associated protein-4 by Treg cells have importance in immune regulation in SCIT.[89] Increase in Treg cell numbers in IL-10 and TGF-β mRNA expression in response to SLIT has been revealed,[90] whereas levels of IL-17 in SLIT have been negatively correlated with the success of SLIT.[91] Immune deviation of Th2 responses to a more protective

Th1 profile as a consequence of SCIT has also been suggested.[89] In response to SCIT, IL-12 mRNA expression in skin macrophages has been found to be increased, together with the presence of Th1 cells and diminished numbers of Th2 cells, which has been correlated with inhibited allergen-induced late cutaneous responses.[92,93] The main difference in SLIT is the use of oral mucosa, which is a site for induction of immune tolerance, namely a protolerogenic site.[94] In summary, SCIT and SLIT induce similar effects, but with some degrees of difference, which requires further studies for conclusive data.

INFLUENCE OF SUBLINGUAL IMMUNOTHERAPY AND SUBCUTANEOUS IMMUNOTHERAPY ON ANTIBODY RESPONSES

Both SCIT and SLIT have influences on antibody responses. AIT decreases allergen-specific IgE production and promotes allergen-specific IgG4 production, which competes with IgE by blocking the binding of allergens to FcεRI on the surface of mast cells and basophils.[95] IL-10 reduces allergen-specific IgE production through IL-4-induced IgE switching by decreasing epsilon transcript expression and enhances allergen-specific IgG4 production by potentiating IL-4-induced IgG4 switching by inducing IL-4-induced gamma4 transcript expression, and also by enhancing growth of cells already committed to produce IgG4.[58,96,97] It has been recently reported that although after grass tablet SLIT allergen-specific IgE and IgG4 responses have been initially upregulated with increased IL-4-producing cell numbers, this phase has then been followed by a shift from Th2 profile toward Th1, with downregulation of allergen-specific IgE production and increased allergen-specific IgG4 production.[98] The long-term tolerance after SLIT has been accompanied by selective persistence of blocking antibodies. After 2 years of successful SLIT, immunotherapy-induced grass pollen–specific IgG1 and IgG4 levels have been normalized to pretreatment levels, and cellular assays that have detected binding of IgE-grass pollen allergen complexes to B cells have shown that inhibitory bioactivity of allergen-specific IgG antibodies has remained unchanged.[53] SLIT also elicits mucosal IgA responses, which may significantly contribute to induction of allergen tolerance.[99] SCIT has similar, but more pronounced effect on antibody responses. Grass pollen SCIT has reduced seasonal increases in serum allergen-specific IgE, whereas 60- to 80-fold increases in allergen-specific IgG and 100-fold increases in allergen-specific IgG4 have been observed.[100] Similarly, inhibitory activity by blocked IgE-facilitated binding of allergen-IgE complexes to B cells has been observed after SCIT.[64] Measuring IgG4 levels has been proposed to be a good indicator of clinical efficacy of AIT during follow-up.

INFLUENCE OF SUBLINGUAL IMMUNOTHERAPY AND SUBCUTANEOUS IMMUNOTHERAPY ON EFFECTOR CELLS

The effector cellular players of allergic inflammation are eosinophils, basophils, and their tissue counterpart mast cells. These cells regulate inflammatory events and anaphylaxis during allergic inflammation. Triggering of mast cells and basophils is responsible for the release of cellular mediators, which increases vascular permeability, edema formation, angiogenesis, and fibrosis development in the long term. Histamine is one of the major mediators released from effector cells. Effects of histamine are mediated by histamine receptors, the four types of which are defined as H1 to H4. Although H1R is known for its proinflammatory and cell-activating properties, H2R is claimed to be involved in establishment of immune tolerance[101,102] by downregulating T-cell and DC responses.[6] Immunosilencing of FcεRI-activated basophils by means of selective suppression mediated by H2 receptors has induced desensitization effect after venom immunotherapy. It has been proposed that early desensitization of FcεRI-bearing mast cells and basophils has been marked in allergen-specific immunotherapy.[103] In addition, basophil expression of diamine oxidase is suggested as a novel biomarker of AIT response.[104] It has been proposed that histamine and leukotrienes are shown to be released without inducing systemic anaphylaxis, probably because their release is under systemic anaphylaxis thresholds during AIT. The granule content of mediators may be depleted and it may become harder to activate mast cells and basophils to emerge anaphylactoid symptoms, which is known to be a short-term effect of AIT.[105–107] However, the number of cutaneous mast cells after immunotherapy has reduced in correlation with the clinical response in terms of seasonal symptoms after grass pollen SCIT.[108] Also, successful grass pollen immunotherapy was associated with inhibition of seasonal increases in basophils and eosinophils in the nasal epithelium.[109]

SUMMARY

AIT has been used for more than 100 years as a desensitizing and immune tolerance–inducing therapy for allergic diseases and represents the only allergen-specific way of treatment. It is a milestone disease-modifying treatment with the possibility of cure of allergic diseases. Its mechanisms of action include changes in memory-type allergen-specific T- and B-cell responses and increased thresholds for mast cells and basophil activation. Besides SCIT and SLIT, novel routes of AIT, such as intralymphatic, epicutaneous, and intranasal immunotherapy, are under investigation.[110] Expanded knowledge in AIT is also expected to contribute to treatment of other immune tolerance–related diseases, such as autoimmune diseases, chronic infection, organ transplantation, and cancer.[2]

REFERENCES

1. Akdis CA, Akdis M. Advances in allergen immunotherapy: aiming for complete tolerance to allergens. Sci Transl Med 2015;7:280ps6.
2. Akdis M, Akdis CA. Mechanisms of allergen-specific immunotherapy: multiple suppressor factors at work in immune tolerance to allergens. J Allergy Clin Immunol 2014;133:621–31.
3. Ozdemir C, Kucuksezer UC, Akdis M, et al. Specific immunotherapy and turning off the T cell: how does it work? Ann Allergy Asthma Immunol 2011;107:381–92.
4. Calderon MA, Casale TB, Nelson HS, et al. An evidence-based analysis of house dust mite allergen immunotherapy: a call for more rigorous clinical studies. J Allergy Clin Immunol 2013;132:1322–36.
5. Cox L, Nelson H, Lockey R, et al. Allergen immunotherapy: a practice parameter third update. J Allergy Clin Immunol 2011;127:S1–55.
6. Akdis CA, Akdis M. Mechanisms of allergen-specific immunotherapy and immune tolerance to allergens. World Allergy Organ J 2015;8:17.
7. Larche M, Akdis CA, Valenta R. Immunological mechanisms of allergen-specific immunotherapy. Nat Rev Immunol 2006;6:761–71.
8. Akdis CA, Blaser K, Akdis M. Genes of tolerance. Allergy 2004;59:897–913.
9. Akdis M, Burgler S, Crameri R, et al. Interleukins, from 1 to 37, and interferon-gamma: receptors, functions, and roles in diseases. J Allergy Clin Immunol 2011;127:701–21.e1-70.
10. Wegrzyn AS, Jakiela B, Ruckert B, et al. T-cell regulation during viral and nonviral asthma exacerbations. J Allergy Clin Immunol 2015;136(1):194–7.e9.

11. Ronka AL, Kinnunen TT, Goudet A, et al. Characterization of human memory CD4 T-cell responses to the dog allergen Can f 4. J Allergy Clin Immunol 2015. [Epub ahead of print].
12. Davies JM, Platts-Mills TA, Aalberse RC. The enigma of IgE+ B-cell memory in human subjects. J Allergy Clin Immunol 2013;131:972–6.
13. Kuo IH, Yoshida T, De Benedetto A, et al. The cutaneous innate immune response in patients with atopic dermatitis. J Allergy Clin Immunol 2013;131:266–78.
14. Ozdemir C, Akdis M, Akdis CA. Role of T cells. In: Bieber T, Leung DY, editors. Atopic dematitis. 2nd edition. New York: Informa; 2009. p. 121–48.
15. Leung DYM. Preface: the epidermal skin barrier: aspects of biology and dysfunction. J Allergy Clin Immunol 2009;124(3 Suppl 2):R1.
16. Akdis M. Healthy immune response to allergens: T regulatory cells and more. Curr Opin Immunol 2006;18:738–44.
17. Akdis CA. Allergy and hypersensitivity: mechanisms of allergic disease. Curr Opin Immunol 2006;18:718–26.
18. Sehmi R, Wardlaw AJ, Cromwell O, et al. Interleukin-5 selectively enhances the chemotactic response of eosinophils obtained from normal but not eosinophilic subjects. Blood 1992;79:2952–9.
19. Akdis M, Verhagen J, Taylor A, et al. Immune responses in healthy and allergic individuals are characterized by a fine balance between allergen-specific T regulatory 1 and T helper 2 cells. J Exp Med 2004;199:1567–75.
20. Wills-Karp M, Luyimbazi J, Xu X, et al. Interleukin 13: central mediator of allergic asthma. Science 1998;282:2258–61.
21. Dardalhon V, Awasthi A, Kwon H, et al. IL-4 inhibits TGF-beta-induced Foxp3+ T cells and, together with TGF-beta, generates IL-9+ IL-10+ Foxp3(-) effector T cells. Nat Immunol 2008;9:1347–55.
22. Veldhoen M, Uyttenhove C, van Snick J, et al. Transforming growth factor-beta 'reprograms' the differentiation of T helper 2 cells and promotes an interleukin 9-producing subset. Nat Immunol 2008;9:1341–6.
23. Sehra S, Yao W, Nguyen ET, et al. T9 cells are required for tissue mast cell accumulation during allergic inflammation. J Allergy Clin Immunol 2015;136(2): 433–40.e1.
24. Brough HA, Cousins DJ, Munteanu A, et al. IL-9 is a key component of memory TH cell peanut-specific responses from children with peanut allergy. J Allergy Clin Immunol 2014;134:1329–38.e10.
25. Prefontaine D, Nadigel J, Chouiali F, et al. Increased IL-33 expression by epithelial cells in bronchial asthma. J Allergy Clin Immunol 2010;125:752–4.
26. Dillon SR, Sprecher C, Hammond A, et al. Interleukin 31, a cytokine produced by activated T cells, induces dermatitis in mice. Nat Immunol 2004;5:752–60.
27. Wang YH, Angkasekwinai P, Lu N, et al. IL-25 augments type 2 immune responses by enhancing the expansion and functions of TSLP-DC-activated Th2 memory cells. J Exp Med 2007;204:1837–47.
28. Nograles KE, Zaba LC, Shemer A, et al. IL-22-producing "T22" T cells account for upregulated IL-22 in atopic dermatitis despite reduced IL-17-producing TH17 T cells. J Allergy Clin Immunol 2009;123:1244–52.e2.
29. Sergejeva S, Ivanov S, Lotvall J, et al. Interleukin-17 as a recruitment and survival factor for airway macrophages in allergic airway inflammation. Am J Respir Cell Mol Biol 2005;33:248–53.
30. Lao-Araya M, Steveling E, Scadding GW, et al. Seasonal increases in peripheral innate lymphoid type 2 cells are inhibited by subcutaneous grass pollen immunotherapy. J Allergy Clin Immunol 2014;134:1193–5.e4.

31. Hogquist KA, Baldwin TA, Jameson SC. Central tolerance: learning self-control in the thymus. Nat Rev Immunol 2005;5:772–82.

32. Sprent J, Kishimoto H. The thymus and negative selection. Immunol Rev 2002; 185:126–35.

33. Soyer OU, Akdis M, Ring J, et al. Mechanisms of peripheral tolerance to allergens. Allergy 2013;68:161–70.

34. Kucuksezer UC, Palomares O, Ruckert B, et al. Triggering of specific Toll-like receptors and proinflammatory cytokines breaks allergen-specific T-cell tolerance in human tonsils and peripheral blood. J Allergy Clin Immunol 2013;131: 875–85.e9.

35. Lukkarinen H, Soderlund-Venermo M, Vuorinen T, et al. Human bocavirus 1 may suppress rhinovirus-associated immune response in wheezing children. J Allergy Clin Immunol 2014;133:256–8.e1-4.

36. Konradsen JR, Fujisawa T, van Hage M, et al. Allergy to furry animals: new insights, diagnostic approaches, and challenges. J Allergy Clin Immunol 2015; 135:616–25.

37. Meiler F, Zumkehr J, Klunker S, et al. In vivo switch to IL-10-secreting T regulatory cells in high dose allergen exposure. J Exp Med 2008;205:2887–98.

38. Platts-Mills TA, Woodfolk JA. Allergens and their role in the allergic immune response. Immunol Rev 2011;242:51–68.

39. Sakaguchi S, Sakaguchi N, Asano M, et al. Immunologic self-tolerance maintained by activated T cells expressing IL-2 receptor alpha-chains (CD25). Breakdown of a single mechanism of self-tolerance causes various autoimmune diseases. J Immunol 1995;155:1151–64.

40. Sun CM, Hall JA, Blank RB, et al. Small intestine lamina propria dendrit's promote de novo generation of Foxp3 T reg cells via retinoic acid. J Exp Med 2007;204:1775–85.

41. Reubsaet L, Meerding J, Giezeman R, et al. Der p 1-induced CD4(+) FOXP3(+)GATA3(+) T cells have suppressive properties and contribute to the polarization of the TH2-associated response. J Allergy Clin Immunol 2013;132:1440–4.

42. Thunberg S, Akdis M, Akdis CA, et al. Immune regulation by CD4+CD25+ T cells and interleukin-10 in birch pollen-allergic patients and non-allergic controls. Clin Exp Allergy 2007;37:1127–36.

43. Chen W, Jin W, Hardegen N, et al. Conversion of peripheral CD4+CD25- naive T cells to CD4+CD25+ regulatory T cells by TGF-beta induction of transcription factor Foxp3. J Exp Med 2003;198:1875–86.

44. Santos AF, James LK, Bahnson HT, et al. IgG4 inhibits peanut-induced basophil and mast cell activation in peanut-tolerant children sensitized to peanut major allergens. J Allergy Clin Immunol 2015;135:1249–56.

45. Begin P, Nadeau KC. Changes in peanut-specific T-cell clonotype with oral immunotherapy. J Allergy Clin Immunol 2015;135:1636–8.e3.

46. van de Veen W, Stanic B, Yaman G, et al. IgG4 production is confined to human IL-10-producing regulatory B cells that suppress antigen-specific immune responses. J Allergy Clin Immunol 2013;131:1204–12.

47. Stanic B, van de Veen W, Wirz OF, et al. IL-10-overexpressing B cells regulate innate and adaptive immune responses. J Allergy Clin Immunol 2015;135: 771–80.e8.

48. Patil SU, Ogunniyi AO, Calatroni A, et al. Peanut oral immunotherapy transiently expands circulating Ara h 2-specific B cells with a homologous repertoire in unrelated subjects. J Allergy Clin Immunol 2015;136(1):125–34.e12.

49. Deniz G, Erten G, Kucuksezer UC, et al. Regulatory NK cells suppress antigen-specific T cell responses. J Immunol 2008;180:850–7.
50. Deniz G, van de Veen W, Akdis M. Natural killer cells in patients with allergic diseases. J Allergy Clin Immunol 2013;132:527–35.
51. Campbell KS, Hasegawa J. Natural killer cell biology: an update and future directions. J Allergy Clin Immunol 2013;132:536–44.
52. Zolkipli Z, Roberts G, Cornelius V, et al. Randomized controlled trial of primary prevention of atopy using house dust mite allergen oral immunotherapy in early childhood. J Allergy Clin Immunol 2015. [Epub ahead of print].
53. James LK, Shamji MH, Walker SM, et al. Long-term tolerance after allergen immunotherapy is accompanied by selective persistence of blocking antibodies. J Allergy Clin Immunol 2011;127:509–16.e1-5.
54. Francis JN, James LK, Paraskevopoulos G, et al. Grass pollen immunotherapy: IL-10 induction and suppression of late responses precedes IgG4 inhibitory antibody activity. J Allergy Clin Immunol 2008;121:1120–5.e2.
55. Wachholz PA, Soni NK, Till SJ, et al. Inhibition of allergen-IgE binding to B cells by IgG antibodies after grass pollen immunotherapy. J Allergy Clin Immunol 2003;112:915–22.
56. Cameron LA, Durham SR, Jacobson MR, et al. Expression of IL-4, Cepsilon RNA, and Iepsilon RNA in the nasal mucosa of patients with seasonal rhinitis: effect of topical corticosteroids. J Allergy Clin Immunol 1998;101:330–6.
57. Kucuksezer UC, Ozdemir C, Akdis M, et al. Mechanisms of immune tolerance to allergens in children. Korean J Pediatr 2013;56:505–13.
58. Akdis CA, Blesken T, Akdis M, et al. Role of interleukin 10 in specific immunotherapy. J Clin Invest 1998;102:98–106.
59. Jutel M, Akdis M, Budak F, et al. IL-10 and TGF-beta cooperate in the regulatory T cell response to mucosal allergens in normal immunity and specific immunotherapy. Eur J Immunol 2003;33:1205–14.
60. Taylor A, Akdis M, Joss A, et al. IL-10 inhibits CD28 and ICOS costimulations of T cells via src homology 2 domain-containing protein tyrosine phosphatase 1. J Allergy Clin Immunol 2007;120:76–83.
61. Radulovic S, Jacobson MR, Durham SR, et al. Grass pollen immunotherapy induces Foxp3-expressing CD4+ CD25+ cells in the nasal mucosa. J Allergy Clin Immunol 2008;121:1467–72, 1472.e1.
62. Tsai YG, Lai JC, Yang KD, et al. Enhanced CD46-induced regulatory T cells suppress allergic inflammation after *Dermatophagoides pteronyssinus*-specific immunotherapy. J Allergy Clin Immunol 2014;134:1206–9.e1.
63. Wambre E, DeLong JH, James EA, et al. Specific immunotherapy modifies allergen-specific CD4(+) T-cell responses in an epitope-dependent manner. J Allergy Clin Immunol 2014;133:872–9.e7.
64. Nouri-Aria KT, Wachholz PA, Francis JN, et al. Grass pollen immunotherapy induces mucosal and peripheral IL-10 responses and blocking IgG activity. J Immunol 2004;172:3252–9.
65. Creticos PS, Adkinson NF Jr, Kagey-Sobotka A, et al. Nasal challenge with ragweed pollen in hay fever patients. Effect of immunotherapy. J Clin Invest 1985;76:2247–53.
66. Vickery BP, Scurlock AM, Kulis M, et al. Sustained unresponsiveness to peanut in subjects who have completed peanut oral immunotherapy. J Allergy Clin Immunol 2014;133:468–75.
67. Shamji MH, Francis JN, Wurtzen PA, et al. Cell-free detection of allergen-IgE cross-linking with immobilized phase CD23: inhibition by blocking antibody

responses after immunotherapy. J Allergy Clin Immunol 2013;132: 1003–5.e1-4.

68. Bohm L, Maxeiner J, Meyer-Martin H, et al. IL-10 and regulatory T cells cooperate in allergen-specific immunotherapy to ameliorate allergic asthma. J Immunol 2015;194:887–97.

69. Nolte H, Maloney J, Nelson HS, et al. Onset and dose-related efficacy of house dust mite sublingual immunotherapy tablets in an environmental exposure chamber. J Allergy Clin Immunol 2015;135:1494–501.e6.

70. Burks AW, Wood RA, Jones SM, et al. Sublingual immunotherapy for peanut allergy: long-term follow-up of a randomized multicenter trial. J Allergy Clin Immunol 2015;135:1240–8.e3.

71. Narisety SD, Frischmeyer-Guerrerio PA, Keet CA, et al. A randomized, double-blind, placebo-controlled pilot study of sublingual versus oral immunotherapy for the treatment of peanut allergy. J Allergy Clin Immunol 2015;135:1275–82.e6.

72. Focke-Tejkl M, Weber M, Niespodziana K, et al. Development and characterization of a recombinant, hypoallergenic, peptide-based vaccine for grass pollen allergy. J Allergy Clin Immunol 2014;135(5). 1207-7.e1-11.

73. von Moos S, Johansen P, Tay F, et al. Comparing safety of abrasion and tape-stripping as skin preparation in allergen-specific epicutaneous immunotherapy. J Allergy Clin Immunol 2014;134:965–7.e4.

74. Ozdemir C. An immunological overview of allergen specific immunotherapy – subcutaneous and sublingual routes. Ther Adv Respir Dis 2009;3:253–62.

75. Moingeon P, Batard T, Fadel R, et al. Immune mechanisms of allergen-specific sublingual immunotherapy. Allergy 2006;61:151–65.

76. Mascarell L, Lombardi V, Louise A, et al. Oral dendritic cells mediate antigen-specific tolerance by stimulating TH1 and regulatory CD4+ T cells. J Allergy Clin Immunol 2008;122:603–9.e5.

77. Frischmeyer-Guerrerio PA, Keet CA, Guerrerio AL, et al. Modulation of dendritic cell innate and adaptive immune functions by oral and sublingual immunotherapy. Clin Immunol 2014;155:47–59.

78. Novak N, Haberstok J, Bieber T, et al. The immune privilege of the oral mucosa. Trends Mol Med 2008;14:191–8.

79. Moingeon P, Mascarell L. Induction of tolerance via the sublingual route: mechanisms and applications. Clin Dev Immunol 2012;2012:623474.

80. Allam JP, Stojanovski G, Friedrichs N, et al. Distribution of Langerhans cells and mast cells within the human oral mucosa: new application sites of allergens in sublingual immunotherapy? Allergy 2008;63:720–7.

81. Allam JP, Wuestenberg E, Wolf H, et al. Immunologic response and safety in birch pollen sublingual versus oral vestibule immunotherapy: a pilot study. J Allergy Clin Immunol 2014;133:1757–9.e3.

82. Palomares O, Ruckert B, Jartti T, et al. Induction and maintenance of allergen-specific FOXP3+ Treg cells in human tonsils as potential first-line organs of oral tolerance. J Allergy Clin Immunol 2012;129:510–20, 520.e1-9.

83. Annunziato F, Romagnani C, Romagnani S. The 3 major types of innate and adaptive cell-mediated effector immunity. J Allergy Clin Immunol 2015;135(3):626–35.

84. Roediger B, Kyle R, Tay SS, et al. IL-2 is a critical regulator of group 2 innate lymphoid cell function during pulmonary inflammation. J Allergy Clin Immunol 2015. [Epub ahead of print].

85. Nagarkar DR, Ramirez-Carrozzi V, Choy DF, et al. IL-13 mediates IL-33-dependent mast cell and type 2 innate lymphoid cell effects on bronchial epithelial cells. J Allergy Clin Immunol 2015;136(1):202–5.

86. Christianson CA, Goplen NP, Zafar I, et al. Persistence of asthma requires multiple feedback circuits involving type 2 innate lymphoid cells and IL-33. J Allergy Clin Immunol 2015;136(1):59–68.e14.
87. Bartemes KR, Kephart GM, Fox SJ, et al. Enhanced innate type 2 immune response in peripheral blood from patients with asthma. J Allergy Clin Immunol 2014;134:671–8.e4.
88. Barlow JL, Peel S, Fox J, et al. IL-33 is more potent than IL-25 in provoking IL-13-producing nuocytes (type 2 innate lymphoid cells) and airway contraction. J Allergy Clin Immunol 2013;132:933–41.
89. Maggi E, Vultaggio A, Matucci A. T-cell responses during allergen-specific immunotherapy. Curr Opin Allergy Clin Immunol 2012;12:1–6.
90. O'Hehir RE, Gardner LM, de Leon MP, et al. House dust mite sublingual immunotherapy: the role for transforming growth factor-beta and functional regulatory T cells. Am J Respir Crit Care Med 2009;180:936–47.
91. Incorvaia C, Frati F, Puccinelli P, et al. Effects of sublingual immunotherapy on allergic inflammation. Inflamm Allergy Drug Targets 2008;7:167–72.
92. Alexander C, Tarzi M, Larche M, et al. The effect of Fel d 1-derived T-cell peptides on upper and lower airway outcome measurements in cat-allergic subjects. Allergy 2005;60:1269–74.
93. Plewako H, Wosinska K, Arvidsson M, et al. Production of interleukin-12 by monocytes and interferon-gamma by natural killer cells in allergic patients during rush immunotherapy. Ann Allergy Asthma Immunol 2006;97:464–8.
94. Novak N, Bieber T, Allam JP. Immunological mechanisms of sublingual allergen-specific immunotherapy. Allergy 2011;66:733–9.
95. Fujita H, Soyka MB, Akdis M, et al. Mechanisms of allergen-specific immunotherapy. Clin Transl Allergy 2012;2:2.
96. Jeannin P, Lecoanet S, Delneste Y, et al. IgE versus IgG4 production can be differentially regulated by IL-10. J Immunol 1998;160:3555–61.
97. Meiler F, Klunker S, Zimmermann M, et al. Distinct regulation of IgE, IgG4 and IgA by T regulatory cells and toll-like receptors. Allergy 2008;63:1455–63.
98. Suarez-Fueyo A, Ramos T, Galan A, et al. Grass tablet sublingual immunotherapy downregulates the TH2 cytokine response followed by regulatory T-cell generation. J Allergy Clin Immunol 2014;133:130–8.e1-2.
99. Scadding GW, Shamji MH, Jacobson MR, et al. Sublingual grass pollen immunotherapy is associated with increases in sublingual Foxp3-expressing cells and elevated allergen-specific immunoglobulin G4, immunoglobulin A and serum inhibitory activity for immunoglobulin E-facilitated allergen binding to B cells. Clin Exp Allergy 2010;40:598–606.
100. Jutel M, Jaeger L, Suck R, et al. Allergen-specific immunotherapy with recombinant grass pollen allergens. J Allergy Clin Immunol 2005;116:608–13.
101. Frei R, Ferstl R, Konieczna P, et al. Histamine receptor 2 modifies dendritic cell responses to microbial ligands. J Allergy Clin Immunol 2013;132(1):194–204.
102. Ferstl R, Frei R, Schiavi E, et al. Histamine receptor 2 is a key influence in immune responses to intestinal histamine-secreting microbes. J Allergy Clin Immunol 2014;134:744–6.e3.
103. Novak N, Mete N, Bussmann C, et al. Early suppression of basophil activation during allergen-specific immunotherapy by histamine receptor 2. J Allergy Clin Immunol 2012;130:1153–8.
104. Shamji MH, Layhadi JA, Scadding GW, et al. Basophil expression of diamine oxidase: a novel biomarker of allergen immunotherapy response. J Allergy Clin Immunol 2015;135:913–21.e9.

105. Eberlein-Konig B, Ullmann S, Thomas P, et al. Tryptase and histamine release due to a sting challenge in bee venom allergic patients treated successfully or unsuccessfully with hyposensitization. Clin Exp Allergy 1995;25:704–12.
106. Jutel M, Müller UM, Fricker M, et al. Influence of bee venom immunotherapy on degranulation and leukotriene generation in human blood basophils. Clin Exp Allergy 1996;26:112–8.
107. Plewako H, Wosinska K, Arvidsson M, et al. Basophil interleukin 4 and interleukin 13 production is suppressed during the early phase of rush immunotherapy. Int Arch Allergy Immunol 2006;141:346–53.
108. Durham SR, Varney VA, Gaga M, et al. Grass pollen immunotherapy decreases the number of mast cells in the skin. Clin Exp Allergy 1999;29:1490–6.
109. Wilson DR, Irani AM, Walker SM, et al. Grass pollen immunotherapy inhibits seasonal increases in basophils and eosinophils in the nasal epithelium. Clin Exp Allergy 2001;31:1705–13.
110. Casale TB, Stokes JR. Immunotherapy: what lies beyond. J Allergy Clin Immunol 2014;133:612–9 [quiz: 620].

Mechanisms Underlying Induction of Tolerance to Foods

M. Cecilia Berin, PhD[a],*, Wayne G. Shreffler, MD, PhD[b]

KEYWORDS

- Tolerance • Treg • Foxp3 • IgE • IgG4 • Immunotherapy • Microbiota

KEY POINTS

- Oral tolerance is mediated by allergen-specific Tregs that are generated by mucosal dendritic cells.
- Factors such as intestinal mucin and cytokines produced by epithelial cells and innate lymphoid cells contribute to tolerance by modifying the phenotype of gastrointestinal dendritic cells.
- Oral tolerance by early dietary introduction can prevent peanut allergy in infants at high risk of peanut allergy.
- Humoral mechanisms, in particular the generation of allergen-specific IgG4, are associated with development of tolerance to foods in humans.
- Clinical tolerance induced by immunotherapy is associated with immune changes in basophils, IgG4, allergen-specific Th2 cells, and allergen-specific cells with regulatory markers.

IMMUNE MECHANISMS OF ORAL TOLERANCE

An early description of the phenomenon of oral tolerance was provided by Wells and Osborne in 1911, when they described a series of studies showing that guinea pigs could not be induced to undergo experimental anaphylaxis to corn or oats if it was a component of the diet.[1] In the intervening century, there has been a growing body of literature defining the immune mechanisms of oral tolerance. Classic oral tolerance experiments are performed by feeding of antigen, either a single high-dose

Disclosure: The authors have no conflicts of interest to disclose.
[a] Pediatric Allergy & Immunology, Mindich Child Health and Development Institute, Immunology Institute, Icahn School of Medicine at Mount Sinai, One Gustave L. Levy Place, Box 1198, New York, NY 10029, USA; [b] Center for Immunology and Inflammatory Diseases, Massachusetts General Hospital, 149 13th Street, Boston, MA 02129, USA
* Corresponding author.
E-mail address: cecilia.berin@mssm.edu

(50–100 mg) feed or multiple low doses (0.5–1 mg) administered daily by gavage or in the drinking water for 5 to 7 days. Oral tolerance is then defined as the suppression of an immune response elicited by immunization, and commonly measured by reduction in cytokine production by lymph node cells re-stimulated with allergen in vitro, delayed type hypersensitivity reaction (ear swelling on injection), or reduction of anaphylaxis or allergic symptoms.

Role of Regulatory T Cells

The appreciation that oral tolerance was an active regulatory immune response rather than solely caused by deletion or anergy of antigen-specific cells came from studies in which tolerance could be transferred to naive animals through the transfer of CD4+ or CD8+ lymphocytes. Weiner and colleagues[2,3] first described a population of cells termed Th3 cells, that express surface transforming growth factor (TGF)-beta and can be identified by staining for latency-associated peptide. These cells do not express CD25 or Foxp3, and suppress by a TGF-beta–dependent mechanism.[4] In addition to these cells, antigen-specific Tregs expressing the transcription factor Foxp3 are also induced in response to antigen feeding, and these iTregs also suppress through a TGF-beta–dependent mechanism.[5,6] Tr1 cells that are interleukin (IL)-10 dependent and suppress through an IL-10–dependent mechanism are involved in the prevention of colitis and microbial-induced inflammation in the intestine,[7] but most studies have shown that IL-10 is dispensable for the induction of tolerance to food antigens.[6,8] Some of this difference in mechanisms may have to do with the site of regulatory responses. The greatest antigenic burden from food occurs in the small intestine, whereas the greatest antigen burden from the microbiota (and subsequent inflammation) occurs in the colon.

Site of Initiation of Tolerance

The mucosal immune system is the largest lymphoid organ in the body, and comprises organized lymphoid structures and a densely packed population of resident immune cells found in the epithelium and underlying lamina propria. Organized structures include Peyer's patches (PP) and isolated lymphoid follicles that are located within the mucosal tissue, as well as mesenteric lymph nodes (MLN) that drain the intestine via lymphatics. The digestive process breaking down food proteins to small peptides and amino acids that can be absorbed by enterocytes begins in the stomach and continues in the duodenum and jejunum. However, a small percentage of intact protein escapes digestion and is absorbed across the mucosal barrier in a form that is immunologically active (ie, that can be presented by antigen-presenting cells). Antigen can be acquired through several different mechanisms. Microfold or M cells are flattened epithelial cells that overlie PP and are specialized for the uptake of particulate antigens such as viruses and bacteria. Some food antigens have also been shown to be selectively sampled through the PP.[9,10] Soluble food antigens are excluded from passing between enterocytes by tight junctions, but are taken up by fluid phase endocytosis and transported to the underlying immune cells. Recently, a novel mechanism of small intestinal antigen uptake was identified through goblet cell–associated antigen passages or GAPs.[11] A conduit was identified in small intestine that rapidly filled with luminal antigen, delivering antigen to lamina propria dendritic cells (DCs). This mechanism of antigen uptake was under the control of cholinergic regulation, showing an important point of control of mucosal immunity by nerves in the gastrointestinal tract.[11] Intestinal mononuclear phagocytes have been shown to extend dendrites between enterocytes, reaching into the lumen and pulling antigen across the epithelium without disrupting the integrity of the tight junctions between cells.[12,13]

The role of different organized lymphoid structures in the development of oral toler-ance has been addressed by several studies, the results of which suggest that PP are dispensable for the induction of oral tolerance, whereas MLN are required.[14–17] These studies have been done using a combination of immunologic ablation of lymphoid structures and surgical interventions such as removal of the MLN or preparation of exteriorized intestinal loops. After induction in the MLN, it is necessary for Tregs to re-circulate in the intestinal lamina propria before being optimally conditioned to sup-press systemic immune responses.[5,18] Migration of Tregs to the lamina propria likely expands these Tregs over a prolonged period of exposure to antigen, and the regula-tory phenotype of antigen-presenting cells in the intestinal lamina propria contributes to this expansion of Tregs.

Role of Gastrointestinal Dendritic Cell Subsets

DCs are essential for priming of naive T cells throughout the body, and this is also true for generation of regulatory T cells from naive T cells in the gastrointestinal tract. Expansion of DCs systemically using the growth factor Flt3L results in enhancement of oral tolerance.[19] Prevention of migration of DCs from lamina propria to MLN by genetic deletion of the chemokine receptor CCR7 abolishes the generation of oral tolerance.[17] Within the intestinal lamina propria are several subsets of DCs, including a population of monocyte-derived CD11b+ CX3CR1+ cells, and DC progenitor-derived CD103+ CX3CR1− cells, which can be CD11b positive or negative.[20–22] The monocyte-derived CX3CR1+ cells extend dendrites between intestinal epithelial cells, do not migrate to the MLN under steady state,[21] and are transcriptionally more similar to macrophages than DCs.[23] These cells express high levels of IL-10 through the influence of the intestinal microbiota. The CD103+ DCs are migratory under ho-meostatic conditions. CD103+ DCs in the MLN of mice and humans express high levels of TGF-beta and the enzyme RALDH, which facilitates the production of retinoic acid (RA) from vitamin A.[24–26] CD103+ cells in the MLN also express the enzyme indo-leamine 2,3-dioxygenase (IDO).[27] TGF-beta, RA, and IDO are factors that actively pro-mote the development of Tregs from naive T cells in the MLN. Responder T cells upregulate $\alpha4\beta7$ and CCR9, receptors responsible for homing back to the lamina propria, which is also preferentially induced by CD103+ DCs in the MLN through an RA-dependent mechanism.[26] CX3CR1+ cells can acquire antigen via their extensions that protrude into the lumen, and this mechanism can contribute to the development of tolerance in 2 ways. These cells transfer antigen to CD103+ DCs that can migrate to the MLN and induce Tregs.[28] In addition, once Tregs have been primed in the MLN and home back to the lamina propria, they interact with the CX3CR1+ cells and are expanded locally.[5] This gut-homing stage of Tregs has been shown to be necessary for full development of oral tolerance.[5,18]

Unique Regulatory Milieu of the Gastrointestinal Tract

Although immune tolerance can be induced at sites beyond the gastrointestinal tract, there are several unique mechanisms that help to maintain the regulatory tone of the intestine. It is well known that the cytokine IL-10 is necessary for the maintenance of immune homeostasis in the gastrointestinal tract, and in the absence of IL-10 there is the development of spontaneous colitis from inappropriate immune reactivity to the commensal microbiota.[29] Many different knockout mice have been described that develop spontaneous colitis, whereas spontaneous models of food allergy have rarely been described (although this may be due to lack of looking for it, as sensitization to food proteins can be found in the absence of frank symptoms). The fact that IL-10 is critical for tolerance to the microbiota but dispensable for oral tolerance to fed protein antigens suggests that different immunoregulatory mechanisms are responsible for tolerance to foods compared with microorganisms.

Sampling of soluble dietary proteins through goblet cells is 1 mechanism that can promote the development of tolerance. The intestinal mucin Muc2 has been shown to act as a tolerogenic adjuvant promoting the development of regulatory T cells to co-administered antigens.[30] Muc2 interacts with CD103+ DCs through a receptor complex composed of galectin-3, dectin-1, and FcγRIIb. Ligation of this receptor complex results in β-catenin signaling that suppresses inflammatory NF-κB signaling. Muc2 enhances the regulatory phenotype of CD103+ DCs by increasing the expression of TGF-beta and RALDH.[30] In the absence of Muc2, tolerance is impaired to fed antigens; exogenous mucin can restore the development of tolerance in Muc2−/− mice. These results suggest that factors that influence intestinal mucin production can alter the regulatory milieu of the gastrointestinal tract.

The regulatory phenotype of CD103+ DCs is also promoted by intestinal production of the cytokine Csf2 (GM-CSF).[31] The primary source of Csf2 in the intestine is innate lymphoid cells (ILCs) present within isolated lymphoid follicles. Production of Csf2 by these ILCs is dependent on signals from the commensal microbiota. The ILCs do not directly respond to the microbiota, but are regulated by intestinal macrophages that produce IL-1β in response to microbial colonization.[31] IL-1β and Csf2 have not traditionally been thought of as regulatory cytokines, but they are essential for the maintenance of the regulatory phenotype of gastrointestinal DCs and, in their absence, the generation of induced Tregs is impaired.

Role of the Commensal Microbiota in Oral Tolerance to Foods

There are conflicting reports in the literature about the role of the intestinal microbiota in the development of oral tolerance to foods using germ-free mice. One difficulty in interpreting studies using germ-free mice is that the mucosal immune system is poorly developed in the absence of microbial colonization and germ-free status may affect different steps of the tolerance response (uptake, presentation, T-cell response) differently. However, it is clear that many components of the regulatory immune network in the intestine are regulated by the intestinal microbiota. As previously mentioned, Csf2 production by ILCs, which drives the generation of iTregs, is under control of the intestinal microbiota.[31] It has been of interest to determine if some microbes are better at generating a regulatory milieu than others, which would have translational implications. Atarashi and colleagues[32,33] identified Clostridia species (isolated from mouse or human) as being potent inducers of colonic Tregs capable of suppressing both colitis and food allergy. Round and Mazmanian[34] showed that polysaccharide A from *Bacteroides fragilis* promoted the generation of Tregs in the gastrointestinal tract, which could suppress colitis. A more general characteristic of the commensal microbiota is their ability to break down dietary fiber into short-chain fatty acids, such as butyrate and priopionate. This category of bacterial metabolite drives Tregs in the colon and contributes to suppression of colitis.[35] The finding that the induction of Tregs is not unique to certain bacterial species was reported by Faith and colleagues,[36] who showed that a broad range of microbes isolated from humans could induce Tregs in the mouse colon.

Impaired Regulatory Responses and Food Allergy

Much of the work on regulation of Tregs has focused on the colon and colitis, and there is less information on the small intestine in the context of tolerance to foods. Stefka and colleagues[37] reported that Clostridia colonization increased Tregs in the colon and enhanced IL-22 expression in both small and large intestine, which in turn enhanced epithelial barrier function and prevented uptake of food allergens. The IL-22-mediated regulation of epithelial barrier function did not influence development of sensitization to peanut, however, suggesting that perhaps the impact on Tregs was responsible for the suppression of sensitization with colonization. Noval Rivas and colleagues[38] have also shown that the intestinal microbiota regulates susceptibility to food allergy, and that there is a unique microbial signature in genetically food allergy-susceptible mice that can transmit food allergy susceptibility when transferred to germ-free mice. A key role for Tregs in controlling food allergy was shown recently by the same group, who identified a Th2-like phenotype in Tregs of food allergic mice.[39] On sensitization, Tregs from susceptible but not resistant mice had a Treg phenotype characterized by expression of the Th2 transcription factor GATA-3 as well as production of IL-4. Genetic deletion of Th2 cytokine production specifically from Foxp3+ cells prevented the development of food allergy. Ohnmacht and colleagues[40] recently published findings that also support this finding that the Treg phenotype is critical to the development of allergy and Th2 immunity. They found that the intestinal microbiota promoted the expression of the transcription factor RORγt in regulatory T cells, and in the absence of RORγt in the Tregs, there is an expansion of Tregs that express GATA-3 as well as conventional Th2 cells. Furthermore, there is a marked increase in IgE production. These studies indicate that the microbiota educates Tregs to be able to appropriate suppress Th2 responses, and in the absence of this education process, Tregs can deviate to a phenotype that not only does not suppress food allergy but contributes to it. **Fig. 1** illustrates the major mechanisms of oral tolerance and how disruptions in these mechanisms can lead to food allergy.

Therapeutic Oral Tolerance for Food Allergy

Using mouse models, beginning with the experiments of Wells and Osborne,[1,5] it has been shown that experimental food allergy and anaphylaxis are prevented by oral tolerance. There is a great deal of current research in mouse models and in clinical trials focusing on determining if oral tolerance can be established after sensitization has occurred. Mice orally sensitized to egg proteins using the mucosal adjuvant cholera toxin to break oral tolerance were subsequently administered egg white in the drinking water or purified allergens by gavage in increasing doses to mimic the build up and maintenance phase of oral immunotherapy.[41] Mice were protected from oral allergen challenge while receiving immunotherapy, but regained clinical reactivity once therapy was stopped. Increasing the duration of immunotherapy did not lead to any increase in sustained effect. These results are consistent with desensitization rather than tolerance. One explanation is that the use of adjuvant permanently alters the milieu of the gastrointestinal tract, although generally adjuvants must be co-administered with antigens to be effective, indicating that their effects are transient. An alternative mechanism was identified by Burton and colleagues,[42] who showed that IgE-dependent activation of mast cells suppressed the development of Tregs. It has previously been shown that mast cell activation can provide adjuvant activity to DCs.[43] Administration of peanut to peanut-allergic mice in the presence but not the absence of Syk inhibitors (to block mast cell activation) resulted in the development of protection against anaphylaxis.[42] The challenge was done 2 weeks after the termination of immunotherapy, suggesting a sustained effect. A significant downstream effect of mast cell activation was shown to be a Th2-deviation of regulatory T cells, rendering them ineffective at suppressing food allergic responses.[39] These studies suggest that sensitization and activation of mast cells in the gastrointestinal tract suppresses the development of oral tolerance, although it remains unclear why desensitization of

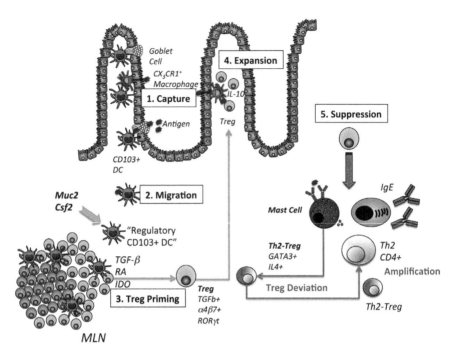

Fig. 1. Mechanism of oral tolerance in food allergy. The main steps in the induction of oral tolerance are (1) capture of antigen by CD103$^+$ DCs via goblet cell–associated passages or indirectly through CX$_3$CR1$^+$ macrophages; (2) CCR7-dependent migration to MLN; (3) priming of Tregs from naive T cells in a mechanism dependent on TGFb, RA, and IDO from "regulatory" CD103$^+$ DCs; (4) expansion of newly generated Tregs in the lamina propria by IL-10 expressing macrophages, and (5) suppression of IgE production, mast cell activation, and Th2 generation. In a prevention strategy, tolerance suppresses food allergy. Once sensitization has occurred, mast cells drive Tregs to a Th2-Treg phenotype characterized by GATA-3 and IL-4 expression. These Th2-Tregs are unable to suppress components of the food allergic response. The intestinal microbiota is a critical regulator of steps 1 to 4, and therefore is a key influence in the development of food allergy.

mast cells by oral immunotherapy does not then pave the way for development of sustained tolerance.

EVIDENCE OF ORAL TOLERANCE IN HUMANS

Companion articles in this issue provide thorough reviews on the routes, protocols, and adjuncts for immunotherapy targeting food allergy. This section of our review focuses on what evidence there is for mechanisms of tolerance to dietary antigens in humans generally and the mechanisms that have been proposed to account for the clinical effects of immunotherapy. Other investigators have also distinguished desensitization from long(er) lasting tolerance, sometimes referred to as sustained unresponsiveness. However, when trying to distinguish immune response correlates to these clinical phenotypes, it is currently uncertain how distinct those phenotypes may be, that they are defined variably, and that even sustained unresponsiveness may be both tenuous and distinct from the natural tolerance of nonallergic individuals, and that state, in turn, may also be distinct from individuals who were once allergic but have become tolerant.

Given the current paradigm that food allergy results from (1) Th2-skewed immunity to food antigens, (2) the production of specific IgE (sIgE) to food antigens, and (3) the sensitization of innate immune cells that express high-affinity IgE receptor (FcERI) with that sIgE, it makes sense that most of the focus on effects of immunotherapy has been on alterations in allergen-specific antibody (eg, less sIgE, more specific IgG or IgA), suppression of FcERI-expressing effector cells (ie, mast cells, basophils), and effects on CD4 T cells, all of which are expected to be significantly interdependent. Even when immunotherapy-induced changes have been studied using unbiased approaches, they have largely focused on these usual suspects (ie, CD4 T cells, basophils, and so forth.) in the hope that multidimensional datasets may provide new mechanistic insights. Furthermore, with technical progress over the past decade, studies on the small subset of antigen-specific cells in the CD4 T-cell and B-cell compartments are now possible with greater precision, but most are still subject to potential artifacts of in vitro activation and all are limited to sampling peripheral blood.

B-Cell Response to Dietary Antigens in Healthy Versus Allergic Individuals

As discussed earlier, animal models of oral tolerance, including adoptive transfer studies, demonstrate that oral tolerance is an active immune state with significant data supporting a key role for Tregs. Consistent with the fact that oral tolerance is not mediated by immune ignorance, anergy, or deletion, dietary antigens are known to induce detectable and benign class-switched immunoglobulin responses in most human individuals beginning within the first year of life,[44–46] which seems to be at least roughly comparable with the kinetics of nonpathologic antibody induction to the gut microbiome.[47,48] Therefore, making at least some specific class-switched antibody to exogenous gut antigens is not a sign of impaired tolerance. However, comparisons between healthy and allergic individuals (with the caveat that some studies do not adequately distinguish the clinically allergic state from the IgE-sensitized state), reveal that allergic individuals generally mount a stronger allergen-specific antibody response.[46,49] Both the prevalence and mean concentrations of non-IgE Ig responses are greater in sensitized individuals and the same is true of IgE levels when comparing allergic versus sensitized but clinically tolerant individuals. Whether the humoral response in allergic individuals is also broadly distinct by other measures of immune progression, such as greater somatic hypermutation and affinity, has yet to be characterized to our knowledge, but that would logically follow as a consequence of impaired tolerance.

Food allergy is also not the only state associated with broadly higher levels of (non-IgE) antibody to dietary antigens. Both inflammatory bowel disease and celiac disease have been associated with the same, even though dietary antigens (with the exception of the gluten-derived trigger of CD) are not directly involved in disease pathogenesis. IgA deficiency is also associated with more IgG to food antigens, although that may be a compensatory effect. Therefore, it is not clear whether higher antibody concentrations to food antigens in food allergy reflects some general disease association, such as poor gut barrier, or is a specific hallmark of a break in immune tolerance. Sensitization, meaning the presence of detectable IgE by serum or skin testing, is also far from uniquely associated with a loss in clinical tolerance, and low levels of food antigen-specific IgE are actually quite common in young children, especially if they have risk factors for atopic disease. Thus, it is arguably unclear how we should think about the sensitized state with respect to immune tolerance. Early sIgE is clearly associated with an increased risk of developing true allergy, but it could be that it is a marker of early loss of immune tolerance allowing for sufficient T-cell help to induce a

Th2-mediated class switch of specific B cells, or rather that the humoral response, including IgE class switch, is to a significant degree autonomous from T-cell tolerance but may then provide an adjuvant signal, perhaps via activation of mast cells as shown in murine models discussed earlier,[42] that subsequently facilitates a true break in tolerance. These 2 scenarios may not be mutually exclusive. So, we do not know to what extent preventing the induction of IgE (eg, by a lack of Th2 help for B cells) or rather preventing its subsequent function (eg, by suppression of mast cells by Treg) is most important for clinical outcomes or whether either might be better regarded as a primary checkpoint of true immune tolerance.

The recently published LEAP (Learning Early about Peanut Allergy) trial provides some insight into the development of antibody responses in a high-risk population with or without oral exposure to the major food allergen, peanut.[50] This was the first randomized controlled intervention to address prevention of peanut allergy. Infants with egg allergy or eczema (and therefore at higher risk for the development of peanut allergy) were randomized to regular consumption of peanut or avoidance and subjected to food challenge at 5 years of age to determine their allergic status. More than 20% (174 of 834) of this population was already sensitized to peanut at less than 11 months of age and before the introduction of peanut to the diet. Only 2% (7 of 319) were confirmed to be clinically allergic at that time, but the true prevalence of peanut allergy was likely to be significantly higher given that 9% (76 of 834) were excluded from further evaluation because the strength of skin test reactivity (>4 mm) was taken as sufficient evidence of established allergy. They found that regular oral exposure (participants were instructed to ingest peanut at least 3 times every week) strongly reduced the risk of being reactive to peanut at year 5 and dramatically induced peanut-specific IgG (mean $\sim$10 μg/mL at 12 months). That level of sIgG to peanut antigen is roughly comparable with that induced by pathogen antigens after vaccination or in convalescence. IgE also increased over time, and the prevalence of low levels (<1 kU/L) of sIgE seems to be induced by consumption, but the development of very high levels of sIgE (>100 kU/L) was completely suppressed. In the control avoidance group, all individuals with sIgE level greater than 10 kU/L were reactive and several individuals developed very high levels of sIgE (>100 kU/L). It remains to be seen whether some of those in the consumption group with moderate levels of sIgE (10–100 kU/L) will prove to be persistently tolerant, and a follow-up study is now in progress to address this, but regular oral consumption suppressed clinical reactivity in concert with high titer sIgE while driving up sIgG, at least transiently.

In murine models of oral tolerance, as discussed earlier, induction of IgG is not generally described and dietary Ag-specific IgG is regarded as a marker of tolerance loss. Burton and colleagues recently demonstrated that when IgE-deficient Il4raF709 mice were subjected to the same feeding regimen that leads to allergic sensitization in IgE-sufficient Il4raF709 mice, allergen-specific IgG was induced, and although not included as a control, this would not be expected in the wt mice. This would be consistent with the interpretation that the higher levels of allergen-specific IgG seen in allergic humans is a sign of impaired tolerance. However, this apparent and potentially significant difference in the immunogenicity of dietary antigens between humans as they introduce solid foods versus murine models of oral tolerance should not be overlooked and may deserve greater attention. Furthermore, although much of the literature regarding antibody function in the context of regulating allergy has focused on its potential to antagonize IgE-mediated effector cell responses, the capacity of food antigen-specific antibody to modulate the mucosal immune response via IgG-FcRn or IgA-pIgR also deserves further study.[51]

T-Cell Response to Dietary Antigens in Healthy Versus Allergic Individuals

Even early studies after the emergence of the Th1/Th2 paradigm, continuing with successive refinement conventional CD4 T-cell subsets, have found evidence of Th2-skewed immunity to food allergens in allergic individuals in contrast to healthy controls, but systematic characterization of T-cell responses to food antigens from an early age are very limited. One recent effort to characterize human T-cell responses in a prospective cohort by Sicherer and colleagues[52] enrolled more than 200 children between 3 and 15 months of age with early reactivity to milk or egg consistent with established allergy and followed them over 5 years. They found that IL-4 in response to allergen stimulation of peripheral blood mononuclear cells (PBMCs) was directly associated with more persistent clinical allergy. There were no healthy controls for comparison. Martino and colleagues[53] conducted a nested case-control study of banked PBMCs from birth and at 1 year comparing 30 children who developed confirmed IgE-mediated food allergy by 1 year of age with 30 healthy controls and stimulated them with allergen and with anti-CD3 and then analyzed cytokine secretion and CD4 transcriptional profiles. Consistent with previous work, they found evidence that, within the allergic group, the CD4 T cells were hyporesponsive to T cell receptor (TCR) stimulation, but that by 1 year the allergic patient cells were predominantly Th2 skewed, although specifically in response to ovalbumin allergen, there was also higher interferon-γ secretion.

Foxp3 expressing Tregs have long been hypothesized as being important for tolerance to food antigens based on murine studies and the observation that mutations in Foxp3 resulting in Immune dysregulation, polyendocrinopathy, enteropathy, X-linked (IPEX) syndrome lead to loss of immune tolerance causing severe autoimmunity but also manifestations of food allergy. This is complemented by the growing literature linking the microbiota and the key metabolites they produce to the normal induction and function of Tregs and the proposed relationship between dysbiosis and the epidemiology of autoimmunity and allergy.[54] Evaluation of Treg responses to dietary antigens in healthy humans, especially at a very young age when sensitization occurs in food allergic individuals, is limited. One of the best evaluations of the Treg phenotype in food allergy, specifically in pediatric patients with milk allergy in contrast to controls (both healthy controls and food allergic but milk tolerant) was reported recently by Noval Rivas and colleagues.[39] One of the key observations is one that has been seen by others in attempted comparisons of allergen-specific T cells in the time frame of already established disease; the frequency of allergen-specific T cells is very low in nonallergic individuals. Noval Rivas and colleagues[39] evaluated the phenotype of allergen-specific Foxp3+ CD4 T cells by characterizing those that proliferated in response to milk allergen (β-lactoglobulin). They found that the percentage of proliferative Foxp3+ cells that expressed IL-4 was significantly higher than in either the healthy or allergic, milk-tolerant controls. In addition, the percentage of total circulating Foxp3+ CD4 T cells was lower in milk allergy and more likely to co-express markers of Th2 deviation: GATA-3 and IRF-4. This may represent an expansion of a population similar to that defined by Miyara and colleagues[55] as cytokine-secreting CD45RA- Foxp3lo nonsuppressive cells, which they found to be poorly demethylated at the STAT5-responsive region of Foxp3 and suggest are likely to be activation-induced Foxp3-expressing cells. Transient Foxp3 expression in activated effector T cells has been shown to occur in human, but not murine, CD4 T-effector cells.[56] Alternatively, as supported by murine experiments presented by the authors, it may represent an in vivo deviation of iTreg cells to a nonsuppressive Th2 population.[39] The latter model would indirectly support the notion that healthy individuals have a population of allergen-specific iTregs, but this was not shown, quite possibly because if they are present, they are not very proliferative to milk allergy under the conditions of the in vitro assay. Further complicating the interpretation of the human data is the observation by others that CD45RA− Tregs have an unstable phenotype with predominantly Th2 differentiation during in vitro culture.[57]

One way to avoid the potential artifacts of in vitro stimulation as a means of identifying antigen-specific T cells is by use of major histocompatibility complex class II (MHCII)–epitope tetramers, which allow for the detection of allergen-specific cells by direct binding of the TCR. So far, little has been published and studies of very young children during the initial immune response to these antigens are technically challenging. What has been reported to date is that there are very low frequencies of antigen-specific T cells of any phenotype in healthy controls but what few cells there are, do not have a Treg phenotype. For example, DeLong and colleagues[58] showed that they could identify Ara h 1-specific T cells from peanut-allergic individuals, that they expressed the Th2-associated chemokine receptor, CCR4, and produced predominantly the Th2 cytokines, IL-4 and IL-5, detected by intracellular staining, as opposed to interferon-γ, IL-10, or IL-17.

Another focus has been to compare those with confirmed food allergy versus those with sensitization (ie, production of allergen-specific IgE) but not clinical reactivity as one way to hone in on those factors that might identify regulatory checkpoints that are downstream of sensitization. Brough and colleagues[59] offer an example of that approach in which they also attempt to evaluate CD4 T-cell subsets (β7-vs CLA-expressing). They first contrast the transcriptome of those 2 CD4 T-cell populations drawn from allergic and nonallergic patients, focusing on those activated (CD69+) by short-term culture with peanut allergen using a microarray. They then validate several genes identified as differentially expressed in a larger number of samples. There are several interesting genes differentially regulated and they focus primarily on IL9, which they validate by quantitative polymerase chain reaction and intracellular cytokine staining. IL-9 is interesting as it plays a role in activating mast cells and is also induced by IL-4 with TGF-beta,[60] suggesting that it may be an important marker of differentiation of peanut-specific cells that might have been induced to become Foxp3+ Treg (a known function of TGF-beta on naive T cells) but instead become Th9 under the influence of IL-4. IL-9 expression was significantly higher in peanut-activated T cells from peanut-allergic versus peanut-sensitized and tolerant; however, it was not unique as such.

Responses to Diet Allergens During Immunotherapy

Another potential way to gain insight into the regulation of tolerance to food allergens could be to evaluate the changes that occur during immunotherapy protocols where the goal of therapy is to restore clinical tolerance. As discussed earlier, there are important questions about whether clinical tolerance achieved after immunotherapy, even for the subset that seem to have some degree of persistent tolerance, is distinct from natural tolerance. Studies of immunotherapy for food allergy have repeatedly shown that IgE increases or stays flat initially, followed by a decline, and that IgG, IgG4, and IgA increase, with the increase in IgG4 tending to be later and more persistent. Vickery and colleagues[61] have also shown that there is a strong increase in the number of epitopes recognized after oral immunotherapy within the IgG4 antibody fraction, suggesting that the IgG4 response is diversified over time with immunotherapy, whereas the number of epitopes that can be detected in the IgE fraction contracts. Burton and colleagues[62] have also recently demonstrated that after oral immunotherapy, serum can block IgE-mediated basophil activation in vitro in a CD32-dependent manner. Consistent with an expansion of the non-IgE response induced by immunotherapy, Patil and colleagues[63] used affinity to Ara h 2 to show that circulating Ara h 2–specific B cells transiently expand in the first several weeks of oral immunotherapy and they and Hoh and colleagues[64] have established this approach as a method to potentially track B-cell repertoire changes induced by oral immunotherapy. What is still lacking, however, is convincing correlation between these changes and clinical outcomes of patients.

Basophils are suppressed by oral immunotherapy ex vivo, as has been reproducibly shown in several studies, and suppression in at least some studies has been correlated with the desensitized state[65,66]; however, 2 groups have now presented data demonstrating reversibility of basophil suppression over time,[67,68] and particularly with withdrawal of regular allergen exposure. This is consistent with an oral immunotherapy-induced anergic effect on basophils reported in the context of oral immunotherapy for peanut allergy,[66] but that has yet to be replicated by other groups, and 1 other study of oral immunotherapy for peanut allergy evaluating basophil reactivity found suppression during treatment but did not find evidence for reversible suppression seen by others.[69]

The T-cell arm of the immune system is affected by immunotherapy as well, although studies have only recently begun to adopt methods to examine the small fraction of antigen-specific T cells. Apart from food allergy, in studies of both mucosal and subcutaneous routes of immunotherapy for allergy to respiratory allergens, there are human data that therapy induces regulatory T cells and decreases Th2 effector cells from peripheral blood[70] and some data that Tregs may be induced at mucosal lymphoid sites[71,72] with local exposure. MHCII tetramer-based studies, although documenting a loss of predominantly Th2-skewed effector cells from the periphery, have failed to find evidence of Treg expansion.[73]

An early study of peanut oral immunotherapy that included measurement of CD4 T-cell responses found a transient expansion of circulating Foxp3+ cells at 6 and 12 months after immunotherapy but not at later time points. The methodology used involved in vitro culture of PBMCs with peanut allergen for 6 days. Given what we now know about the promiscuity of Foxp3 expression in activated human T cells, it is difficult to know if this represents an expansion of bona fide iTreg or simply antigen-specific T cells more generally.[74] Most studies of food allergy immunotherapy in which T cells have been evaluated in some manner have found evidence of diminished Th2 responses (eg, by cytokine secretion in allergen-stimulated PBMCs). Syed and colleagues[69] reported outcomes of a nonrandomized phase I trial of peanut oral immunotherapy in peanut allergy that followed participants (median age, 10 years; range, 5–45 years) who were successfully desensitized through a period of avoidance (up to 6 months). They found that allergen-specific CD4+ CD25+ Foxp3+ (defined variably by either proliferation or upregulation of activation markers after stimulation with in vitro peanut allergen), but not total Treg percentages, as well as the level of Foxp3 transcript, increased significantly in those study participants who had the most sustained clinical benefit (complete tolerance after 3 months of avoidance, n = 7 of 20 who completed the study). Furthermore, they reported that within the antigen-specific Treg compartment, methylation of the Foxp3 locus decreased dramatically in those individuals with persistent clinical improvement compared with those who achieved only desensitization. Similar to the discussion regarding the phenotypes of Foxp3-expressing CD4 T cells, the true nature of cells with lower levels of Foxp3 expression (less suppressive capacity, a more methylated Foxp3 locus, and stronger association with allergy outcomes) and whether they are more likely to be an activated effector population transiently expressing Foxp3 or a deviated Treg population might be addressed by TCR repertoire analyses. In the results reported by

Syed and colleagues,[69] however, it does seem that persistent clinical tolerance was associated with the induction of a Treg population, not simply a reduction of effector T cells.

SUMMARY

Data from animal models have clearly highlighted the central role of antigen-specific regulatory T cells in the maintenance of tolerance to antigens encountered orally. The understanding of the immune basis of tolerance to foods in humans is more limited. Food allergen-specific IgG antibodies seem to play a central role in oral tolerance in humans, including tolerance induced during primary prevention or during immunotherapy to induce clinical tolerance to foods. Recent reports in mice and humans suggest that an altered Treg phenotype may contribute to the lack of tolerance to foods in food allergy, however further study is required to dissect the contribution of Th2 cells and true Tregs in the generation of tolerance to foods.

REFERENCES

1. Wells HG, Osborne TB. The biological reactions of the vegetable proteins. I. Anaphylaxis. J Infect Dis 1911;8:66–124.
2. Chen Y, Kuchroo VK, Inobe J, et al. Regulatory T cell clones induced by oral tolerance: suppression of autoimmune encephalomyelitis. Science 1994;265:1237–40.
3. Fukaura H, Kent SC, Pietrusewicz MJ, et al. Induction of circulating myelin basic protein and proteolipid protein-specific transforming growth factor-beta1-secreting Th3 T cells by oral administration of myelin in multiple sclerosis patients. J Clin Invest 1996;98:70–7.
4. Weiner HL, Cunha AP, da Quintana F, et al. Oral tolerance. Immunol Rev 2011; 241:241–59.
5. Hadis U, Wahl B, Schulz O, et al. Intestinal tolerance requires gut homing and expansion of FoxP3+ regulatory T cells in the lamina propria. Immunity 2011; 34:237–46.
6. Mucida D, Kutchukhidze N, Erazo A, et al. Oral tolerance in the absence of naturally occurring Tregs. J Clin Invest 2005;115:1923–33.
7. Asseman C, Mauze S, Leach MW, et al. An essential role for interleukin 10 in the function of regulatory T cells that inhibit intestinal inflammation. J Exp Med 1999; 190:995–1004.
8. Gonnella PA, Waldner HP, Kodali D, et al. Induction of low dose oral tolerance in IL-10 deficient mice with experimental autoimmune encephalomyelitis. J Autoimmun 2004;23:193–200.
9. Chambers SJ, Wickham MSJ, Regoli M, et al. Rapid in vivo transport of proteins from digested allergen across pre-sensitized gut. Biochem Biophys Res Commun 2004;325:1258–63.
10. Roth-Walter F, Berin MC, Arnaboldi P, et al. Pasteurization of milk proteins promotes allergic sensitization by enhancing uptake through Peyer's patches. Allergy 2008;63:882–90.
11. McDole JR, Wheeler LW, McDonald KG, et al. Goblet cells deliver luminal antigen to CD103+ dendritic cells in the small intestine. Nature 2012;483:345–9.
12. Niess JH, Brand S, Gu X, et al. CX3CR1-mediated dendritic cell access to the intestinal lumen and bacterial clearance. Science 2005;307:254–8.
13. Rescigno M, Urbano M, Valzasina B, et al. Dendritic cells express tight junction proteins and penetrate gut epithelial monolayers to sample bacteria. Nat Immunol 2001;2:361–7.

14. Kraus TA, Brimnes J, Muong C, et al. Induction of mucosal tolerance in Peyer's patch-deficient, ligated small bowel loops. J Clin Invest 2005;115:2234–43.

15. Spahn TW, Fontana A, Faria AM, et al. Induction of oral tolerance to cellular immune responses in the absence of Peyer's patches. Eur J Immunol 2001;31: 1278–87.

16. Spahn TW, Weiner HL, Rennert PD, et al. Mesenteric lymph nodes are critical for the induction of high-dose oral tolerance in the absence of Peyer's patches. Eur J Immunol 2002;32:1109–13.

17. Worbs T, Bode U, Yan S, et al. Oral tolerance originates in the intestinal immune system and relies on antigen carriage by dendritic cells. J Exp Med 2006;203: 519–27.

18. Cassani B, Villablanca EJ, Quintana FJ, et al. Gut-tropic T cells that express integrin $\alpha 4\beta 7$ and cCR9 are required for induction of oral immune tolerance in mice. Gastroenterology 2011;141:2109–18.

19. Viney JL, Mowat AM, O'Malley JM, et al. Expanding dendritic cells in vivo enhances the induction of oral tolerance. J Immunol 1998;160:5815–25.

20. Bogunovic M, Ginhoux F, Helft J, et al. Origin of the lamina propria dendritic cell network. Immunity 2009;31:513–25.

21. Schulz O, Jaensson E, Persson EK, et al. Intestinal CD103+, but not CX3CR1+, antigen sampling cells migrate in lymph and serve classical dendritic cell functions. J Exp Med 2009;206:3101–14.

22. Varol C, Vallon-Eberhard A, Elinav E, et al. Intestinal lamina propria dendritic cell subsets have different origin and functions. Immunity 2009;31:502–12.

23. Miller JC, Brown BD, Shay T, et al, Immunological Genome Consortium. Deciphering the transcriptional network of the dendritic cell lineage. Nat Immunol 2012;13: 888–99.

24. Coombes JL, Siddiqui KRR, Arancibia-Cárcamo CV, et al. A functionally specialized population of mucosal CD103+ DCs induces Foxp3+ regulatory T cells via a TGF-beta and retinoic acid-dependent mechanism. J Exp Med 2007;204: 1757–64.

25. Jaensson E, Uronen-Hansson H, Pabst O, et al. Small intestinal cD103+ dendritic cells display unique functional properties that are conserved between mice and humans. J Exp Med 2008;205:2139–49.

26. Johansson-Lindbom B, Svensson M, Pabst O, et al. Functional specialization of gut CD103+ dendritic cells in the regulation of tissue-selective T cell homing. J Exp Med 2005;202:1063–73.

27. Matteoli G, Mazzini E, Iliev ID, et al. Gut CD103+ dendritic cells express indoleamine 2,3-dioxygenase which influences T regulatory/T effector cell balance and oral tolerance induction. Gut 2010;59:595–604.

28. Mazzini E, Massimiliano L, Penna G, et al. Oral tolerance can be established via gap junction transfer of fed antigens from CX3CR1+ macrophages to CD103+ dendritic cells. Immunity 2014;40:248–61.

29. Kühn R, Löhler J, Rennick D, et al. Interleukin-10-deficient mice develop chronic enterocolitis. Cell 1993;75:263–74.

30. Shan M, Gentile M, Yeiser JR, et al. Mucus enhances gut homeostasis and oral tolerance by delivering immunoregulatory signals. Science 2013;342:447–53.

31. Mortha A, Chudnovskiy A, Hashimoto D, et al. Microbiota-dependent crosstalk between macrophages and ILC3 promotes intestinal homeostasis. Science 2014;343:1249288.

32. Atarashi K, Tanoue T, Oshima K, et al. Treg induction by a rationally selected mixture of Clostridia strains from the human microbiota. Nature 2013;500:232–6.

33. Atarashi K, Tanoue T, Shima T, et al. Induction of colonic regulatory T cells by indigenous Clostridium species. Science 2011;331:337–41.
34. Round JL, Mazmanian SK. Inducible Foxp3+ regulatory T-cell development by a commensal bacterium of the intestinal microbiota. Proc Natl Acad Sci U S A 2010; 107:12204–9.
35. Furusawa Y, Obata Y, Fukuda S, et al. Commensal microbe-derived butyrate induces the differentiation of colonic regulatory T cells. Nature 2013;504:446–50.
36. Faith JJ, Ahern PP, Ridaura VK, et al. Identifying gut microbe-host phenotype relationships using combinatorial communities in gnotobiotic mice. Sci Transl Med 2014;6:220ra11.
37. Stefka AT, Feehley T, Tripathi P, et al. Commensal bacteria protect against food allergen sensitization. Proc Natl Acad Sci U S A 2014;111:13145–50.
38. Noval Rivas M, Burton OT, Wise P, et al. A microbiota signature associated with experimental food allergy promotes allergic sensitization and anaphylaxis. J Allergy Clin Immunol 2013;131:201–12.
39. Noval Rivas M, Burton OT, Wise P, et al. Regulatory T cell reprogramming toward a Th2-cell-like lineage impairs oral tolerance and promotes food allergy. Immunity 2015;42:512–23.
40. Ohnmacht C, Park J-H, Cording S, et al. The microbiota regulates type 2 immunity through RORγt+ T cells. Science 2015. http://dx.doi.org/10.1126/science.aac4263.
41. Leonard SA, Martos G, Wang W, et al. Oral immunotherapy induces local protective mechanisms in the gastrointestinal mucosa. J Allergy Clin Immunol 2012;129:1579–87.e1.
42. Burton OT, Noval Rivas M, Zhou JS, et al. Immunoglobulin E signal inhibition during allergen ingestion leads to reversal of established food allergy and induction of regulatory T cells. Immunity 2014;41:141–51.
43. McLachlan JB, Shelburne CP, Hart JP, et al. Mast cell activators: a new class of highly effective vaccine adjuvants. Nat Med 2008;14:536–41.
44. Hofmaier S, Hatzler L, Rohrbach A, et al. 'Default' versus 'pre-atopic' IgG responses to foodborne and airborne pathogenesis-related group 10 protein molecules in birch-sensitized and nonatopic children. J Allergy Clin Immunol 2015;135:1367–74.e1–8.
45. Hochwallner H, Schulmeister U, Swoboda I, et al. Patients suffering from non-IgE-mediated cow's milk protein intolerance cannot be diagnosed based on IgG subclass or IgA responses to milk allergens. Allergy 2011;66:1201–7.
46. Rowntree S, Cogswell JJ, Platts-Mills TA, et al. Development of IgE and IgG antibodies to food and inhalant allergens in children at risk of allergic disease. Arch Dis Child 1985;60:727–35.
47. Christmann BS, Abrahamsson TR, Bernstein CN, et al. Human seroreactivity to gut microbiota antigens. J Allergy Clin Immunol 2015. http://dx.doi.org/10.1016/j.jaci.2015.03.036.
48. Simón-Soro Á, D'Auria G, Collado MC, et al. Revealing microbial recognition by specific antibodies. BMC Microbiol 2015;15:132.
49. Shek LPC, Bardina L, Castro R, et al. Humoral and cellular responses to cow milk proteins in patients with milk-induced IgE-mediated and non-IgE-mediated disorders. Allergy 2005;60:912–9.
50. Toit G, du Roberts G, Sayre PH, et al. Randomized trial of peanut consumption in infants at risk for peanut allergy. N Engl J Med 2015;372:803–13.
51. Berin MC. Mucosal antibodies in the regulation of tolerance and allergy to foods. Semin Immunopathol 2012;34:633–42.

52. Sicherer SH, Wood RA, Vickery BP, et al. The natural history of egg allergy in an observational cohort. J Allergy Clin Immunol 2014;133:492–9.
53. Martino DJ, Bosco A, Mckenna KL, et al. T-cell activation genes differentially expressed at birth in CD4+ T-cells from children who develop IgE food allergy. Allergy 2012;67:191–200.
54. Maslowski KM, Mackay CR. Diet, gut microbiota and immune responses. Nat Immunol 2011;12:5–9.
55. Miyara M, Yoshioka Y, Kitoh A, et al. Functional delineation and differentiation dynamics of human CD4+ T cells expressing the FoxP3 transcription factor. Immunity 2009;30:899–911.
56. Gavin MA, Torgerson TR, Houston E, et al. Single-cell analysis of normal and FOXP3-mutant human T cells: FOXP3 expression without regulatory T cell development. Proc Natl Acad Sci U S A 2006;103:6659–64.
57. Hansmann L, Schmidl C, Kett J, et al. Dominant Th2 differentiation of human regulatory T cells upon loss of FOXP3 expression. J Immunol 2012;188:1275–82.
58. Delong JH, Hetherington Simpson K, Wambre E, et al. Ara h 1-reactive T cells in individuals with peanut allergy. J Allergy Clin Immunol 2011;127(5):1211–8.e3.
59. Brough HA, Cousins DJ, Munteanu A, et al. IL-9 is a key component of memory TH cell peanut-specific responses from children with peanut allergy. J Allergy Clin Immunol 2014;134:1329–38.e10.
60. Schmitt E, Germann T, Goedert S, et al. IL-9 production of naive CD4+ T cells depends on IL-2, is synergistically enhanced by a combination of TGF-beta and IL-4, and is inhibited by IFN-gamma. J Immunol 1994;153:3989–96.
61. Vickery BP, Lin J, Kulis M, et al. Peanut oral immunotherapy modifies IgE and IgG4 responses to major peanut allergens. J Allergy Clin Immunol 2013;131:128–34.e1-3.
62. Burton OT, Logsdon SL, Zhou JS, et al. Oral immunotherapy induces IgG antibodies that act through FcγRIIb to suppress IgE-mediated hypersensitivity. J Allergy Clin Immunol 2014;134(6):1310–7.e6.
63. Patil SU, Ogunniyi AO, Calatroni A, et al. Peanut oral immunotherapy transiently expands circulating Ara h 2-specific B cells with a homologous repertoire in unrelated subjects. J Allergy Clin Immunol 2015;136(1):125–34.e12.
64. Hoh RA, Joshi SA, Liu Y, et al. Single B-cell deconvolution of peanut-specific antibody responses in allergic patients. J Allergy Clin Immunol 2015. http://dx.doi.org/10.1016/j.jaci.2015.05.029.
65. Burks AW, Jones SM, Wood RA, et al. Oral immunotherapy for treatment of egg allergy in children. N Engl J Med 2012;367:233–43.
66. Thyagarajan A, Jones SM, Calatroni A, et al. Evidence of pathway-specific basophil anergy induced by peanut oral immunotherapy in peanut-allergic children. Clin Exp Allergy 2012;42:1197–205.
67. Gorelik M, Narisety SD, Guerrerio AL, et al. Suppression of the immunologic response to peanut during immunotherapy is often transient. J Allergy Clin Immunol 2015;135:1283–92.
68. Kulis MD, Burk C, Yue X, et al. Basophil hyporesponsiveness following six months of Peanut Oral Immunotherapy (OIT) is associated with suppression of syk phosphorylation. J Allergy Clin Immunol 2015;134:AB24.
69. Syed A, Garcia MA, Lyu S-C, et al. Peanut oral immunotherapy results in increased antigen-induced regulatory T-cell function and hypomethylation of forkhead box protein 3 (FOXP3). J Allergy Clin Immunol 2014;133:500–10.
70. Akdis CA, Akdis M. Advances in allergen immunotherapy: aiming for complete tolerance to allergens. Sci Transl Med 2015;7:280ps6.

71. Palomares O, Rückert B, Jartti T, et al. Induction and maintenance of allergen-specific FOXP3+ Treg cells in human tonsils as potential first-line organs of oral tolerance. J Allergy Clin Immunol 2012;129:510–20, 520.e1–9.

72. Scadding GW, Shamji MH, Jacobson MR, et al. Sublingual grass pollen immunotherapy is associated with increases in sublingual Foxp3-expressing cells and elevated allergen-specific immunoglobulin G4, immunoglobulin A and serum inhibitory activity for immunoglobulin E-facilitated allergen binding to B cells. Clin Exp Allergy 2010;40:1–9.

73. Wambre E, Delong JH, James EA, et al. Specific immunotherapy modifies allergen-specific CD4(+) T-cell responses in an epitope-dependent manner. J Allergy Clin Immunol 2014;133:872–9.e7.

74. Jones SM, Pons L, Roberts JL, et al. Clinical efficacy and immune regulation with peanut oral immunotherapy. J Allergy Clin Immunol 2009;124:292–7.

Allergen Immunotherapy
Vaccine Modification

Peter Socrates Creticos, MD[a,b]

KEYWORDS

- Allergic rhinitis • Allergen immunotherapy • Vaccine modification

KEY POINTS

- New modalities of allergen immunotherapy may allow effective immunization with shorter treatment regimens, improved patient compliance, and the potential of safer agents.
- Toll receptors on specific regulatory cells provide a unique pathway to initiate regulatory pathways capable of down-regulating the untoward allergic diathesis.
- Synthetic peptides offers the ability to immunize allergic subjects with a concise 4-injection intradermal regimen. The smaller peptides are less likely to trigger crosslinking of IgE on mast cells, thereby minimizing the risk of allergic reactions and anaphylaxis.

OVERVIEW

Allergic rhinitis (AR) is a common clinical condition; both its incidence and prevalence seem to be increasing in North America, perhaps reflective of population shifts, climate changes, and genetic susceptibility. Demographic surveys identity up to 20% to 40% of the population as sufferers of AR/conjunctivitis and approximately 8% troubled with asthma.[1–4]

Allergen immunotherapy (AIT) comes to the forefront in our therapeutic approach to immunoglobulin E (IgE)–mediated diseases (allergic rhinoconjunctivitis, allergic asthma, food allergy, venom sensitivity, and possibly even atopic eczema), as it affords a means of redirecting the untoward immune response, reestablishing immunologic tolerance, and accomplishing long-term clinical remission.

Although effective, current immunotherapy regimens are burdened by tedious treatment regimens that not only negatively impact on patient adherence and compliance but also serve as barriers to limit access to this form of disease-modifying therapy. Furthermore, systemic reactions to immunotherapy, although infrequent, can be severe and potentially life threatening.

Thus, there is a recognized need for newer therapeutic agents that improve the safety of AIT, provide an ease of delivery to patients that fosters compliance and

[a] Division of Allergy & Clinical Immunology, Johns Hopkins Medicine, Baltimore, MD 21287, USA; [b] Creticos Research Group, 1300 Saint Paul's Way, Crownsville, MD 21032, USA
E-mail address: psocrates@comcast.net

Immunol Allergy Clin N Am 36 (2016) 103–124
http://dx.doi.org/10.1016/j.iac.2015.08.010   immunology.theclinics.com

allows access to a greater proportion of the allergic population that could benefit from this disease-modifying treatment, and achieves an acceptable therapeutic benefit for most patients committing to the course of treatment.

Through the years, various chemical modifications of allergens have been tried in an attempt to enhance efficacy, improve safety, and foster adherence with AIT. In many cases, these previous approaches have been viewed as unsuccessful, or only partially successful, in that the allergenicity and immunogenicity have either decreased, or increased in tandem, with no resultant efficacy/safety benefit ratio realized. However, recent clinical trials have led to promising results in immunization approaches with modified allergens, including immune-stimulatory adjuvants, recombinant allergens, and T-cell-tolerizing constructs, as well as with alternate routes of delivery, including oral and sublingual, intralymphatic, and epicutaneous methods, as vehicles for immunization in allergic respiratory disease[5-11] (**Box 1**).

MODIFIED ALLERGEN APPROACHES
Background

Through the years, various groups have attempted to improve AIT through a variety of techniques through which the allergen is modified. In the 1970s to 1980s, efforts by Norman and Marsh at Hopkins modified grass and ragweed (RW) allergens by partially denaturing them in formalin; this led to allergens with markedly reduced allergenicity; but unfortunately, the immunogenicity of allergoids, as judged by the IgG antibody response, was also decreased, as was the clinical effectiveness.[12,13] Sehon and Lee attempted to modify and decrease allergenicity by coupling the allergens to a polyethylene glycol backbone. Again, the result was the same: allergenicity and immunogenicity decreased together.[14,15]

Box 1
Modified AIT constructs

Injectable immunotherapy approaches

Alum salts (SQ)

Chemical modifications (SQ)
  Allergoids/polymerized allergens
  Novel adjuvants (SQ; IM)

DNA vaccines
  TLR-9 (CpG oligonucleotides) (SQ)

    Linked to allergen; cocombined

    Nanoparticle-based VLPs
  TLR-4 (MPL) (SQ)
  Lysosomal plasmids (IM)

Peptides (T-cell epitopes) (ID)

Recombinant allergens (SQ)

Alternate routes for immunization

Sublingual immunotherapy

Intralymphatic

Epicutaneous

Abbreviations: ID, intradermal; IM, intramuscular; MPL, monophosphoryl lipid A; SQ, subcutaneous; VLPs, viral-like particles.

Then Patterson developed polymerized allergens, wherein a glutaraldehyde-linked polymerization rendered an allergen product that in animal studies was shown to be less reactive on immunization but maintained immunogenicity. Studies of allergic patients with polymerized grass and RW allergens demonstrated efficacy and tolerability in double-blind placebo-controlled clinical trials. However, this project was fraught with regulatory issues related to standardization of the allergen.[16–18]

Subsequently, in the mid-90s, Gefter developed synthetic T-cell tolerizing peptides from cat Fel d 1 and RW Amb a 1. The concept was based on the recognition that specific peptide sequences (epitopes) form the whole allergen and were capable of inducing what was thought to be anergy or, in fact, tolerance.[19,20]

In collaborative studies with cat peptides and RW peptides, Norman and colleagues demonstrated peptide immunization significantly reduced clinical symptoms without an increased IgG antibody response. Although significant therapeutic results were observed, the effects were less than that achieved with unmodified AIT; furthermore, patients experienced late-onset adverse symptoms that mimicked natural allergen exposure.[21–24]

During this same time, groundbreaking work demonstrated that bacterial DNA could have profound effects on the humoral and cellular limbs of the immune system and that this could be used to advantage to manipulate the immune response to proteins and, hence, allergens.[25–38]

Capitalizing on the potential to induce T-cell tolerance with long-term suppression of the allergic diathesis, Raz and colleagues[39–46] demonstrated first, in animal models, and then in human studies that allergen vaccination with immune-stimulatory DNA was capable of redirecting the untoward Th2:Th1 allergic diathesis.

These novel approaches are discussed below.

Immunostimulatory Adjuvants

CpG oligonucleotide conjugated to ragweed Amb a 1

An adjuvant approach, developed by Dynavax Technologies, Inc., in which immune-stimulatory DNA is conjugated to the principal allergic moiety of RW (Amb a 1) (Amb a 1–immunostimulatory complex [AIC]; synonymously termed Toll-Like Receptor 9 [TLR-9] vaccine) has been shown to greatly enhance the Amb a 1–specific Th1 immune response in animals and is capable of diminishing RW-induced pulmonary hyperreactivity in mice. AIC has been shown to be demonstrably less allergenic than unconjugated Amb a 1 or RW extract. This combination of decreased allergenicity and enhanced Amb a 1–specific immune response with AIC was thought to afford an opportunity to use an allergen modification capable of simultaneously providing improved clinical efficacy, an enhanced safety profile, and a more convenient dosing regimen. The basis for enhancement of Th1 response by immune-stimulatory DNA sequences is derived from the recognition that bacterial DNA induces an immune response (through its toll-like receptor ligand on plasmacytoid dendritic cells) that is characterized by a potent interleukin (IL)-12 activation of Th1 cells to secrete interferon (IFN)-gamma and a much lower level of activation of Th2 cells secreting IL-4 and IL-5.

Initial phase 1-2 safety and dose-ranging studies by Creticos and colleagues[47,48] in the early 2000s demonstrated that the vaccine was well tolerated and induced the expected immunologic changes in humans. In 2006, Creticos and colleagues reported the proof-of-concept study for this TLR-9 agonist in a 2-year double-blind placebo-controlled clinical study of 25 RW-allergic subjects immunized with a brief 6-injection regimen (0.06–12.0 mcg AIC; administered before the first RW season only). The mean peak-season rhinitis symptoms, as measured by a standard visual analog scale (VAS), were significantly improved in both RW seasons (year 1: 68% [$P = .006$]; year 2: 72%

[*P* = .02]) in the TLR-9 vaccine group versus Placebo. Similar findings were observed for the peak-season daily nasal symptom diary scores (year 1: 55% [*P* = .02]; year 2: 53% [*P* = .02]). These data provided consistent evidence that the vaccine conferred meaningful long-term clinical efficacy, which extended over the 2 RW seasons under study.[49]

Furthermore, the vaccine blunted the typical seasonal increase in Amb a 1–specific IgE antibody in the first RW season and markedly suppressed the IgE antibody titer in the following RW season, providing evidence for long-term immune tolerance (as defined by suppression of the allergic antibody, IgE). In addition, a reduction in the number of IL-4–positive basophils in AIC-treated patients correlated with lower VAS scores (r = 0.49; *P* = .03)—an important corollary, as IL-4 is a key cytokine involved in B-cell class switching to IgE antibody.[49]

In a separate DBPC Canadian study (n = 57 RW-AR subjects), a subset (n = 19) consented to nasal provocation and biopsy. Tulic and colleagues[50] reported that the 6-week injection course with the TLR-9 vaccine (administered before the first RW season) modified the nasal inflammatory immune response to allergen challenge after RW season; the study findings showed that treatment significantly reduced the increase in nasal eosinophilia (*P* = .02) and IL-4 mRNA-positive cells (*P* = .008), which was paralleled by an increase in number of IFN-gamma mRNA-positive cells (*P* = .002) as compared with PL-treated subjects. A positive trend in nasal symptom score improvement was observed by the second RW season in the vaccine-treated group.

Based on the findings from these clinical studies, Dynavax explored both a higher immunization dose (30 µg) and a booster regimen (30 µg × 2 before the second RW season). The high-dose phase 1 safety study by Vaishnav and Creticos provided the safety data needed for the subsequent performance of the first large-scale multi-center clinical trial. Findings from this study also demonstrated a significant decrease in the late-phase skin test reaction in the AIC-treated group versus PL (*P* = .008), and a significant increase in both anti-RW and anti-Amb a 1 IgG antibody compared with baseline and PL (*P*<.05), with no significant increase in IgE allergic antibody levels, findings reaffirming the premise that AIC's mechanism of action involves redirection of the untoward Th2 inflammatory response.[51]

The subsequent phase 2/3 multicenter clinical trial of the TLR-9 vaccine (TOLAMBA) (n = 462 RW-allergic patients), conducted from 2004 to 2006 and encompassing 2 RW seasons, was reported at the 2006 American Academy of Allergy, Asthma, and Immunology (AAAAI) annual meeting by Busse. Active-treated patients reported improvement in the defined efficacy end point total nasal symptom scores (TNSS) reported as change from baseline compared with PL during the peak RW season (treatment effect: year 1: 21.0% [*P* = .04]; year 2: 28.5% [*P* = .02]). However, subjects in the booster arm of the study did not achieve significant improvement in their TNSS (treatment effect: 13.5%; *P* = .28). After discussion with regulatory authorities, Dynavax commenced to undertake a second DBPC multicenter phase 2/3 clinical trial.[52]

In 2007, Dynavax announced that their second large-scale 2-year multicenter trial with the TLR-9 vaccine (n = 716 patients) was being halted after the first year based on their preliminary analyses of the 1-year data, which unfortunately showed that the TNSS in the overall study population provided an insufficient level of symptoms that could be ascribed to ragweed in the enrolled patients, thus making it impossible to demonstrate a meaningful therapeutic effect between the active arms and the PL-treated group, if the study were to continue.[53]

In 2008, the company reported the findings from their Canadian environmental exposure chamber (EEC) study (n = 253 patients) in which, although a measureable clinical effect on TNSS (in the chamber) was observed, the primary end point did not achieve statistical significance (treatment effect [intention to treat]: 41% vs PL; $P = .09$).[54]

Based on the company's concerns about the subjective nature of assessing efficacy by symptom scores, Dynavax decided to discontinue their clinical development program for the RW allergy vaccine program. However, the company continues to pursue its TLR-9 agonist program in hepatitis and cancer, its collaborative TLR agonist program in asthma and COPD with AstraZeneca, and its collaborative ventures with GlaxoSmithKline in autoimmune diseases.

Monophosphoryl lipid A adjuvant

Another novel toll-like receptor vaccine under development for North America is Allergy Therapeutics' TLR-4 adjuvant (Pollenex Quattro). This compound is a novel therapeutic extract wherein the native allergen (eg, grass; RW) is modified in 3 ways to achieve a safe and effective immune-modifying vaccine: it capitalizes on adsorbing a glutaraldehyde-modified allergoid (chemical modification that reduces the allergen's inherent IgE reactivity but preserves its immunogenicity) onto an L-tyrosine absorbent (to enhance slow-release kinetics), combined with the immunostimulatory adjuvant (monophosphoryl lipid A [MPL]). MPL is derived from detoxified lipopolysaccharide (originating from gram negative bacterium *Salmonella minnesota*), a Th1–inducing adjuvant. The clinical trials have demonstrated clinical efficacy with an *ultrashort* 4-injection preseason regimen.[55–59]

Their major DBPC randomized multicenter grass study conducted in 84 centers in North America, the United Kingdom, and Austria (1028 patients; aged 18–59 years) compared grass modified allergen tyrosine adsorbate–MPL (MATA-MPL) (n = 514) with placebo (n = 514). The vaccine-treated patients reported significant improvement (reduction) in their symptom and medication usage scores as compared with the PL-treated group on analysis of their electronic diary-recorded data over the 4 peak weeks of the 2007 grass pollen season (difference between MATA-MPL versus PL in mean combined symptom medication score: 13.6%; $P = .0038$). Subgroup analysis provided evidence for a greater benefit in patients with more severe symptoms (16.6%; $P = .0023$), sites with higher allergen burden (31%; $P<.0001$), and European subjects (27.4%; $P = .0341$). Serum grass-specific IgG increased 6.5-fold from baseline in the MATA-MPL-treated patients and was significantly elevated versus PL ($P<.001$). Overall, the treatment was well tolerated (Treatment-Related Adverse Events leading to dropout: 2.5% vs 0.4% PL); 92% of subjects completed the study. The most commonly reported adverse events (AEs) were injection site reactions, and there was the occurrence of one severe systemic reaction (generalized erythema in an MATA-MPL subject). However, after treatment, one study subject was reported to have developed transverse myelitis (>4 weeks after the final MATA-MPL injection) (see *clinical hold* notation). Of note, the 95.7% compliance attests to the patients' willingness to adhere to a short (3–4 weeks) 4-injection regimen.[58]

A parallel randomized DBPC multicenter RW clinical study was also initiated in North America in 2007; however, because of a subsequent clinical hold (now lifted), this trial only had 381 of the planned 993 subjects receive all 4 study injections. Even so, a clinical effect was observed in the primary end point for the RW MATA-MPL–treated group versus PL (12%; $P<.05$).[59]

More recently, in 2013, Allergy Therapeutics published their Canadian EEC study with their MPL adjuvant. This allergen preparation contains a glutaraldehyde-modified RW allergoid absorbed onto tyrosine combined with the aforementioned immune-stimulatory adjuvant (MPL) derived from gram-negative bacterium (*Salmonella minnesota*).

RW allergic subjects (n = 228 adults) were randomized in a double-blind placebo-controlled fashion to either active therapy (MATA-MPL, administered in 4 weekly injections) or placebo. Controlled RW pollen exposure (3500 ±500 pollen grains per cubic meter) in the EEC was performed at baseline (before treatment) and again at 3 weeks after the completion of treatment.

Study subjects that received the MPL-adjuvant vaccine showed a relative mean improvement in their total symptom scores (TSS) (48%; $P<.05$). The 4-injection regimen was well tolerated, and no serious AEs (SAEs) occurred in the study; nonetheless, 94.7% of the subjects in the MPL-adjuvant group and 67.7% in the placebo group reported AEs. The difference between the active and placebo groups was significant but mainly due to injection-site reactions of swelling (77% vs 16%), pruritus (80% vs 5%), pain (60% vs 33%), and warmth (27% vs 2%).[60]

The company markets in Europe a dust mite (DM) allergoid product in which purified allergens from *Dermatophagoides pteronyssinus* are modified through treatment with glutaraldehyde and combined with the L-tyrosine absorbent for the treatment of perennial mite allergy. In a clinical trial comparing the safety and efficacy of conventional (administered over 3 weeks) versus clustered dosing of the DM allergoid in 30 adult patients with persistent perennial AR, no AEs were recorded. Improvements in nasal challenge symptom scores and nasal peak inspiratory flow and an increase in IgG4-specific antibody were observed. In a 1-year follow-up study reported at the 2015 European Academy of Allergy and Clinical Immunology (EAACI)–Barcelona meeting, investigators reported a 50% reduction (improvement) in symptom scores on the nasal challenge, a sustained increase in IgG4, and a treatment-induced IL-10, a recognized marker of clinical tolerance.[61,62] Based on these findings, the company is also focused on development of an ultrashort course DM allergoid incorporating the MPL adjuvant.

Nanoparticle-based immunomodulation with viral-like particles

Cytos Biotechnology Ltd has focused on a nanoparticle-based immunomodulator. Their construct uses viral-like particles (VLPs) to deliver synthetic cytosine deoxynucleotide phosphorylated to guanine deoxynucleotide (CpG) oligonucleotide (G10) contained in a bacteriophage Qb capsid VLP admixed to allergen (eg, house dust mite [HDM]) or administered independent of allergen (TLR-9 agonist alone).[63]

In an initial safety and dose-ranging study, Kundig and colleagues[64] studied a VLP construct in which allergen (a synthetic 16 amino acid sequence of *Der p 1*) was incorporated into a VLP derived from bacteriophage, Qbeta (QB) (*QB-Der p 1*). This study assessed 24 healthy volunteers who were randomly assigned to varying dosing regimens (10 vs 50 mcg) and routes of immunization (intramuscular [IM] vs subcutaneous [SQ]). The *QB-Der p 1* vaccine was well tolerated in this single-injection study design, and no SAEs or systemic reactions were observed. The 50-mcg single dose, regardless of route of administration, was more efficient at generating an IgG antibody titer (1:2000); this robust B-cell response in humans is consistent with the observations made by the group in mice. The study demonstrated that a VLP could be used as a carrier to efficiently deliver allergen to antigen-presenting cells (APCs), inducing high titers of antibody without requiring the use of an adjuvant.[64]

This study was followed by an open-label study by Senti and colleagues[65] in which 20 HDM-allergic adult volunteers were immunized with *QB-Der p 1* to which the CpG oligonucleotide (*G10*) was admixed. The treatment regimen used a dose-escalating cluster schedule that led to a *fixed* 6 SQ injection regimen administered at 1- to 2-week intervals. The QbG10 adjuvant was well tolerated, abrogated the response to allergen challenge in the CPT, significantly attenuated both rhinoconjunctivitis and asthma symptoms, and demonstrated expected shifts in IgG antibody and skin test reactivity.[65]

In 2011, Klimek and colleagues[66] reported the findings from a phase 2b clinical trial of the TLR-9 agonist construct in which 299 patients with perennial HDM allergy were randomized in a double-blind placebo-controlled fashion to 2 different dosing regimens of the QbG10 adjuvant (6 weekly SQ injections of either 0.5 or 1.0 mg CYT003-QbG10) or placebo.

The clinical study findings demonstrated that the higher-dose vaccine regimen improved rhinoconjunctivitis symptom medication scores (0.31 vs 0.52; $P = .04$ vs placebo), positively shifted conjunctival provocation (10-fold increase in allergen tolerance), and was generally well tolerated. However, although no drug-related SAEs were reported, 16 patients discontinued the study (8 because of AEs, of which 6 were defined as treatment-related AEs).[66]

Based on subsequent data that demonstrated that QbG10 acted through an allergen-independent mechanism of action and that combination with an allergen did not result in any benefit over allergen alone, Cytos halted work in AR and instead focused on pursuing persistent allergic asthma requiring long-term treatment with inhaled corticosteroids (ICS).

In 2013, Cytos reported the midstage results with their CYT003-QbG10 compound in a small phase 2a asthma study (n = 63). They reported that treatment resulted in maintained asthma control and pulmonary function in patients with Global Initiative for Asthma (GINA)-defined persistent asthma even with the reduction in ICS in the stepdown phase of the study.[67]

However, in April 2014, the company reported that their larger phase 2b asthma study (n = 360 patients with moderate to severe persistent allergic asthma) did not meet its primary end point. Specifically, the study was not able to show *clinically relevant improvement* in asthmatic patients treated with CYT003-QbG10 versus PL for the primary end point of the study (improvement in the Asthma Control Questionnaire score at week 12 of therapy). Of note, a confounding observation was that a clinical improvement was observed in PL and all dose levels of the investigational drug. Furthermore, additional secondary end points, including pulmonary function, likewise failed to show a significant difference versus PL.[68]

Following this setback, Cytos announced that they had terminated the 1-year study and have halted further development of the program.

Lysosomal-associated membrane protein

Immunomic (ITI) has focused on developing a novel vaccine that acts through the innate immune system to achieve immune modulation. The concept takes advantage of lysosomal processing of antigens with major histocompatibility complex (MHC) class II presentation thereby promoting an efficient means of upregulating the innate immune system through a glycoprotein found on the lysosomal membrane (lysosomal-associated membrane protein [LAMP]).

Animal studies provide evidence that in the presence of modified allergen (eg, bacterial DNA encoded into the lysosome), natural killer cells are primed to secrete IFN-gamma, which acts on DCs to secrete IL-12 and IFN-gamma through a T-box transcription factor (T-bet)–mediated process that favorably orients the immune response to Th1 differentiation with attenuation of the Th2 inflammatory profile.

Initial studies in Japanese red cedar (JRC)–allergic subjects have demonstrated that a 4 IM injection regimen with the LAMP construct (CrJ2 nucleotide sequence from JRC inserted into LAMP) was well tolerated and resulted in induction of allergen-specific IgG to JRC; suppression and subsequent elimination of skin test reactivity to JRC, mountain cedar, and Cry 12; and conversion of skin test–positive subjects to nonreactors (skin test negative).[69–71]

Further phase 2 studies are underway.

Synthetic Peptides

T-cell–tolerizing peptides

As noted, initial studies carried out by Gefter and colleagues in the mid-1990s provided evidence that synthetic T-cell-tolerizing peptides could be used to suppress IgE-mediated allergic diseases, such as AR and asthma, through induction of immune tolerance. Their laboratory developed both cat (two 27 amino acid peptides derived from Fel d 1) and RW (short amino acid sequences derived from Amb a 1) T-cell–tolerizing peptides.[20]

Subsequent collaborative studies with Norman and colleagues at Johns Hopkins and Mass General used a cat-room challenge model to demonstrate that varying doses of SQ-injected cat peptides could improve clinical symptoms on natural cat-room exposures.[21,22] Creticos and colleagues undertook 2 large multicenter trials with varying doses and dosing regimens with the RW peptide vaccine, which provided evidence for modest clinical improvement but reduced the need for rescue medication to relieve breakthrough nasal symptoms in the RW season.[23,24]

However, these first-generation peptides did not achieve the expected degree of clinical benefit and, perhaps because the peptides were too large or given in high SQ doses, were observed to induce delayed-onset AEs, such as chest tightness. This developmental program was terminated in the late 1990s.

Synthetic peptide immunoregulatory epitopes

A new class of synthetic peptides, termed synthetic peptide immunoregulatory epitopes (SPIREs) emanated from the laboratories of Barry Kay and Mark Larché at Imperial College in London.

These synthetic T-cell–tolerizing peptides were designed as smaller peptide units (eg, cat: 7 peptides, 13–17 amino acids in length), are assembled from different T-cell epitopes, are administered in much smaller quantities than the Gefter's laboratory's molecules (75 µg vs 750 µg), and are administered intradermally, thereby more efficiently interacting with resident antigen-presenting cells. Following acquisition of the technology from Imperial College, Circassia Ltd has further refined the formulation of these peptides to prevent dimer formation and, hence, preserve bioactivity of the peptides.

These novel immunoregulatory peptides are designed to induce immunologic tolerance by binding to MHC class II molecules on antigen-presenting cells, thereby inducing the upregulation of regulatory T cells. The smaller size of these synthetic peptides is an inherent advantage, as the peptides should be of insufficient length to trigger cross-linking of IgE on mast cells and basophils, thus significantly reducing the risk of IgE-mediated allergic reactions and anaphylaxis.[72–80]

CAT–SYNTHETIC PEPTIDE IMMUNOREGULATORY EPITOPES

The lead compound for Circassia is their Cat-SPIRE construct. It consists of 7 separate small peptides (13–17 AA in length) derived from Fel d 1, the major cat allergenic moiety. After reconstitution, it is administered as a series of 4 intradermal (ID) injections into the dermis.

The selection of peptides in Cat-SPIRE was defined based on MHC class II binding studies in conjunction with T-cell proliferation and histamine release assays performed on ex vivo blood samples from cat allergic volunteers. The T-cell proliferative responses to an *internal standard* allergen extract of cat dander and Cat-SPIRE were closely correlated and provided confirmatory evidence that most of the T-cell reactivity to cat dander could be ascribed to the 7 synthetic peptide epitopes selected for Cat-SPIRE. As further evidence for an optimal peptide mix, the peptides induced in vitro IL-10 release from peripheral blood mononuclear cells in greater than 90% of cat-allergic subjects.

The peptide construct's IgE-binding activity was evaluated through performance of basophil histamine release assays on whole blood from cat-allergic individuals. These assays affirmed that Cat-SPIRE had significantly less capability than whole allergen to cross-link IgE and induce histamine release.[72–80]

The antiinflammatory properties ascribed to the cat peptides are most well defined in a study of transgenic mice by Campbell and colleagues[76] in which treatment with a single peptide in Cat-SPIRE resulted in reductions in bronchoalveolar lavage total cells and eosinophils, reductions in pulmonary and systemic TH2 inflammatory cytokines, reduced recruitment of TH2 inflammatory cells to the lungs, and reduced proliferative responses to cat Fel d 1.

Furthermore, administration of an anti–IL-10 monoclonal antibody (immediately after treatment with the peptide) blocked these effects, thereby emphasizing the potential critical regulatory interaction between the T-cell–tolerizing peptide and IL-10, a critical cytokine in the underlying mechanism of action ascribed to SPIREs for reestablishment of immune tolerance.[76]

Cat–Synthetic Peptide Immunoregulatory Epitopes Clinical Studies

Phase 1/2a safety and efficacy trial

In 2011, Worm and colleagues[78] published their initial safety and efficacy findings on the cat Fel d 1 peptide. Eighty-eight volunteers were randomized to (single-dose) escalating ID injections or to SQ injections of the peptide. The primary end point for the study was safety and tolerability. The Cat-SPIRE construct was well tolerated in doses up to 12 nmol (ID) and 20 nmol (SQ) (the ID dose was equivalent to 150 mcg of Fel d 1). No SAEs were observed, and no subject withdrew from the study because of an AE. The study also assessed the effect of the drug on the late-phase skin test response, a recognized surrogate clinical end point for efficacy of immunotherapy; although not statistically significant, the 3-nmol ID peptide dose resulted in a 40% reduction in the late phase skin response (vs 10% for placebo). This initial study demonstrated that the cat-peptide could be administered at an effective dose that might obviate the buildup phase required for Subcutaneous immunotherapy.

Phase 2b environmental chamber study

The phase 2 dose-ranging studies with Cat-SPIRE were performed using an EEC methodology, as this model provides a controlled setting in which to evaluate AIT. As such, it avoids many of the pitfalls that can plague natural field trials (eg, weather change, outdoor pollution, exposure to confounding allergens). Furthermore, in a chamber setting, it is possible to expose patients to predefined allergen levels that are known to cause symptoms of sufficient severity to allow assessment of *drug effect*.

In the study design, subjects had a baseline EEC challenge that consisted of 4 consecutive days on which patients were exposed for 3 hours each day in the chamber. The subjects returned at 18 to 22 weeks after the start of treatment and underwent a repeat 4-day chamber challenge. The primary end point for the study was the Total Rhinitis Symptom Score (TRSS) (defined as the difference in TRSS at each time point on each day between baseline and posttreatment challenge).

One hundred twenty-one (121) subjects who met a qualifying *threshold* symptom score were randomized to one of 4 treatment arms or placebo: (1) 3 nmol × 4 ID injections, 2 weeks apart; (2) 6 nmol × 4 ID injections, 2 weeks apart; (3) 3 nmol × 4 ID injections, 4 weeks apart; (4) 3 nmol × 8 ID injections, 2 weeks apart; (5) placebo × 8 ID injections.

Dosing over 12 to 14 weeks, as opposed to 6 weeks, demonstrated a greater shift in the TRSS. Subgroup analysis showed that those patients who received 8 ID injections of 3 nmol of peptide 2 weeks apart had the greatest reduction in TRSS (reduction of symptoms versus baseline: −4.8 points versus PL: 3.1 points [P<.05]). Although not significant, the 6-nmol dose showed a magnitude of improvement that was superior to the 3-nmol dose. An interesting corollary was that improvement in clinical scores was greater on later challenge days, whereas scores in the placebo group remained largely unchanged; this would be consistent with the findings from the late phase skin response in the Worm study.[78]

No SAEs were observed with any of the 4 treatment regimens, and respiratory system treatment-emergent AEs (TEAEs) occurred at a low frequency in all groups, with no difference between active groups or placebo.[81,82]

This EEC study provided preliminary evidence that a sustained treatment effect could be achieved with Cat-SPIRE. The positive effect observed in the EEC at 18 to 22 weeks is consistent with the cat-room exposure study by Norman and colleagues,[21] which showed a stronger effect at approximately 26 weeks than at any earlier time point.

Phase 2b Cat–synthetic peptide immunoregulatory epitopes environmental exposure chamber trial with 1-year follow-up

The focus of the study by Patel and colleagues[83] was to further explore whether a persistent treatment effect could be achieved with Cat-SPIRE in patients with cat-induced AR.

This randomized DBPC trial used the same baseline challenge methodology as the earlier cited study and had patients undergo the cat-allergen challenge in the EEC at 18 to 22 weeks and at 50 to 54 weeks after the start of treatment. The primary end point was defined as the change in TRSS (posttreatment vs baseline EEC challenges) at 1 to 3 hours on days 2 to 4 in the chamber.

A total of 202 cat-allergic patients were randomize to (1) 4 ID doses of 6-nmol cat peptide, 4 weeks apart (n = 66); (2) 8 ID doses of 3-nmol cat peptide, 2 weeks apart (n = 67); or (3) placebo (n = 69).

At the 18- to 22-week chamber challenge, a distinct treatment effect was observed on all chamber exposure challenge days in the nonasthmatic (per protocol) population with the 6 nmol × 4 ID injections, 4-weeks-apart regimen of Cat-SPIRE versus placebo (median change: −5.77 versus −3.67; mean change: −5.56 versus −3.52; Least square means change: −5.52 versus −3.56; [P value (analysis of covariance) = .05]). The treatment was well tolerated.

In phase 2 of this clinical trial, patients were reconsented to continue in the study and undergo a repeat chamber exposure to cat at 1-year (50–54 weeks). Treatment with Cat-SPIRE was shown to provide a treatment effect that persisted at 1 year after the start of treatment compared with placebo (6 nmol × 4 ID injections, 4 weeks apart versus 3 nmol × 8 ID injections, 2 weeks apart [P = .0342]; 6 nmol × 4 ID injections, 4 weeks apart versus placebo [P = .0104]). Furthermore, the effect on the TRSS at the 1-year challenge was heightened in comparison with the changes observed at the phase 1 (18–22 week) challenge (**Fig. 1**).

A distinct treatment effect was observed at all time points after 1 hour on days 2 to 4 in EEC at the 50- to 54-week challenge in the nonasthmatic population for the 6 nmol × 4

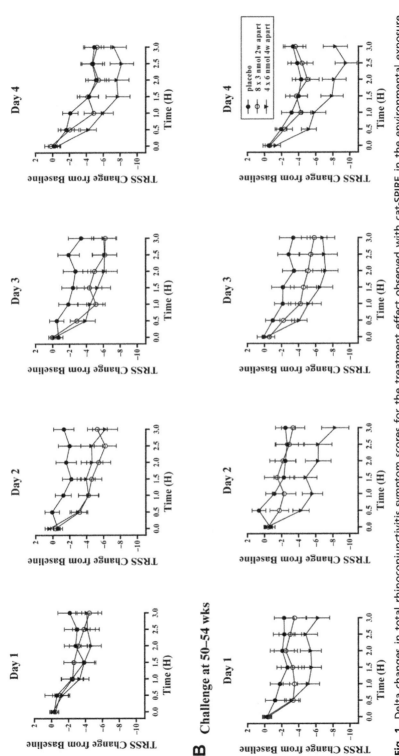

Fig. 1. Delta changes in total rhinoconjunctivitis symptom scores for the treatment effect observed with cat-SPIRE in the environmental exposure chamber. (*From* Creticos PS. Advances in synthetic peptide immuno-regulatory epitopes. World allergy Organ J 2014;7:30.)

dose regimen versus placebo. Furthermore, the clinical effects were similar when assessing all patients (including patients with asthma) with the 6 nmol $\times$ 4 dose regimen versus placebo.

An important corollary from this work is that the mean level of airborne Fel d 1 allergen content in the EEC (48 ng/m^3) is within the range reported in homes with cats (10–200 ng/m^3); hence, the EEC unit provides a real-world assessment of the disease. Furthermore, the improvement in TRSS with Cat-SPIRE in the EEC (~4 units change) compares favorably with allergen chamber studies of sublingual immunotherapy cat allergy drops (1.6 units change) and a chamber study of the anti-histamine fexofenadine, 180 mg (1.3 units change).[79]

Another important outcome from this study was the finding that no significant changes in cat-specific IgE levels were observed after the 1-year follow-up visit for any of the treatment regimens when compared with the baseline EEC visit. This finding is reassuring based on the premise that the peptides should be of insufficient size to cross-link IgE on mast cells and basophils.

In these trials, Cat-SPIRE was reasonably well tolerated. Of note, there were no asthma-related SAEs in the asthmatic subset of patients. Most of the TEAEs were mild in severity, and no TEAEs were rated as severe on patient diaries. Six subjects dropped out of the study because of a TEAE; except for one patient who experienced a hypersensitivity reaction to the drug, none of the other patient withdrawals were as-sesses as study drug related.

With respect to respiratory TEAEs, there were no reductions in forced expiratory volume in the first second of expiration greater than 30% (the prospectively defined cutoff in the study). Three study patients who received (6 nmol) peptide experienced an episode of dyspnea, bronchospasm, or asthma, whereas 14 subjects who received 3 nmol and 11 subjects who received placebo reported similar symptoms.[83]

These data from the 1-year follow-up study demonstrate a persistence of effect with the initial 4-injection peptide treatment regimen. The findings from this study extended the observations made in the earlier EEC clinical trial and provide evidence that a long-lasting effect on symptoms can be achieved through immunization with Cat-SPIRE in cat-allergic individuals.

Phase 2b Cat–synthetic peptide immunoregulatory epitopes clinical trial: 2-year environmental exposure chamber follow-up

Of the 86 patients who completed all visits at the 1-year follow-up trial with Cat-SPIRE, 51 agreed to reconsent, remain blinded, and enroll in the 2-year follow-up study. No further treatment was administered to study patients.

Study patients underwent repeat chamber challenge at the 2-year time point (102–106 weeks) with the same protocol challenge methodology (4 consecutive days of 3-hour allergen exposures in the EEC).

A sustained improvement in mean TRSS (from baseline) was observed for the pa-tient group who received 6 nmol (−5.87) versus the 3-nmol group (−3.05) versus the placebo group (−2.02) at the 2-year (102–106 weeks) posttreatment challenge. Although this positive trend did not reach significance for the primary end point ($P = .13$), a statistically significant difference was observed for the prespecified sec-ondary end point that assessed effect at the time point when the cumulative allergen challenge was greatest (day 4, third hour) ($P = .02$).[84]

The third-year posttreatment data presented at the EAACI 2015 meeting provided evidence for persistence of the treatment effect in the subgroup of patients with higher baseline symptoms and in which the 6-nmol dose had been administered.[85]

The encouraging findings from these EEC studies provided the basis for undertaking the first large-scale clinical trial with Cat-SPIRE in patients who live with cats in their home environment. This global study is currently ongoing, and clinical trial results should be available within 1 to 2 years.

Other Peptide Constructs

Circassia also has ongoing clinical trials with peptide constructs of grass, RW, and house DM in various stages of clinical development. The initial trials have again focused on the environmental chamber model to ascertain efficacy and safety in a controlled setting.[80,86–88]

Summary

The work by Durham and colleagues[89] with SCIT in which a 3-year course of immuno-therapy with a modified standardized grass extract can induce sustained benefit, serves as the benchmark for new immunotherapy constructs. The potential for synthetic peptide immune-regulatory epitopes to achieve long-lasting clinical benefit, safely and with a concise treatment regimen, is certainly a desired goal in AIT.

OVERLAPPING PEPTIDES

Anergis uses its technology of contiguous overlapping peptides (COP) for the development of allergy vaccines. Products based on COP reproduce the complete amino acid sequence of the allergen in separate synthetic long peptides, designed to provide the complete allergen sequence covering all T-cell epitopes, but to not cross-react with IgE, and thereby avoid the early phase response. The objective is ultrafast allergy desensitization after only 2 months of treatment.[90,91]

In 2014, Spertini reported data from a phase 2b study for AllerT, a birch pollen allergy vaccine candidate. In this placebo-controlled, double-blind, randomized multi-center trial, a total of 239 subjects were divided into 3 groups (placebo, AllerT 50 µg, and AllerT 100 µg, respectively). From November 2012 to March 2013, the subjects received 5 injections over a period of 2 months as a preseasonal treatment. During the subsequent 2013 birch pollen season, compared with the placebo group, the combined Rhinoconjunctivitis Symptom and Medication Score (RSMS, primary end point) was reduced by 30% ($P = .024$, statistically significant) with AllerT 50 µg and by 19% ($P = .190$; NS) with AllerT 100 µg. Both AllerT doses were associated with similar statistically significant improvements in the total score of the Rhinoconjunctivitis Quality of Life Questionnaire (Mini-RQLQ) and in the rhinoconjunctivitis symptom score throughout the birch pollen season.[92]

Previous data showed that both AllerT doses induced highly significant increases in anti-Bet v 1 IgG4 antibody ($\sim$20-fold; $P<.0001$) versus PL in season 1. In the 2014 trial, the sustained efficacy of AllerT was assessed in the same group of birch-allergic study patients during a second follow-up season without additional treatment. Study results showed persistence of the anti-Bet v 1 IgG4 antibody biomarker, which was accompanied by sustained improvement in clinical parameters of efficacy (RSMS; Mini-RQLQ; nighttime nasal symptom score). These immunologic data provide the first observation that antibody responses to a peptide epitope could be distinguished from natural allergen. As a corollary, no significant difference was observed in Bet v 1–specific IgE levels between active-treated and PL patients. AllerT was safe and well tolerated throughout the 2-month preseasonal treatment.[93,94]

Intralymphatic Immunotherapy

Another intriguing approach to immunization of allergic patients is that of intralymphatic injection (ILIT) of the allergen, which was being developed by Imvision Therapeutics. The premise was based on animal and human investigations which have demonstrated that RNA, DNA, oligopeptides, proteins, and adjuvants can be delivered directly to the regional lymph nodes where they are capable of strongly enhancing immune responses.[11,95–98]

With respect to allergic conditions, ILIT has been investigated in studies of seasonal allergic conditions (birch and grass) and cat allergy. Senti and colleagues[95] performed an open-label, single-center study of ILIT versus SCIT in 165 patients with grass pollen-induced rhinoconjunctivitis in which subjects were randomized to SCIT (54 injections over 3 years; cumulative standardized quality units (SQ-U) dose: 4,031,540 units) or 3 ILITs (at 4-week intervals; cumulative dose: 3000 SQ-U). ILIT resulted in attenuate of hay fever symptoms, inhibition of skin test reactivity to grass pollen, a decrease in serum-specific IgE, and a positive shift in nasal responsivity on nasal provocation. ILIT was well tolerated and resulted in fewer AEs as contrasted with SCIT. Most relevant, the nasal provocation procedures, performed at 4 months, 12 months, and 3 years, demonstrated attenuation to grass challenge within 4 months.[95]

The cat study reported by Senti and colleagues[97] evaluated 20 cat-allergic subjects who were randomized to either placebo or active therapy with a modified recombinant allergen rFel d 1 (recombinant of major cat allergen) fused to a translocator peptide trans-activating transcription factor (TAT) and to part of the human invariant chain (Ii), to generate a modular antigen transporter (MAT) vaccine (MAT-Fel d 1). The product was administered via injection using a conventional needle and syringe directly into lymph nodes in the groin.[97]

This initial study demonstrated that the active vaccine was well tolerated, with no AEs related to the 3-injection procedure other than reports of swelling and itching in the lymph node in the groin used for injection. Furthermore, the MAT-Fel d 1 vaccine increased cat-specific IgG4 6-fold ($P = .003$); the IgG4 response positively correlated with IL-10 production ($P = .026$); and the threshold for nasal provocation to cat was significantly shifted (74-fold vs <3-fold; $P<.001$).[97]

Hylander and colleagues performed a hybrid open-label (followed by DBPC phase) study in birch-allergic patients. Seven birch-allergic patients received birch SCIT (Alutard; ALK) over 3 years (14-week buildup phase to achieve 100,000 SQ-U administered every 6–8 weeks during the 3-year maintenance phase of the study) and served as open-label controls. Twenty-one patients (6 on open-label ILIT; 15 in a cohort randomized to receive ILIT [n = 7] or PL [n = 8]) received 3 ultrasound-guided IL injections of either birch or grass ILIT (1000 SQ-U) or PL. Patients on ILIT were shown to have an improvement on nasal provocation, which was associated with a decrease in inflammatory cells in nasal lavage fluids. Albeit a small number of patients were undergoing treatment, ILIT was well tolerated; patients reported improvement in their seasonal allergic symptoms (scored on a 10-point VAS: 0 [unchanged] to 10 [total symptom relief]) (SCIT: 6.1 [$P = .03$]; ILIT: 5.5 [$P = .05$] versus baseline, respectively).

As opposed to SCIT, ILIT did not result in an increase in IgG4. However, peripheral T-cell activation was evaluated with flow cytometry that showed upregulated expression of CD69 ($P = .02$) and CD98 ($P = .04$) on CD4+ lymphocytes with ILIT but not with PL. However, this cellular activation of peripheral CD4+ T cells was not accompanied by IL-10 secretion.[98]

At the 2015 AAAAI annual meeting, Patterson and colleagues[99] presented the first trial with the 3-injection (50/100/250 protein nitrogen units; ≥4 weeks apart) ultrasound-guided ILIT with a commercially available US grass extract (*Phleum pratense*) in 15 young adults with grass pollen–induced allergic rhinoconjunctivitis with or without intermittent asthma. The ILIT was well tolerated (100% completed all injections), with the total safety score (TSS) showing no difference between active treatment and PL ($P = .8$).[99]

The ability to deliver allergen directly to antigen-processing cells in the lymphoid tissue residing in a regional lymph node (eg, inguinal node) provides an attractive approach: it allows immunization to be accomplished with a smaller dose; it achieves long-lasting benefit with a minimal number of injections; and it seems to be well tolerated.

Epicutaneous Immunotherapy

Another approach that attempts to capitalize on ease of access to antigen-presenting cells is that of epicutaneous delivery of allergen. Studies in the early allergy literature attempted to introduce allergen through ID inoculation or scarification techniques (cutaneous quadrille ruling) in an attempt to circumvent the problem of anaphylaxis associated with subcutaneous injections of allergens. Interestingly, some of this early work demonstrated a positive benefit; however, patient discomfort and imprecise allergen delivery led to discontinued interest in this approach. However, with the development of modern transcutaneous delivery systems, this method of immunization has again generated increased interest as a means of possibly effectively administering allergens.

Senti and colleagues[100–103] have studied allergen patches prepared with grass allergen extract derived from respective pollen species (*Phleum*, *Dactylis*, *Lolium*, *Poa*, *Festuca*, *Holcus*).

Recombinant Vaccines

Natural recombinant vaccines (wild type) have been studied in DBPC clinical trials in grass- and birch-allergic patients.[104,105] A study by Jutel and colleagues[106] with a recombinant timothy grass pollen extract demonstrated significant improvement in the combined symptom medication score and quality of life; however, allergen-specific IgE was not suppressed. Pauli and colleagues[106,107] compared recombinant Bet v 1a, purified Bet v 1, and standard birch pollen extract and showed similar improvements with all 3 treatments in symptom medication diary scores; IgG1/IgG2/IgG4 antibody increases were observed in all 3 treatment groups. Again, no significant shift was observed in the safety profile, and injection site swelling was more frequently observed in the group that received the recombinant birch vaccine.

Subsequent interest has focused on hypoallergenic recombinant allergens wherein conformational changes are inserted onto the native allergen's IgE epitopes to reduce the allergen's inherent allergenicity.

An environmental chamber study (n = 36) by Meyer and colleagues[108] with a novel hypoallergenic recombinant birch extract, administered as 10 weekly injections, demonstrated significant improvement in patient-reported EEC symptoms (pretreatment vs posttreatment score) and was accompanied by the expected increase in allergen-specific IgG1. The investigators, however, reported that grade II AEs were more frequently observed in patients receiving the 2 higher dosing regimens.[108]

Valenta and colleagues[104,105] have focused on studies with recombinant fragments and in a series of studies have shown that, as opposed to intact allergen, the fragments did not induce allergen-specific IgE, did increase protective IgG and IgA antibody, inhibited facilitated antigen binding, and attenuated nasal sensitivity on nasal allergen provocation. However, subsequent DBPC trials could not demonstrate significant improvement in clinical outcomes, including symptom diary scores and relief medication usage.

Valenta in association with Biomay have recently focused their research and development on a recombinant B-cell epitope vaccine (BM32). This vaccine is a peptide carrier fusion vaccine that contains linear peptides that are part of B-cell epitopes; these peptides are fused to an immunogenic carrier element and, using recombinant technology, are expressed as fusion proteins. A peptide carrier fusion vaccine is capable of inducing allergen-specific IgG that is directed against parts of the IgE epitope and blocks the binding of IgE.[105,109,110]

In a 2-year European phase 2b DBPC trial of the fusion vaccine (BM32), 181 patients were randomized to receive either of 2 doses of BM32 or the matching placebo. The treatment phase consisted of 3 subcutaneous injections administered over the 2 months before the 2013 grass pollen season, followed by a fall boost injection and 3 additional doses before the 2014 season. (The Data Monitoring Committee reviewed the safety data after the completion of the first year of treatment and recommended that all actively treated patients should receive the lower vaccine dose [20 μg of each of the 4 protein components]).[109,110]

Several of the study's secondary clinical outcomes provided statistically significant evidence for therapeutic efficacy with the vaccine, including a 25% difference between active drug and PL in the Rhinoconjunctivitis Symptom Score during the peak pollen season in the second treatment year ($P = .042$) and improvement on the VAS ($P = .014$) and the Rhinoconjunctivitis Quality of Life Questionnaire ($P<.005$). A measureable positive trend was observed for the primary end point (Combined Symptom and Medication Score) versus placebo (22% difference; $P = .085$).[109,110]

The positive clinical findings were paralleled by a sustained induction of allergen-specific IgG antibody, and the vaccine did not boost IgE antibody. The treatment was well tolerated; most side effects were mild to moderate and short-lived (resolving in a short period after drug administration).[109,110]

The company also has a strategic focus for the development of birch, RW, house DM, and cat peptide-carrier fusion proteins.

SUMMARY

There is a recognized need for newer therapeutic agents that improve the safety of AIT, provide an ease of delivery to patients that fosters compliance and allows access to a greater proportion of the allergic population that could benefit from this disease-modifying treatment, and achieve an acceptable therapeutic benefit for most patients committing to the course of treatment.

The recent advances in sublingual AIT are most encouraging, as this now offers patients a noninjectable form of treatment of inhalant allergies.[111]

Furthermore, the continued research and development of the novel therapeutic constructs discussed in this article holds the promise of accomplishing the aforementioned goals in the not-so-distant future.

REFERENCES

1. Arbes SJ Jr, Gergen PJ, Elliott L, et al. Prevalence of positive skin test responses to 10 common allergens in the US population: results from the third National Health and Nutrition Examination Survey. J Allergy Clin Immunol 2005;116: 377–83.

2. Akinbami LJ, Moorman JE, Liu X. Asthma prevalence, health use, and mortality: U.S., 2005-2009. National Health Statistics Report; no 32, 32. Washington, DC: National Center for Health statistics; 2011. p. 1–14.
3. Bousquet J, Khaltaev N, Cruz AA, et al. Allergic Rhinitis and Its Impact on Asthma (ARIA) 2008 update (in collaboration with the World Health Organization, GA(2)LEN and AllerGen). Allergy 2008;63(Suppl 86):8–160.
4. Wallace D, Dykewicz M, Bernstein D, et al. The diagnosis and management of rhinitis: an updated practice parameter. J Allergy Clin Immunol 2008;122:S1–84.
5. Broide DH. Immunomodulation of allergic disease. Annu Rev Med 2009;60: 279–91.
6. Valenta R, Ferreira F, Focke-Tejkl M, et al. From allergen genes to allergy vaccines. Annu Rev Immunol 2010;28:211–41.
7. Focke M, Swoboda I, Marth K, et al. Developments in allergen-specific immunotherapy: from allergen extracts to allergy vaccines bypassing allergen-specific immunoglobulin E and T cell reactivity. Clin Exp Allergy 2010;40:385–97.
8. Canonica GW, Bousquet J, Casale T, et al. Sublingual immunotherapy: World Allergy Organization position paper 2009. Allergy 2009;64(Suppl 91):1–59.
9. Akdis M, Akdis C. Therapeutic manipulation of immune tolerance in allergic disease. Nat Rev Drug Discov 2009;8:640–60.
10. Creticos PS. Sublingual and oral immunotherapy for allergic rhinitis. Waltham (MA): UpToDate; 2015.
11. Cox L, Compalati E, Kundig T, et al. New directions in immunotherapy. Curr Allergy Asthma Rep 2013;13:178–95.
12. Marsh DG, Belin L, Bruce CA, et al. Rapidly released allergens from short ragweed pollen. I. Kinetics of release of known allergen in relation to biological activity. J Allergy Clin Immunol 1981;67:206–16.
13. Norman P, Lichtenstein L, Marsh D. Studies on allergoids from naturally occurring allergens. IV. Efficacy and safety of long-term allergoid treatment of ragweed hay fever. J Allergy Clin Immunol 1981;59:314–9.
14. Wie SI, Wie CW, Lee WY, et al. Suppression of reaginic antibodies with modified allergens. III. Preparation of tolerogenic conjugates of common allergens with monomethoxypolyethylene glycols of different molecular weights by the mixed anhydride method. Int Arch Allergy Appl Immunol 1981;64:84–99.
15. Sehon AH, Wy Lee. Suppression of IgE antibodies with modified allergens. J Allergy Clin Immunol 1979;64(4):242–50.
16. Patterson R, Suszko IM, Pruzansky JJ, et al. Polymerization of mixtures of grass allergens. J Allergy Clin Immunol 1977;59:314–9.
17. Grammer LC, Zeiss CR, Suszko IM, et al. A double-blind placebo-controlled trial of polymerized whole ragweed for immunotherapy of ragweed allergy. J Allergy Clin Immunol 1982;69(6):494–9.
18. Grammer LC, Shaughnessy MA, Suszko IM, et al. A double-blind histamine placebo-controlled trial of polymerized whole grass for immunotherapy of grass allergy. J Allergy Clin Immunol 1983;72(5 Pt 1):448–53.
19. Briner TJ, Kuo MC, Keating KM, et al. Peripheral T-cell tolerance induced in naive and primed mice by subcutaneous injection of peptides from the major cat allergen Fel d I. Proc Natl Acad Sci U S A 1993;90:7608–12.
20. Wallner BP, Gefter ML. Immunotherapy with T-cell-reactive peptides derived from allergens. Allergy 1994;49:302–8.
21. Norman PS, Ohman JL Jr, Long AA, et al. Treatment of cat allergy with T cell epitope containing peptides. Am J Respir Crit Care Med 1996;154:1623–8.

22. Norman PS, Nicodemus CF, Creticos PS, et al. Clinical and immunologic effects of component peptides in Allervax® Cat. Int Arch Allergy Immunol 1997;113:1–3.

23. Creticos PS, Hebert J, Philip G, Allervax® Ragweed Study Group. Efficacy of Allervax® ragweed in the treatment of ragweed-induced allergy. J Allergy Clin Immunol 1997;99(No. 1, Part 2):S401(1631).

24. Creticos PS. Peptide downregulation of the immune response. Chapter 30. In: Marone G, Austen KF, Holgate ST, et al, editors. Asthma and allergic diseases. San Diego: Academic Press; 1998. p. 407–15.

25. Bird AP. DNA methylation and the frequency of CpG in animal DNA. Nucleic Acids Res 1980;8(7):81499–504.

26. Tokunaga T, Yamamoto H, Shimada S, et al. Antitumor activity of deoxyribonucleic acid fraction from Mycobacterium bovis BCG: I: isolation, physiochemical characterization, and antitumor activity. J Natl Cancer Inst 1981;72:955–62.

27. Yamamoto S, Yamamoto T, Shimada S, et al. DNA from bacteria, but not from vertebrates, induces interferons, activates natural killer cells and inhibits tumor growth. Microbiol Immunol 1992;36:983–97.

28. Yamamoto T, Yamamoto S, Kataoka T, et al. Synthetic oligonucleotides with certain palindromes stimulate interferon production of human peripheral blood lymphocytes in vitro. Jpn J Cancer Res 1994;85:775–9.

29. Pisetsky DS. Immune activation by bacterial DNA: a new genetic code. Immunity 1996;5:303–10.

30. Krieg AM, Yi AK, Matson S, et al. CpG motifs in bacterial DNA trigger direct B-cell activation. Nature 1995;374:546–9.

31. Wagner H. Toll meets bacterial CpG-DNA. Immunity 2001;14(5):499–502.

32. Bauer S, Kirschning CJ, Häcker H, et al. Human TLR9 confers responsiveness to bacterial DNA via species-specific CpG motif recognition. Proc Natl Acad Sci U S A 2001;98(16):9237–42.

33. Klinman DM, Yi AK, Beaucage SL, et al. CpG motifs present in bacterial DNA rapidly induce lymphocytes to secrete interleukin6-, interleukin 12, and interferon gamma. Proc Natl Acad Sci U S A 1996;93:2879–83, 124.

34. Klinman DM, Yamshchikov G, Ishigatsubo Y. Contributions of CpG motis to the immunogenicity of DNA vaccines. J Immunol 1980;158:3635–9.

35. Messina JP, Gilkeson GS, Pisetsky DS. Stimulation of in vitro murine lymphocyte proliferation by bacterial DNA. J Immunol 1991;147:1759–64.

36. Sato Y, Roman M, Tighe H, et al. Immunostimulatory DNA sequences necessary for effective intradermal gene immunization. Science 1996;273:352–4.

37. Cowdery JS, Chace JH, Yi AK, et al. Bacterial DNA induces NK cells to produce IFN-gamma in vivo and increases the toxicity of lipopolysaccharides. J Immunol 1996;156:4570–5.

38. Halpern MD, Kurlander RJ, Pisetsky DS. Bacterial DNA induces murine interferon-gamma production by stimulation of interleukin-12 and tumor necrosis factor-alpha. Cell Immunol 1996;167:72–77.8.

39. Raz E, Carson DA, Parker SE, et al. Intradermal gene immunization: the possible role of DNA uptake in the induction of cellular immunity to viruses. Proc Natl Acad Sci U S A 1994;91:9519–23.

40. Raz E, Tighe H, Sato Y, et al. Preferential induction of a T_H1 immune response and inhibition of specific IgE antibody formation by plasmid DNA immunization. Proc Natl Acad Sci U S A 1996;93:5141–5.

41. Tighe H, Takabayashi K, Schwartz D, et al. Conjugation of immunostimulatory DNA to the short ragweed allergen Amb a 1 enhances its immunogenicity and reduces its allergenicity. J Allergy Clin Immunol 2000;105:124–34.

42. Van Nest G, Eiden JJ, Tuck SF, et al. Conjugation of immunostimulatory DNA (ISS) to the major short ragweed allergen, Amb a 1, enhances immunogenicity and reduces allergenicity. J Allergy Clin Immunol 2000;105:S70.
43. Horner AA, Van Uden JH, Zubeldia JM, et al. DNA-based immunotherapeutics for the treatment of allergic disease. Immunol Rev 2001;179:102–18.
44. Broide D, Schwarze J, Tighe H, et al. Immunostimulatory DNA sequences inhibit IL-5, eosinophilic inflammation, and airway hyperresponsiveness in mice. J Immunol 1998;161(12):7054–62.
45. Tighe H, Takabayashi K, Schwartz D, et al. Conjugation of immunostimulatory DNA to the short ragweed allergen Amb a 1 enhances its immunogenicity and reduces its allergenicity. J Allergy Clin Immunol 2000;106(1 Pt 1):124–34.
46. Marshall JD, Abrahi S, Eiden JJ, et al. Immunostimulatory sequences (ISS) DNA linked to Amb a 1 allergen promotes Th1 cytokine expression while downregulating Th2 cytokine expression in PBMC's from ragweed-allergic humans. J Allergy Clin Immunol 2001;108:191–7.
47. Creticos PS, Eiden JJ, Balcer SL, et al. Immunostimulatory oligonucleotides conjugated to Amb a 1: safety, skin test reactivity, and basophil histamine release. J Allergy Clin Immunol 2000;105:S70.
48. Creticos PS, Balcer SL, Schroeder JT, et al. Initial immunotherapy trial to explore the safety, tolerability, and immunogenicity of subcutaneous injections of an Amb a 1 immunostimulatory oligonucleotide conjugate in ragweed-allergic adults. J Allergy Clin Immunol 2001;107:S216.
49. Creticos PS, Schroeder JT, Hamilton RG, et al. Immunotherapy with a ragweed-toll-like receptor 9 agonist vaccine for allergic rhinitis. N Engl J Med 2006;355:1445–55.
50. Tulic M, Fiset P, Christodoulopoulos P, et al. Amb a 1-immunostimulatory oligodeoxynucleotide conjugate immunotherapy decreases the nasal inflammatory response. J Allergy Clin Immunol 2004;113:235–41.
51. Vaishnav AR, Whaley SB, Hamilton R, et al. Evaluation of safety and clinical efficacy of higher dose immunotherapy with AIC (immunostimulatory DNA conjugated with Amba 1) in patients with ragweed-induced seasonal allergic rhinitis (SAR). J Allergy Clin Immunol 2005;115(No.2):S65–260.
52. Busse W, Gross G, Korenblat P, et al. Phase 2/3 study of the novel vaccine Amb a 1 immunostimulatory oligodeoxyribonucleotide conjugate AIC in ragweed allergic adults. J Allergy Clin Immunol 2006;117(No.2):S88–9.
53. Bernstein DI, Segall N, Nayak A, et al. Safety and efficacy of the novel vaccine TOLAMBA™ in ragweed allergic adults, a dose finding study. J Allergy Clin Immunol 2007;119(No 1):S78–9.
54. Dynavax press release. May 16, 2008: Tolamba TM chamber study misses primary endpoint.
55. Drachenberg KJ, Wheeler AW, Stuebner P, et al. A well-tolerated grass pollen specific allergy vaccine containing a novel adjuvant, monophosphoryl lipid A (MPL), reduces allergic symptoms after only four preseasonal injections. Allergy 2001;56:498–505.
56. Drachenberg KJ, Heinzkill M, Urban E, et al. Efficacy and tolerability of short-term specific immunotherapy with pollen allergoids adjuvanted by monophosphoryl lipid A (MPL) for children and adolescents. Allergol Immunopathol (Madr) 2003;31(5):270–7.
57. Mothes N, Heinzkill M, Drachenberg KJ, et al. Allergen-specific immunotherapy with a monophosphoryl lipid A-adjuvanted vaccine: reduced seasonally

boosted immunoglobulin E production and inhibition of basophil histamine release by therapy-induced blocking antibodies. Clin Exp Allergy 2003;33: 1198–208.

58. DuBuske L, Frew A, Horak F, et al. Ultrashort-specific immunotherapy successfully treats seasonal allergic rhinoconjunctivitis to grass pollen. Allergy Asthma Proc 2011;32:239–47.

59. Baldrick P, Richardson D, Woronjecki SR, et al. Pollinex Quattro® ragweed: safety evaluation of a new allergy vaccine adjuvanted with monophosphoryl lipid A (MPL®) for the treatment of ragweed pollen allergy. J Appl Toxicol 2007;27(4): 399–409.

60. Patel P, Holdich T, Weikersthal-Drachenberg K, et al. Efficacy of a short course of specific immunotherapy in patients with allergic rhinoconjunctivitis to ragweed pollen. J Allergy Clin Immunol 2014;133:121–9.

61. Roger A, Depreux M, Jurgens Y, et al. A novel and well tolerated mite allergoid subcutaneous immunotherapy: evidence of clinical and immunologic efficacy. Immun Inflamm Dis 2014;2(2):92–8.

62. Roger A, Depreux M, Jurgens Y, et al. An observational post authorisation 1 year follow-up study of the safety, tolerability, satisfaction and effectiveness of a modified mite-allergoid subcutaneous immunotherapy. Barcelona (Spain): EAACI Abstract; 2015.

63. Storni T, Ruedl C, Schwarz K, et al. Nonmethylated CpG motifs packaged into virus-like particles induce protective cytotoxic T cell responses in the absence of systemic side effects. J Immunol 2004;172(3):1777–85.

64. Kundig TM, Senti G, Schnetzler G, et al. Der p 1 peptide on virus-like particles is safe and highly immunogenic in healthy adults. J Allergy Clin Immunol 2006; 117:1470–6.

65. Senti G, Johansen P, Haug S, et al. Use of A-type CpG oligonucleotides as an adjuvant in allergen- specific immunotherapy in humans: a phase 1/2 clinical trial. Clin Exp Allergy 2009;39:62–70.

66. Klimek L, Willers J, Hammann-Haenni A, et al. Assessment of clinical efficacy of CYT003-QbG10 in patients with allergic rhinoconjunctivitis: a phase 2b study. Clin Exp Allergy 2011;41:1305–12.

67. Beeh K, Kanniess F, Wagner F, et al. The novel TLR-9 agonist QbG10 shows clinical efficacy in persistent asthma. J Allergy Clin Immunol 2013;131:866–74.

68. Casale T, Cole J, Beck E, et al. CYT003, a TLR9 agonist, in persistent asthma – a randomized placebo-controlled phase 2b study. Allergy 2015;22. http://dx.doi.org/10.1111/all.12663.

69. Arruda LB, Sim D, Priya R, et al. Dendritic cell-lysosomal associated membrane protein (DC-LAMP0- and LAMP-1-Gag chimeras have distinct cellular trafficking pathways and prime T- and B-cell responses to a diverse repertoire of epitopes. J Immunol 2006;177:2265–75.

70. Weiner L, Heiland T, Mackler B, et al. Phase 1 study of JRC-LAMP-Vax, a DNA immunotherapy vaccine to treat Japanese red cedar allergy. Ann Allergy Asthma Immunol 2013;111:A8–9.

71. Weiner L, Mackler B, Heery B, et al. A DNA vaccine immunotherapy for Japanese red cedar. World Allergy Organ J 2014;7(Suppl):23.

72. Oldfield W, Larche M, Kay AB. Effect of T-cell peptides derived from Fel d 1 on allergic reactions and cytokine production in patients sensitive to cats: a randomised controlled trial. Lancet 2002;360:47–53.

73. Smith T, Alexander C, Kay AB, et al. Cat allergen peptide immunotherapy reduces CD4 T cell responses to cat allergen but does not alter suppression by

CD4 CD25 T cells: a double-blind placebo-controlled study. Allergy 2004;59: 1097–101.

74. Verhoef A, Alexander C, Kay AB, et al. T cell epitope immunotherapy induces a CD4(+) T cell population with regulatory activity. PLoS Med 2005;2:e78.
75. Larche M. Immunotherapy with allergen peptides. Allergy Asthma and Cx Immunol 2007;3(2):53–9.
76. Campbell J, Buckland K, McMillan S, et al. Peptide immunotherapy in allergic asthma generates IL-10-dependent immunological tolerance associated with linked epitope suppression. J Exp Med 2009;206:1535–47.
77. Larche M, Moldavar D. Immunotherapy with Peptides. Allergy 2011;66:784–91.
78. Worm M, Lee HH, Kleine-Tebbe J, et al. Development and preliminary evaluation of a peptide immunotherapy vaccine for cat allergy. J Allergy Clin Immunol 2011;127:89–97.
79. Worm M, Patel D, Creticos PS. Cat peptide antigen desensitisation for treating Cat allergic rhinoconjunctivitis. Expert Opin Investig Drugs 2013;22(10):1347–57.
80. Creticos PS. Advances in synthetic peptide immune-regulatory epitopes. World Allergy Organ J 2014;7:30.
81. Larche M, Patel D, Patel P, et al. Safety and efficacy of Fel d 1-derived peptide immunotherapy in a DBPC environmental exposure chamber study [ECACI Abstract]. Allergy 2012;67(Suppl 96).
82. Hafner R, Patel P, Salapatek A, et al. Fel d 1 peptide antigen desensitization safety and efficacy in a DBPC EEC study [WAO Abstract]. World Allergy Organ J 2013;6(Supp):150.
83. Patel D, Couroux P, Hickey P, et al. Fel d 1-derived peptide antigen desensitization shows a persistent treatment effect 1 year after the start of dosing: a randomized, placebo-controlled study. J Allergy Clin Immunol 2013;131:103–9.
84. Hafner R, Couroux P, Armstrong K, et al. Two year persistent treatment effect achieved after 4 doses of cat-peptide antigen desensitization in an EEC model of cat allergy. J Allergy Clin Immunol 2013;131(2):AB147.
85. Couroux P, Patel D, Armstrong K, et al. Fel d 1-derived synthetic peptide immune-regulatory epitopes show a long-term treatment effect in cat allergic subjects. Clin Exp Allergy 2015;45:974–81.
86. Hafner R, Salapatek AM, Patel D, et al. Validation of peptide immunotherapy as a new approach in the treatment of allergic rhinoconjunctivitis: the clinical benefits of treatment with Amb a 1 derived T cell epitopes. J Allergy Clin Immunol 2012;129(2):AB368.
87. Hafner R, Salapatek AM, Larche M, et al. Comparison of the treatment effect of house dust mite synthetic peptide immune-regulatory epitopes in the environmental exposure chamber and field setting two years after a short course of treatment. EAACI-2015 abstract, in press.
88. Gliddon DR, Kim YW, Shannon CP, et al. Whole blood immune transcription profiling reveals systemic pathways associated with the mechanism of action of cat-synthetic peptide immune-regulatory epitopes. EAACI-2015 abstract, in press.
89. Durham SR, Walker SM, Varga EM, et al. Long-term clinical efficacy of grass-pollen immunotherapy. N Engl J Med 1999;341:468–75.
90. Pellaton C, Perrin Y, Boudousquie C, et al. Novel birch pollen specific immunotherapy formulation based on contiguous overlapping peptides. Clin Transl Allergy 2013;3:17.
91. Fallrath JM, Kettner A, Dufour N, et al. Allergen-specific T-cell tolerance induction with allergen-derived long synthetic peptides: results of a phase 1 trial. J Allergy Clin Immunol 2003;111(4):854–6.

92. Spertini F, de Blay F, Jacobsen L, et al. Ultra-fast hypoallergenic birch pollen allergy vaccine AllerT is efficient and safe: results of a phase 2b study. J Allergy Clin Immunol 2014;133(2 Suppl):AB290.
93. Spertini F, Jutel M, Jacobsen L, et al. Sustained efficacy of AllerT allergy vaccine after a second birch pollen season: a phase 2b. J Allergy Clin Immunol 2015; 135(2 Suppl):AB143.
94. Reymond C, Kettner A, Boand V, et al. Persistence of anti-Bet 1 v IgG4 prior and during a second pollen season after AllerT ultra-fast immunotherapy (phase 2b follow up). EAACI-2015 abstract, in press.
95. Senti G, Prinz Vavricka BM, Erdmann I, et al. Intralymphatic allergen administration renders specific immunotherapy faster and safer: a randomized controlled trial. Proc Natl Acad Sci U S A 2008;105:17908–12.
96. Senti G, Johansen P, Kundig TM. Intralymphatic immunotherapy. Curr Opin Allergy Clin Immunol 2009;9:537–43.
97. Senti G, Crameri R, Kuster D, et al. Intralymphatic immunotherapy for cat allergy induces tolerance after only 3 injections. J Allergy Clin Immunol 2012;129: 1290–6.
98. Hylander T, Latif L, Petersson U, et al. Intralymphatic allergen-specific immunotherapy: an effective and safe alternative treatment route for pollen-induced allergic rhinitis. J Allergy Clin Immunol 2013;131:412–20.
99. Patterson AM, Bonny AE, Shiels WE, et al. Safety of 3-injection immunotherapy protocol for treating grass pollen-induced rhinoconjunctivitis in adolescents/ young adults. J Allergy Clin Immunol 2015;135(2 Suppl):AB388.
100. Senti G, Graf N, Haug S, et al. Epicutaneous allergen administration as a novel method of allergen-specific immunotherapy. J Allergy Clin Immunol 2009;124: 997–1002.
101. Agostinis F, Forti S, Di Berardino F. Grass transcutaneous immunotherapy in children with seasonal allergic rhinitis. Allergy 2010;65:410.
102. Senti G, von Moos S, Kündig T. Epicutaneous allergen administration: is this the future of allergen specific immunotherapy? Allergy 2011;66(6):798–809.
103. Senti G, von Moos S, Tay F, et al. Epicutaneous allergen-specific immunotherapy ameliorates grass pollen-induced rhinoconjunctivitis: a double-blind, placebo-controlled dose escalation study. J Allergy Clin Immunol 2012;129:128.
104. Valenta R, Niederberger V. Recombinant allergens for immunotherapy. J Allergy Clin Immunol 2007;119:826–30.
105. Valenta R, Linhart B, Swoboda I, et al. Recombinant allergens for allergen-specific immunotherapy: 10 years anniversary of immunotherapy with recombinant allergens. Allergy 2011;66:775–83.
106. Jutel M, Jaeger L, Suck R, et al. Allergen-specific immunotherapy with recombinant grass pollen allergens. J Allergy Clin Immunol 2005;116:608–13.
107. Pauli G, Larsen TH, Rak S, et al. Efficacy of recombinant birch pollen vaccine for the treatment of birch-allergic rhinoconjunctivitis. J Allergy Clin Immunol 2008; 122:951–60.
108. Meyer W, Narkus A, Salapatek AM, et al. Double-blind, placebo-controlled, dose-ranging study of new recombinant hypoallergenic Bet v 1 in an environmental exposure chamber. Allergy 2013;68:724–31.
109. Biomay Press Release. (28 January 2015). Clinicaltrials.gov identifier NCT1538979.
110. Valenta R. Clinical efficacy of a recombinant B-cell epitope based grass pollen allergy vaccine - a phase 2b proof of concept study. EAACI-2015 Abstract, in press.
111. Nelson HS, Makatsori M, Calderon MA. SCIT and SLIT: comparative efficacy, current and potential indications-and warnings-US vs. Europe.

The Use of Adjuvants for Enhancing Allergen Immunotherapy Efficacy

 CrossMark

Julie Chesné, PhD, Carsten B. Schmidt-Weber, PhD*,
Julia Esser von-Bieren, PhD

KEYWORDS

- Allergen-specific immunotherapy • Immune tolerance • Adjuvants

KEY POINTS

- Allergen-specific immunotherapy currently represents the only curative treatment for allergy, but its broader application requires safer and more efficacious treatment protocols.
- Adjuvants can improve the efficacy of allergen-specific immunotherapy, and a variety of promising immunomodulatory adjuvants are currently being developed.
- Innovative strategies have been proposed to simplify immunization and to achieve long-term tolerance.

INTRODUCTION

Allergic diseases are characterized by the seasonally recurring production of T helper 2 (T_H2) cytokines (eg, Interleukin [IL]-4, IL-5, and IL-13), which drive the production of allergen-specific type-E immunoglobulin (IgE) by B cells and the recruitment and sensitization of effector cells such as eosinophils, basophils, and mast cells.[1] Long-time surviving specific memory T cells and B cells generate a pool of cells that quickly expand upon rechallenge thereby forming an immunologic memory that allows quick responses against pathogens but unfortunately also seasonal recurrence of allergic symptoms. A key factor in the early-phase symptoms is that allergen-specific IgE binds to the high affinity IgE receptor, FcεR1, on the surface of mast cells, basophils,

Disclosure Statement: The author is consulting companies involved in the generation of vaccines (PLS-Design, LETI Pharma) and its institution receives grant support (PLS-Design, Allergopharma). The author is holding shares from PLS Design and is co-authoring patents on the use of immunomodulators for specific immunotherapy.
Center of Allergy & Environment (ZAUM), Technical University of Munich and Helmholtz Center, Biedersteiner Street 29, Munich 80802, Germany
* Corresponding author.
E-mail address: csweber@tum.de

eosinophils, and dendritic cells (DCs) resulting in the rapid release of proinflammatory mediators such as histamine, prostaglandins, and leukotrienes, which elicit allergic symptoms such as itching, swelling and bronchoconstriction.[1] Late-phase reactions are mediated by infiltrating T cells that release T_H2 cytokines triggering additional tissue inflammation.

Allergen-specific immunotherapy (SIT) is currently the only curative treatment able to change the seasonal recurring natural course of IgE-mediated allergies and to induce long-term remission.[2] By exposing allergic patients to increasing doses of allergen, this therapeutic strategy aims to re-educate the immune system to promote a tolerogenic response toward a specific allergen.[3] This tolerogenic response is thought to be mediated by a change in immunologic memory. Effective immunotherapy is associated with the induction of distinct subsets of regulatory T cells (Tregs) that induce peripheral tolerance by increased secretion of IL-10 and transforming growth factor (TGF)-β, which increase the production of IgG4 and IgA antibodies.[4] In clinical settings, successful SIT is defined by a marked reduction in symptom duration and severity at the time of allergen exposure, a decrease in the use of antiallergic drugs, and an overall improvement in the quality of life of affected patients.[1]

However, despite great progress in the last decade, SIT faces several problems regarding its efficacy, side effects, low patient adherence, and the high cost owing to the long duration (3–5 years) of treatment.[5] It is estimated that less than 5% of all allergic patients, who could potentially benefit from allergy immunotherapy, actually undergo this treatment. Thus, finding new strategies to enhance SIT safety, more compact treatment regimens, and improved efficacy represents major objectives of current research efforts, which will be instrumental for improving a broader implementation of SIT in the clinic.

Factors that influence the safety and efficacy of SIT include the pattern of sensitization, the nature of the allergen preparation (allergen extracts, adjuvants, and conjugated molecules), and the route of administration (subcutaneous or sublingual). Thus, the optimization of allergen/adjuvant formulations and their mode of administration is currently a bottle neck in specific immunotherapy.[6] Subcutaneous immunotherapy (SCIT) is the most commonly used form of SIT and is found to be effective in adults and children suffering from allergies to house dust mites, animal dander, and pollen.[7] However SCIT requires frequent injections and can be associated with allergic side effects, including fatal airway obstruction and anaphylaxis. Other alternative methods of delivery such as epicutaneous, intralymphatic, oral, or sublingual immunotherapies have been proposed and are currently being evaluated.[8] Because of its noninvasive character and good efficacy, sublingual immunotherapy is now considered a promising alternative to SCIT for respiratory allergies to grass and tree pollen or house dust mite allergens.[9]

In recent years, considerable research effort has been put into the chemical modification of allergens to improve the efficacy and safety of SIT, but also the demand of drug authorities to standardize allergen preparations has consolidated the available allergen preparations. Various strategies have been developed to modify allergenic molecules into safer hypoallergenic derivatives to limit adverse IgE-mediated reactions while maintaining their immunogenic properties.[10–13] Current research shows that allergenic peptides and various forms of recombinant allergens (hypoallergens, dimers, trimers, fusion proteins) can be efficient in controlling allergic inflammation and inhibiting symptoms of asthma notably by inducing the production of inhibitory antibodies.[12,14,15]

The use of appropriate immunomodulatory adjuvants is a particularly promising strategy to improve the safety and efficacy of current SIT protocols, because a stimulated immune system may require less allergen and thus reduce side effects by avoiding allergen–IgE complexes. In the treatment of infectious diseases, adjuvants traditionally are added to vaccines to boost immunization against purified or recombinant pathogen antigens. Because adjuvants can skew the immune response toward T helper 1 (T_H1) known to downregulate allergic T_H2 inflammation, their use in SIT may provide a clear benefit.[16] An optimal adjuvant for specific immunotherapy should reduce the allergen dose, thereby decreasing local side effects and improving the overall safety of SIT, does not induce T_H2 cells, and provides long-lasting tolerogenic memory.

Several adjuvants, from alum (aluminum hydroxide) adjuvants to toll-like receptor (TLR) agonists, probiotics, and nanoparticles were developed and studied in the last decades.[17] This review describes adjuvants currently in use or under development and their role in enhancing the efficacy of allergen immunotherapy. This review summarizes immunologic mechanisms involved in successful allergen-specific immunotherapy and thus targets of adjuvant action and discusses therapeutic effects of current adjuvants and their role in the establishment of allergen tolerance.

IMMUNOLOGIC MECHANISMS OF SUCCESSFUL ALLERGEN-SPECIFIC IMMUNOTHERAPY

Allergen-specific immunotherapy can modulate cellular and humoral responses leading to a significant reduction in the recruitment and activation of inflammatory effector cells at sites of allergen encounter.[18] The long-term allergen-specific immune tolerance triggered by SIT can be divided into rapid, intermediate, and late treatment responses (**Fig. 1**).[4,19]

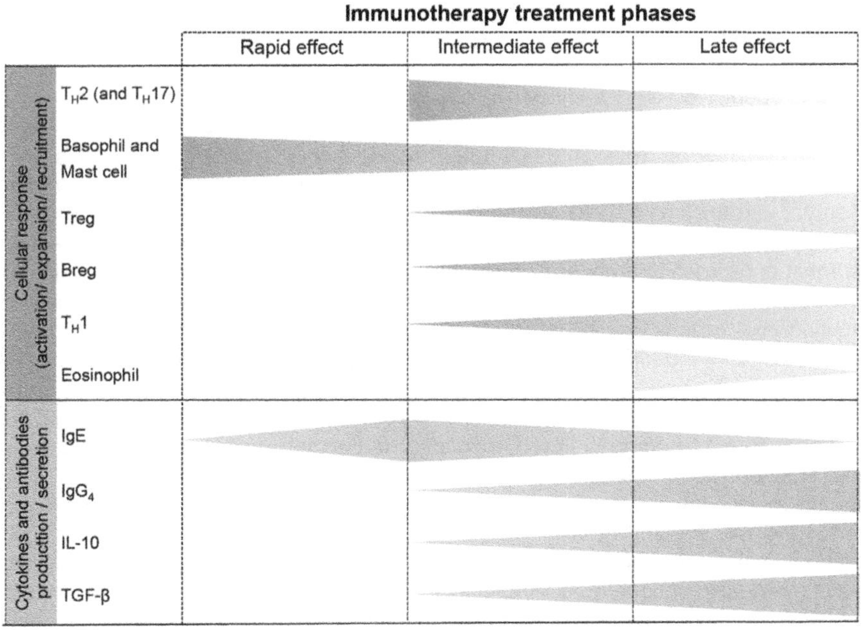

Fig. 1. Immunotherapy treatment phases.

Rapid Treatment Response

The first allergen administration during SIT induces a decrease in basophil and mast cell activation (ie, degranulation and proinflammatory mediator production), thereby reducing the capacity of these cells to induce anaphylaxis.[20,21] During this early phase, mast cells and basophils become unable to respond to environmental proteins despite the presence of specific IgE.[4,22] In a process referred to as *desensitization*, mast cells are rendered hyporesponsive to an activating challenge by exposure to low or high doses of allergen.[4] However, the molecular mechanisms responsible for this rapid desensitization are not yet completely elucidated. A recent study described the rapid upregulation of the histamine receptor 2 (H2R) on the surface of basophils from patients undergoing venom immunotherapy.[23] H2R was found to strongly suppress FcεR1-induced basophil activation and mediator release. Thus, a rapid increase in the surface expression of immunoregulatory receptors such as H2R might be instrumental in early protective mechanisms of SIT, particularly within the first few hours during the repetitive administration of venom protein (build-up phase).

Intermediate Treatment Response

The administration of progressively increasing allergen doses during the course of SIT will then influence adaptive immune responses, resulting in the generation of allergen-specific regulatory T (Treg) and B (Breg) cells and the simultaneous decrease in T_H2 cells. In the last 2 decades, several studies found that Tregs play a major role in the induction and the maintenance of tolerance during SIT.[24–26] After allergen-specific immunotherapy and subsequent allergen challenge, FOXP3$^+$IL-10$^+$ T cells along with single FOXP3$^+$IL-10$^-$ or FOXP3$^-$IL-10$^+$ T cells are detectable in the nasal tissue and are absent in the placebo-treated group.[26] The generation of these Tregs during SIT is associated with the production of the anti-inflammatory cytokines TGF-β and IL-10, which have the capacity to inhibit the activation and migration of effector T_H2 and T helper 17 (T_H17) cells, which are central players in allergic reactions.[27–34]

More recently, a TGF-β and IL-10–producing B-cell subset was identified and found to play an important role in suppressing T_H2 as well as T_H17 immunity while promoting the maintenance of Tregs.[4,35,36] Of note, this regulatory B-cell population has been implicated in the induction of tolerance during SIT in the context of bee venom allergy.[37] Expansion of IL-10 secreting suppressive B cells can promote the emergence of IgG4, an inhibitory antibody isotype suspected to play a key role in the establishment of allergen tolerance.[7,19] One study further suggested that the production of IgG4 is restricted to the regulatory B cells compartment.[37] IgG4 class switch recombination in B cells is caused by co-stimulation with IL-4 and IL-10, whereby IL-10 decreases IL-4–induced IgE class switching, but increases IL-4-induced IgG4 production.[38,39]

The emergence of IgG4 antibodies is of particular importance for SIT because this isotype is found to dampen FcεR1-mediated degranulation of mast cells, basophils, and eosinophils.[18,40] The competition of allergen-specific IgG4 and mast cell–bound–specific IgE antibodies for allergen has been proposed as a central mechanism underlying the efficacy of SIT.[19,41] By competing with IgE, allergen-specific IgG4 antibodies may also decrease the reactivity of antigen-presenting B cells to allergen, thereby reducing antigen presentation to T cells.[41] As serum IgG4 levels dramatically increase after prolonged SIT and remain stable over years after SIT treatment, high-avidity IgG4 has been proposed as a marker of SIT-induced immune tolerance[42];

however generally allergen-specific IgG4 of all avidities is not correlating with clinical success of the therapy.

Late Treatment Response

The long-term efficacy of SIT is associated not only with a significantly reduced immediate response to allergen provocation but also with a blunted late-phase response (LPR) in the affected end organ (eg, skin or respiratory tract).[4,43] The mechanisms driving the late-phase response differ from the mast cell–mediated early-phase response and involve a strong bronchial or nasal hyperreactivity and the recruitment and activation of eosinophils and effector T cells at sites of allergen exposure.[44] This late phase of the allergic response can be modulated by IL-10–producing regulatory B cells and T cells able to inhibit the recruitment and activation of eosinophils and the differentiation and proliferation of T_H2 cells.[42] Because T_H2 cells and eosinophils are central players in tissue remodeling, SIT approaches should induce mechanisms to efficiently control these cells or limit their clonal expansion, thereby avoiding the development of irreversible end organ hyperreactivity.[4]

ADJUVANTS AS MEANS TO OVERCOME LIMITATIONS OF ALLERGEN-SPECIFIC IMMUNOTHERAPY

SIT has been a controversial treatment for allergic diseases.[6] Despite proven efficacy in many clinical studies,[45] concerns regarding the long-term efficacy and safety of SIT currently limit its clinical use.

Because SIT requires the application of high allergen doses and repeated injections (in the case of SCIT), local side effects but also systemic allergic reactions with the risk of severe or fatal anaphylaxis can occur. To reduce the administered allergen dose, allergens can be applied in combination with an adjuvant to boost the immunologic response toward the allergen. Adjuvants are traditionally added to vaccines to reduce the frequency of injections or the dose of antigen owing to their capacity to induce strong and sustained immunity against pathogens. An adjuvant (Latin, *adiuvare:* to aid) is functionally defined as a compound that enhances the specific immune response against an antigen in vivo.[46] On a cellular level it is anticipated that allergen vaccination is inducing de novo T-cell differentiation of naïve T cells into the helper T cells (Th1, T_H2, Tregs etc). In allergy, co-administration of antigen (allergen) with adjuvants can drive T_H1 responses to compete with T_H2-mediated hypersensitivity, actively suppress T_H2 type inflammation. The choice of adjuvant crucially depends on the antigen (allergen) as well as the route of immunization and is limited by the extent of adverse reactions in response to the chosen combination. Ideally, an adjuvant should be cost effective, biodegradable, non-toxic, stable for extended periods of time *in vivo* and induce an appropriate immune response.[47] Unfortunately, the use of adjuvants is hampered by issues such us toxicity and side-effects, limiting a broad application in immunotherapy. Thus, a major aim of current research is to design and develop new adjuvants with improved safety and efficacy profiles.

CURRENT ADJUVANTS AND THEIR EFFECTS ON ALLERGEN-SPECIFIC IMMUNOTHERAPY

To date, alum, an aluminum-based compound discovered more than 80 years ago, still remains the predominant adjuvant for human vaccines. However recent advances in the understanding of immunologic mechanisms underlying immunotherapy may foster the design of new effective adjuvants with improved immunologic profiles. Current adjuvants able to enhance the efficacy of allergy immunotherapy include (!)

Table 1
Immunopotentiators for allergy immunotherapy

Adjuvants	Allergen	Route	Properties	Application in Clinic (Yes/No)
Aluminium hydroxide	Various clinical vaccines	Subcutaneous	Aluminium triggers a depot effect (slow release of the allergen) favoring the interaction with the immune system. Alum facilitates the shift away from T_H2 response through the generation of inhibitory antibodies and Treg response Alum acts as a danger signal and induces IL-1 family cytokines.	Yes (the most used in SIT)
TLRs agonists (MPL, CpG-ODNs, others)	OVA, Amb a 1, grass pollen	Subcutaneous, intradermal, sublingual	CpG-ODNs (TLR9) have good efficacy in immunotherapy mouse models (subcutaneous, intradermally) with ragweed/grass pollen allergens. In mice and humans, a synthetic CpG conjugated to Amb a 1 showed good efficacy when used during SCIT. Other ligands particularly Pam3Csk4 and LP40 (TLR2), imidazoquinolines (TLR7, 8) are found to induce Treg and T_H1 responses in preclinical models	Yes (MPLs, CpGs)

Probiotics	OVA, Bet v1, peanut	Sublingual, oral	Bacteria such as *L plantarum* or *Bifidobacterium plantarum* showed efficacy in the treatment of allergic mice against Bet v1 and OVA. A recent clinical trial found a reduction of IgE and induction of IgG4 in peanut allergic children after oral immunotherapy in combination with probiotics.	Yes (with the probiotic *Lactobacillus rhamnosus*)
Bacteria products (*M vaccae, CTB*)	Mite, birch pollen	Intradermal, subcutaneous, mucosal (oral or nasal, intratracheal)	*M vaccae and CTB* decrease airway inflammation and modulate the immune system (Treg, T$_H$1, IgA) in mice when injected with antigen (house dust mite or birch pollen). Although some benefits have been found in mice, no clinical trials have yet evaluated the effect of *CTB* and *M vaccae* during immunotherapy in humans.	No
Vit D	OVA, grass pollen, house dust mite	Sublingual, subcutaneous	The administration of Vit D alone or in combination with glucocorticosteroids during OVA-specific immunotherapy in mice reduces T$_H$2-driven airway inflammation and airway hyperreactivity. An expansion of Treg and activation of DCs has been reported in response to Vit D. Preliminary promising results have been described after treatment with Vit D in combination with SCIT in mite allergic patients.	Yes (with mite allergen)

Abbreviations: CpG-ODNs, CpG oligodeoxynucleotides; *CTB, Cholera toxin B*; MPL, Monophosphoryl lipid A; OVA, Ovalbumin.

synthetic or biological immunopotentiators reinforcing allergen-specific T_H1 or regulatory T cell responses through a direct activation of T cells, dendritic cells, or epithelial cells (**Table 1**) and (2) nanoparticle delivery systems promoting allergen uptake and presentation by antigen presenting cells (APC) in the oral mucosa but also protecting the encapsulated active product (allergen) (**Table 2**).[9]

Immunopotentiators

Aluminium-based adjuvants

Aluminium-based adjuvants have been used successfully in prophylactic vaccinations for almost 100 years. Aluminum hydroxide or aluminum phosphate are the most widely used adjuvants in allergy immunotherapy to boost immune responses to the injected allergens.[48] Approximately 75% of all adjuvant-based therapies include an aluminum salt.[49] The vaccine preparation is primarily composed of micrometer-sized clusters of nano-sized primary particles of the aluminum salt to which the antigen is adsorbed.[50] The injection of alum-adsorbed allergens has proven efficacious and safe in a variety of SCIT studies and in studies using other parenteral routes.[49] Classically, alum adjuvants have been proposed to promote immune responses through the so-called depot effect, that is, by allowing for the slow release of the antigen from the salt particles, thereby maintaining the stimulation of the immune response at the inoculation site. Several hypotheses regarding alum's mechanisms of action have been proposed.[51] The first immunization with alum-adsorbed allergen was further shown to induce an early cytokine response, including the IL-1 family member IL-18, facilitating IL-4 production.[52] The induction of IL-18 by alum adjuvants has been shown to depend on the activation of the NLRP3 inflammasome.[53,54] After prolonged and repeated immunization, alum was reported to skew the immune response toward a Treg/T_H1 response and to reduce T_H2 activation by increasing IgE-blocking IgG antibodies.[51] Thus, the use of aluminum adjuvants in allergen immunotherapy is a useful tool to trigger a modified T_H2 response with protective character.[55] To date, the use of alum-adsorbed allergen extracts has improved symptoms in the case of aeroallergens and venom immunotherapy. However, aluminum adjuvants have important limitations, particularly with regard to their profound T_H2-biasing effects and their potential implication in neurologic pathologies.[50,56–58] The T_H2 induction is considered an unwanted side effect, possibly related to an increase of allergen-specific IgE after the initiation of immunotherapy, before a blunted IgE response in the following season and decrease after prolonged immunotherapy. Current research aims to develop new adjuvant formulations able to induce tolerance by avoiding the induction or amplification of T_H2 responses.

Toll-like receptor agonists

TLRs are key components of the innate immune system able to elicit an inflammatory response in response to pathogen-associated molecular patterns. Pathogen-associated molecular patterns include lipid, protein, lipoprotein, carbohydrate, and nucleic acidstructures found exclusively on microbes (bacteria, viruses, fungi, and parasites) but absent from host cells. The addition of TLR agonists to immunotherapy has shown some benefits, which were linked to their potential to induce mixed T_H1/Treg responses, reversing established allergic inflammation.[59] The prototypic bacterial lipopolysaccharide (LPS) induces the TLR4-dependent activation of APCs resulting in the induction of a strong specific T_H1 response against co-administered antigens.[60] However, because of the toxicity of LPS, it remains a poor choice for a therapeutic adjuvant.[17] MPL, a derivative of LPS, has been shown to exhibit reduced toxicity while maintaining immunomodulatory properties.[61]

Table 2
Nanoparticle delivery systems for allergy immunotherapy

Adjuvants	Allergen	Route	Properties	Application in Clinic (Yes/No)
Liposomes (OML, nanoliposome)	OVA, Cry j 1, grass pollen, Der p1	Intranasal, intradermal	OML loaded with OVA or Cry j 1 (pollen) improves the allergic features in allergic mouse models by modulating the humoral (control of IgE elevation) and cellular immunity (Tregs CD4+ and Tregs CD8+, T_H1). In humans, cutaneous administration of liposomes loaded with allergen has shown benefits in asthmatic patients (high specific IgGs levels; reduction of sputum eosinophils and serum ECP levels). However, prolonged immunization causes side effects.	Yes (grass pollen, Der p1)
VLPs	Der p 1, Phl 1	Subcutaneous, intramuscular	VLPs are described as effective adjuvants in immunotherapy against mite and grass pollen. VLPs loaded with CpGs only (without allergen) are immunomodulatory.	Yes (Phl p 1, Der p1)
ISCOMs	OVA, PLA2	Subcutaneous, intranasal	In animals, the administration of ISCOMs together with allergen elicits humoral and cellular responses. This system is powerful in activating DCs and inducing antigen-specific cytotoxic CD8+ T cells. ISCOM-based vaccines are found to promote long-lasting immune responses.	No (preclinical)
Polymeric nanoparticles (Chitosan NPs, PLGA, others)	OVA, mite, Bet v1, profilin, peanut	Intranasal, sublingual, subcutaneous, intravenous, oral, intradermal	The therapeutic effect of chitosan-based NPs loaded with allergen or with plasmids encoding allergen has been proven in allergic mice during immunotherapy. Subcutaneously or intravenously administered PLGA NPs containing allergen alone (Bet v1, profilin) or CpG-allergen (mite) in mice enhances the tolerance. Other polymeric NPs are described in mice as potential adjuvants for OIT: (1) Gantrez NPs combined with LPS from *Brucella ovis* stimulating the production of IgG2a antibodies and IL-10; (2) PVM/MA NPs formulated with peanut protein triggering a pro-T_H1 immune response; (3) the copolymer PHEA loaded with a hybrid molecule expressing the pollen allergens (Par j1 and 2) promoting a high T_H1/T_H2 ratio	No (preclinical)

Abbreviations: copolymer PHEA, α,β-Poly(N-2-hydroxyethyl)-d,l-aspartamide; ECP, Eosinophil cationic protein; NPs, nanoparticles; PLA2, phospholipase A2; PLGA, poly(lactic-co-glycolic acid); PVM/MA, poly(methyl vinyl ether-co-maleic anhydride).

Through TLR4 signaling, MPL is able to induce potent immune deviation toward T_H1/Treg response.[62] The use of MPL as adjuvant has been tested in clinical phase II and III studies and was approved for subcutaneous and sublingual immunotherapy (Pollinex Quattro).[63] The formulation allergen-MPL (especially grass pollen) is well tolerated and results in a significant reduction of symptom scores and serum IgE levels while increasing the T_H1 polarization and the production of allergen-specific IgG4.[63]

DNA or CpG-ODNs have been described as immune modulators and as potential vaccine adjuvants.[64] CpG-ODNs interact with TLR9 localized in the endosomes of APCs resulting in the production of a series of cytokines including Interferon-γ and IL-12 favoring the shift of human allergen-specific T_H2 cells toward a T_H1/T_H0 phenotype.[65] In subcutaneously sensitized mice, injection of a mix of grass pollen/CpG-ODN reduced T_H2 inflammation and IgE secretion with conflicting effects on T_H1 stimulation.[66] The clinical use of CpG-ODNs in SIT against ragweed allergy has shown variable effects possibly owing to differences in the efficacy of different types of CpG.[17] Recently, an innovative approach has been developed based on the conjugation of immunostimulatory DNA to allergenic proteins. In both animal and human studies, a synthetic CpG oligonucleotide conjugated to the major allergen of ragweed Amb a 1 has been shown to improve allergic symptoms after subcutaneous administration.[67,68]

Other TLR agonists have been identified in vitro or in vivo as potential adjuvants in allergen immunotherapy. Among these the TLR7 agonists imiquimod (R-837) and resiquimod (R848) (imidazoquinoline class) are of special interest in allergy immunotherapy because in addition to inhibiting T_H2 cell differentiation, they can induce T_H1 responses.[69] However, as imidazoquinolines induce serious side effects (vomiting, alteration of blood cells), their use has been limited to experimental models.[61] Other natural adjuvants signaling through TLR 7, 8, or 9 are currently being investigated, for example, modified 8 OH-adenines as a future adjuvant for use in oral immunotherapy.[70] Additionally, the use of lipopeptides such as the TLR2 agonists Pam3CSK4 and LP40 in SIT has been proposed because of the potential of these compounds to induce Treg and T_H1 responses.[71,72]

Probiotics

The healthy human microbiome is increasingly recognized as a rich source of immunomodulatory compounds, with a great potential to protect from allergy, particularly early in life.[73] Thus, the use of immunomodulatory live micro-organisms (probiotics) has been suggested as a new strategy to improve SIT. Bacteria such as *Lactobacillus plantarum* or *Bifidobacterium bifidum* were found to modulate systemic cytokine production and decrease allergen-specific IgE production following sublingual immunotherapy in mice sensitized to OVA or Bet v1.[74,75] In humans, most clinical trials using selected probiotics as a stand-alone therapy have failed to show clinically relevant beneficial effects on allergy.[76,77]

Attenuated mycobacteria, bacterial products

Because of their immunostimulatory properties, bacterial toxins such as *CTB* and heat-killed *Mycobacterium vaccae* were described as potential adjuvants. The administration of *CTB* (oral or nasal route) or *M vaccae* (intratracheal, subcutaneous) along with antigen (dust mite, birch pollen) in mouse models of allergic airway inflammation is reported to result in a marked reduction in classical features of airway inflammation.[9] *M vaccae* or *CTB* adjuvant was found to prevent T_H2 response by enhancing Treg and T_H1 responses and by inducing the production of IgA antibodies.[78–80] In clinical settings, intradermal injection of *M vaccae* has shown beneficial outcomes in children with atopic dermatitis or asthma. In contrast, *M vaccae* or *CTB* have not yet been tested in combination with allergens in allergic patients.

Vitamin D

Vitamin D is a natural hormone able to prevent various allergic diseases by stimulating tolerogenic processes of the immune system.[10] The active form of vitamin D3 (VitD3),1,25-dihydroxyvitamin D3, is found to promote the migration of DC and the development of Tregs leading to the suppression of allergen-specific T_H2 cells in vitro and in vivo.[81] Studies in mouse models have described VitD3 as a potent adjuvant with the capacity to enhance beneficial effects of immunotherapy and to promote the long-term efficacy of SIT.[82] Deficiency or insufficiency of VitD3 is correlated with an increased risk of allergy and asthma and VitD3 supplementation may enhance the efficacy of SIT.[82,83] The administration of VitD3 in combination with SCIT showed some minor favorable outcomes in asthmatic children sensitized to house dust mite.[84] Ongoing clinical trials are currently evaluating the additive effect of VitD3 in SIT in grass- and birch pollen–allergic patients.

Nanoparticle Delivery Systems

Recently, nanoparticle-based delivery systems such as viruslike particles, liposomes, immunostimulating complex (ISCOMs), and polymeric nanospheres have received attention as potential adjuvants for allergen immunotherapy.[85] These generally well-established carrier systems are found to boost the efficacy of allergy vaccines.[10] Encapsulation in the nanoparticle delivery system allows for the protection of the antigen from environmental influences (eg, pH, humidity, temperature), thereby maintaining or even enhancing the immunogenicity of the allergen cargo. Because of the particle nature the antigen-uptake is limited to those cells that are enabled to phagocytize respective particles.

Liposomes

Liposomes are synthetic spheres made of lipid bilayers that can encapsulate hydrophilic antigens and act as adjuvants.[47] Liposomes increase the half life of antigens in blood ensuring a sustained antigen exposure to APCs after vaccination. Intranasal immunization with OVA encapsulated in oligomannose-coated liposomes (OML) was found to induce a Treg response and an improvement of allergic symptoms in a murine food allergy model.[86] Similar results have been obtained after intradermal immunization of pollen-allergic mice with Cry j 1 (Japanese cedar major allergen) encapsulated in OML.[87] More recently, this system has been used to improve the delivery of other adjuvants—particularly CPG-ODN—for which extensive preclinical and clinical evaluation had previously confirmed an immunomodulatory potential in allergy. Co-encapsulation of OVA antigen with CpG-ODN adjuvant in nanoliposomes is found to profoundly increase antigen-specific T_H1 immune responses in vitro.[88] In humans, the cutaneous injection of liposome-encapsulated mite or grass pollen allergens was well tolerated[89] but found to induce delayed local reactions.[9] Furthermore, the use of liposome adjuvants in humans is limited by their low stability and manufacturing problems.[90] Liposomal delivery systems with improved stability and tailored immunologic properties are currently being developed for a future application in allergen immunotherapy. Of note, phosphatidyl serine containing liposomes mimic vesicles derived from apoptotic cells, and their phagocytosis was found to promote tolerogenic immune responses.[91]

Viruslike particles

Viruslike particles (VLP) are self-assembling nanoparticles formed of biocompatible capsid proteins.[92] VLPs have the potential to interact with the immune system while avoiding pathologic effects caused by the absence of viral pathogenicity factors. Currently, some of these vectors have been evaluated in humans via parental routes (subcutaneously or intramuscularly).[92] The administration of VLPs from Qβ phage conjugated with peptides derived from *Dermatophagoïdes* pteronyssinus (Der p) 1 mite allergen was shown to induce a strong IgG response in healthy volunteers.[93] Clinical trials have evaluated the therapeutic effect of Qβ-derived VLPs loaded with CpGs or the allergen (eg, mite, mite extracts) in adult allergic patients.[94] After 6 weekly injections, allergy symptoms improved with increased levels of IgG antibodies observed in the group receiving VLP/CpGs/allergen but also VLP/CpGs alone. The good efficacy of VLPs loaded with CpGs alone has been confirmed in allergic rhinitis patients undergoing SIT treatment.[95] More recently, a rhinovirus-derived VP1 protein loaded with peptide from Phleum pratense (Phl) 1 grass pollen has also been proposed as a candidate vaccine for grass pollen allergies.[96] Because of their good safety and efficacy profile VLP-encapsulated allergens represent promising candidates for immunotherapy of allergic disorders.

Immunostimulating complex

ISCOMs are spherical complexes about 40 nm in size, composed of saponin adjuvant Quil A, cholesterol, phospholipids, and protein antigen.[90] ISCOMs are able to trap the antigen by apolar interactions and to elicit strong humoral, cellular, and mucosal T_H1 responses after subcutaneous or intranasal immunization.[97] The particularity of ISCOMs is the generation of antigen-specific $CD8^+$ cytotoxic cells, observed after immunization in mice.[98] Although ISCOMs have been proposed as potential vaccine vectors in vaccination with influenza or human immunodeficiency virus, no study has yet evaluated the effect of ISCOMs as adjuvants in allergen immunotherapy.

Polymeric nanoparticles

Several NPs have been developed in recent years, and particularly biodegradable polymeric carriers have shown great potential as new drug delivery systems.[90] In addition, the application of polymeric nanoparticles has yielded promising results in systemic and mucosal immunotherapy.[99] Biodegradable polymers can be of natural (eg, collagen, albumin, chitosan) or synthetic (eg, poly [lactic acids], PLA; poly [lactide-co-glycolic acids], PLGA; poly [methyl methacrylate], PVMA; poly [anhydride] nanoparticles, PHE; poly [hydroxyethyl] aspartamide) origin.[90] Two of the most extensively investigated polymers in allergen immunotherapy is chitosan and PLGA.

Chitosan is a natural mucoadhesive polysaccharide derived from crustacean shells.[6] Chitosan-based nanoparticles have been widely studied because of their biocompatibility, biodegradability, nontoxic nature, and their ability to enhance the penetration of macromolecules across the mucosa.[90] Intranasal application of Der f entrapped in chitosan microparticles in sensitized mice attenuated bronchial hyperreactivity, lung inflammation, and mucus production.[100] The immunotherapeutic efficacy of chitosan microparticles has also been shown during sublingual immunization with OVA in a murine model of allergic airway inflammation.[100–102] Several studies found that chitosan polymers improve the uptake of antigen by mucosal DCs, thereby enhancing tolerance induction during intranasal or sublingual immunotherapy.[101,102] Other studies indicate that the oral administration of chitosan NPs formulated with plasmid DNA encoding the dust mite allergens Der p1 and Der p2 or with the Ara h2 allergen (major peanut allergen) in mice could trigger a significant reduction in allergic symptoms.[103–105] A recent study found that the treatment of mice with chitosan DNA NPs loaded with OVA led to a transferable antigen-specific tolerance, which involved Treg cells.[106]

Poly (lactic-co-glycolic acid) (PLGA) is a polyester widely used for the preparation of NPs. This polymer has been approved for several clinical applications in humans owing to its well-established biocompatibility, safety, and biodegradability.[10] In recent years, the PLGA nanoparticles have received great attention for the therapy of allergies.[107] Subcutaneous immunization of mice with PLGA particles formulated with Bet v1 (major birch pollen allergen) was found to decrease the T_H2 response to Bet v1 and to increase immunomodulatory immunoglobulins and cytokines.[108] Similar results were obtained after the immunization of allergic mice with PLGA particles composed of recombinant birch profilin (protein identified as allergen in pollen, latex, and plant food).[109] Moreover, a recent study has reported an alternative co-delivery method resulting in the successful tolerization of mice using CpG and PLGA loaded with a major house dust mite allergen (Der p2).[110,111] This approach using PLGA particles containing CpG and Der p2 resulted in the reduction of allergen-specific IgE while enhancing class switching to IgG2a. More recently, intravenous or subcutaneous immunization using tolerogenic PLGA nanoparticles loaded with peptide or antigen and the immunosuppressant rapamycin was found to induce sustained antigen-specific tolerance in animals.[112] In this study, co-administration of rapamycin was crucial for inducing both antigen-specific humoral and cellular immunity. As an alternative to PLGA polymer particles, new polymer-based adjuvant systems are being developed, including an injectable hydrogel composite comprising PLGA-PEG (poly [ethylene glycol]) copolymers. Although this system has never been tested in allergen immunotherapy, it could be a new approach to improve the efficacy of SCIT.[113]

Other polymeric nanoparticles have recently provided positive results in allergy immunotherapy in animal models including the Gantrez nanoparticles combined with lipopolysaccharide from Brucella Ovis,[114] the PVMA nanoparticles loaded with peanut,[115] and the copolymer PHEA (α,β-poly [N-2-hydroxyethyl]-DL-aspartamide) loaded with pollen extracts.[116] Currently, none of those polymeric systems have been tested in the context of mucosal allergy vaccines in humans.

SUMMARY AND FUTURE OUTCOMES

SIT currently represents the only curative treatment for allergic diseases. Despite its proven efficacy in a considerable proportion of allergy patients, SIT has been constrained by adverse events requiring either prophylactic or rescue medications. To overcome this, innovative strategies have been proposed to simplify immunization and to achieve long-term tolerance. Among these strategies, the co-administration of immunomodulatory adjuvants during SIT is of central importance. Thus, new adjuvant systems are currently under development that will hopefully overcome the limitations of traditionally used adjuvants such as alum. Although a variety of candidate adjuvants are found to induce tolerance during SIT protocols in murine models, a limited number of these compounds have been tested in humans (**Fig. 2**). Thus, additional studies are urgently needed to show the true potential of these new adjuvants in SIT. Deeper insights into the immunologic mechanisms underlying allergy have resulted in the development and approval of targeted therapies. Monoclonal antibodies targeting IgE and T_H2 cytokines (IL-4, IL-13, IL-5) are already in clinical use for the treatment of severe allergic inflammation and have recently been proposed as an alternative to improve SIT.[117,118] Omalizumab (anti-IgE) is the first immunomodulatory drug shown to

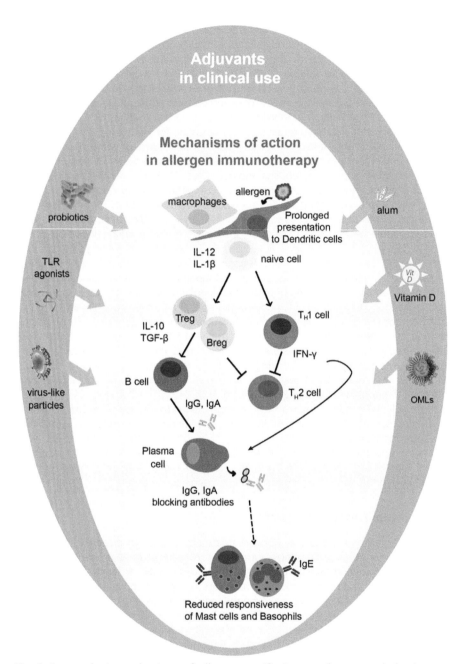

Fig. 2. Immunologic mechanisms of allergen-specific immunotherapy and the immune pontentiators or adjuvants used in clinic.

improve the efficacy and safety of SIT in humans when administered orally or subcutaneously.[119] It is hoped that future research on immunomodulatory adjuvants will result in safer and more efficacious allergen immunotherapy protocols, instrumental in fighting the ever-worsening allergy epidemic.

REFERENCES

1. Cuppari C, Leonardi S, Manti S, et al. Allergen immunotherapy, routes of administration and cytokine networks: an update. Immunotherapy 2014;6:775–86.
2. Bousquet J, Lockey R, Malling HJ. Allergen immunotherapy: therapeutic vaccines for allergic diseases. A WHO position paper. J Allergy Clin Immunol 1998;102:558–62.
3. Akdis CA, Akdis M. Advances in allergen immunotherapy: aiming for complete tolerance to allergens. Sci Transl Med 2015;7:280ps6.
4. Akdis M, Akdis CA. Mechanisms of allergen-specific immunotherapy: multiple suppressor factors at work in immune tolerance to allergens. J Allergy Clin Immunol 2014;133:621–31.
5. Akdis CA. Therapies for allergic inflammation: refining strategies to induce tolerance. Nat Med 2012;18:736–49.
6. Ye Y-L, Chuang Y-H, Chiang B-L. Strategies of mucosal immunotherapy for allergic diseases. Cell Mol Immunol 2011;8:453–61.
7. Matsuoka T, Shamji MH, Durham SR. Allergen immunotherapy and tolerance. Allergol Int 2013;62:403–13.
8. Ponda P, Hochfelder JL. Allergen immunotherapy: routes, safety, efficacy, and mode of action. Immuno Targets and Therapy 2013;61–71.
9. Moingeon P. Adjuvants for allergy vaccines. Hum Vaccin Immunother 2012;8: 1492–8.
10. Jongejan L, van Ree R. Modified allergens and their potential to treat allergic disease. Curr Allergy Asthma Rep 2014;14:478.
11. Moldaver D, Larché M. Immunotherapy with peptides. Allergy 2011;66:784–91.
12. Marth K, Focke-Tejkl M, Lupinek C, et al. Allergen peptides, recombinant allergens and hypoallergens for allergen-specific immunotherapy. Curr Treat Options Allergy 2014;1:91–106.
13. Valenta R, Vrtala S, Focke-Tejkl M, et al. Synthetic and genetically engineered allergen derivatives for specific immunotherapy of type I allergy. Clin Allergy Immunol 2002;16:495–517.
14. Bouchaud G, Braza F, Chesné J, et al. Prevention of allergic asthma through Der p 2 peptide vaccination. J Allergy Clin Immunol 2015;136(1):197–200.e1.
15. Vrtala S. From allergen genes to new forms of allergy diagnosis and treatment. Allergy 2008;63:299–309.
16. Jacobsen L, Wahn U, Bilo MB. Allergen-specific immunotherapy provides immediate, long-term and preventive clinical effects in children and adults: the effects of immunotherapy can be categorised by level of benefit -the centenary of allergen specific subcutaneous immunotherapy. Clin Transl Allergy 2012;2:8.
17. Smarr CB, Bryce PJ, Miller SD. Antigen-specific tolerance in immunotherapy of Th2-associated allergic diseases. Crit Rev Immunol 2013;33:389–414.
18. Shamji MH, Durham SR. Mechanisms of immunotherapy to aeroallergens. Clin Exp Allergy 2011;41:1235–46.
19. Álvaro M, Sancha J, Larramona H, et al. Allergen-specific immunotherapy: update on immunological mechanisms. Allergol Immunopathol (Madr) 2013;41: 265–72.
20. Sullivan TJ. Antigen-specific desensitization of patients allergic to penicillin. J Allergy Clin Immunol 1982;69:500–8.
21. Ozdemir O. Any defining role of mast cell or mast cell density in oral squamous cell carcinoma? Ann Med Health Sci Res 2014;4:975–7.

22. Plewako H, Wosińska K, Arvidsson M, et al. Basophil interleukin 4 and interleukin 13 production is suppressed during the early phase of rush immunotherapy. Int Arch Allergy Immunol 2006;141:346–53.

23. Novak N, Mete N, Bussmann C, et al. Early suppression of basophil activation during allergen-specific immunotherapy by histamine receptor 2. J Allergy Clin Immunol 2012;130:1153–8.e2.

24. Jutel M, Akdis M, Budak F, et al. IL-10 and TGF-beta cooperate in the regulatory T cell response to mucosal allergens in normal immunity and specific immunotherapy. Eur J Immunol 2003;33:1205–14.

25. Francis JN, Till SJ, Durham SR. Induction of IL-10+CD4+CD25+ T cells by grass pollen immunotherapy. J Allergy Clin Immunol 2003;111:1255–61.

26. Radulovic S, Jacobson MR, Durham SR, et al. Grass pollen immunotherapy induces Foxp3-expressing CD4+ CD25+ cells in the nasal mucosa. J Allergy Clin Immunol 2008;121:1467–72, 1472.e1.

27. Stelmaszczyk-Emmel A. Respiratory physiology & neurobiology. Respir Physiolo Neurobiol 2015;209:59–63.

28. Chesné J, Braza F, Chadeuf G, et al. Prime role of IL-17A in neutrophilia and airway smooth muscle contraction in a house dust mite-induced allergic asthma model. J Allergy Clin Immunol 2015;135(6):1643–1643.e3.

29. Chesné J, Braza F, Mahay G, et al. IL-17 in Severe Asthma. Where Do We Stand? Am J Respir Crit Care Med 2014;190:1094–101.

30. Palomares O, n-Fontecha MMI, Lauener R, et al. Regulatory T cells and immune regulation of allergic diseases: roles of IL-10 and TGF-b. Genes Immun 2014;15: 511–20.

31. Palomares O, Yaman G, Azkur AK, et al. Role of Treg in immune regulation of allergic diseases. Eur J Immunol 2010;40:1232–40.

32. Eyerich S, Onken AT, Weidinger S, et al. Mutual antagonism of T cells causing psoriasis and atopic eczema. N Engl J Med 2011;365:231–8.

33. Mantel P-Y, Schmidt-Weber CB. Transforming growth factor-beta: recent advances on its role in immune tolerance. Methods Mol Biol 2011;677: 303–38.

34. Schmidt-Weber CB, Akdis M, Akdis CA. TH17 cells in the big picture of immunology. J Allergy Clin Immunol 2007;120:247–54.

35. Braza F, Chesne J, Castagnet S, et al. Regulatory functions of B cells in allergic diseases. Allergy 2014;69(11):1454–63.

36. Fujita H, Soyka MB, Akdis M, et al. Mechanisms of allergen-specific immunotherapy. Clin Transl Allergy 2012;2:2.

37. van de Veen W, Stanic B, Yaman G, et al. IgG4 production is confined to human IL-10-producing regulatory B cells that suppress antigen-specific immune responses. J Allergy Clin Immunol 2013;131:1204–12.

38. Jeannin P, Lecoanet S, Delneste Y, et al. IgE versus IgG4 production can be differentially regulated by IL-10. J Immunol 1998;160:3555–61.

39. Akdis CA, Blesken T, Akdis M, et al. Role of interleukin 10 in specific immunotherapy. J Clin Invest 1998;102:98–106.

40. Santos AF, James LK, Bahnson HT, et al. IgG4 inhibits peanut-induced basophil and mast cell activation in peanut-tolerant children sensitized to peanut major allergens. J Allergy Clin Immunol 2015;135:1249–56.

41. Wachholz PA, Durham SR. Mechanisms of immunotherapy: IgG revisited. Curr Opin Allergy Clin Immunol 2004;4:313–8.

42. Jutel M, Akdis CA. Immunological mechanisms of allergen-specific immunotherapy. Allergy 2011;66:725–32.

43. Larsen GL. Late-phase reactions: observations on pathogenesis and prevention. J Allergy Clin Immunol 1985;76:665–9.
44. Larché M, Akdis CA, Valenta R. Immunological mechanisms of allergen-specific immunotherapy. Nat Rev Immunol 2006;6:761–71.
45. Passalacqua G. Recommendations for appropriate sublingual immunotherapy clinical trials. World Allergy Organ J 2014;7:1–5.
46. Pfaar O, Cazan D, Klimek L, et al. Adjuvants for immunotherapy. Curr Opin Allergy Clin Immunol 2012;12:648–57.
47. Petrovsky N, Aguilar JC. Vaccine adjuvants: current state and future trends. Immunol Cell Biol 2004;82:488–96.
48. Jensen-Jarolim E. Aluminium in allergies and allergen immunotherapy. World Allergy Organ J 2015;8:1–7.
49. Exley C. Aluminium adjuvants and adverse events in sub-cutaneous allergy immunotherapy. Allergy Asthma Clin Immunol 2014;10:4.
50. Kramer MF, Heath MD. Aluminium in allergen-specific subcutaneous immunotherapy – A German perspective. Vaccine 2014;32:4140–8.
51. Hogenesch H. Mechanism of immunopotentiation and safety of aluminum adjuvants. Front Immunol 2013;3:1–13, 406.
52. Grun JL, Maurer PH. Different T helper cell subsets elicited in mice utilizing two different adjuvant vehicles: the role of endogenous interleukin 1 in proliferative responses. Cell Immunol 1989;121:134–45.
53. Marrack P, McKee AS, Munks MW. Towards an understanding of the adjuvant action of aluminium. Nat Rev Immunol 2009;9:287–93.
54. Kool M, Soullié T, van Nimwegen M, et al. Alum adjuvant boosts adaptive immunity by inducing uric acid and activating inflammatory dendritic cells. J Exp Med 2008;205:869–82.
55. Wilcock LK, Francis JN, Durham SR. Aluminium hydroxide down-regulates T helper 2 responses by allergen-stimulated human peripheral blood mononuclear cells. Clin Exp Allergy 2004;34:1373–8.
56. Lindblad EB. Aluminium compounds for use in vaccines. Immunol Cell Biol 2004;82:497–505.
57. Brewer JM, Conacher M, Satoskar A, et al. In interleukin-4-deficient mice, alum not only generates T helper 1 responses equivalent to freund's complete adjuvant, but continues to induce T helper 2 cytokine production. Eur J Immunol 1996;26:2062–6.
58. De Sole P, Rossi C, Chiarpotto M, et al. Possible relationship between Al/ferritin complex and Alzheimer's disease. Clin Biochem 2013;46:89–93.
59. Casale TB, Stokes JR. Immunotherapy: what lies beyond. J Allergy Clin Immunol 2014;133:612–20.
60. Hoebe K, Janssen EM, Kim SO, et al. Upregulation of costimulatory molecules induced by lipopolysaccharide and double-stranded RNA occurs by Trif-dependent and Trif-independent pathways. Nat Immunol 2003;4:1223–9.
61. Filì L, Cardilicchia E, Maggi E, et al. Immunology letters. Immunol Lett 2014;161: 207–10.
62. Puggioni F, Durham SR, Francis JN. Monophosphoryl lipid A (MPL) promotes allergen-induced immune deviation in favour of Th1 responses. Allergy 2005; 60:678–84.
63. Drachenberg KJ, Wheeler AW, Stuebner P, et al. A well-tolerated grass pollen-specific allergy vaccine containing a novel adjuvant, monophosphoryl lipid A, reduces allergic symptoms after only four preseasonal injections. Allergy 2001;56:498–505.

64. Bode C, Zhao G, Steinhagen F, et al. CpG DNA as a vaccine adjuvant. Expert Rev Vaccines 2011;10:499–511.

65. Hemmi H, Takeuchi O, Kawai T, et al. A toll-like receptor recognizes bacterial DNA. Nature 2000;408:740–5.

66. Hessenberger M, Weiss R, Weinberger EE, et al. Transcutaneous delivery of CpG-adjuvanted allergen via laser-generated micropores. Vaccine 2013;31: 3427–34.

67. Tighe H, Takabayashi K, Schwartz D, et al. Conjugation of immunostimulatory DNA to the short ragweed allergen amb a 1 enhances its immunogenicity and reduces its allergenicity. J Allergy Clin Immunol 2000;106:124–34.

68. Simons FER, Shikishima Y, Van Nest G, et al. Selective immune redirection in humans with ragweed allergy by injecting Amb a 1 linked to immunostimulatory DNA. J Allergy Clin Immunol 2004;113:1144–51.

69. Brugnolo F, Sampognaro S, Liotta F, et al. The novel synthetic immune response modifier R-848 (Resiquimod) shifts human allergen-specific CD4+ TH2 lymphocytes into IFN-gamma-producing cells. J Allergy Clin Immunol 2003;111:380–8.

70. Hirota K, Kazaoka K, Niimoto I, et al. Discovery of 8-hydroxyadenines as a novel type of interferon inducer. J Med Chem 2002;45:5419–22.

71. Tsai Y-G, Yang KD, Niu D-M, et al. TLR2 agonists enhance CD8+Foxp3+ regulatory T cells and suppress Th2 immune responses during allergen immunotherapy. J Immunol 2010;184:7229–37.

72. Lombardi V, Van Overtvelt L, Horiot S, et al. Toll-like receptor 2 agonist Pam3CSK4 enhances the induction of antigen-specific tolerance via the sublingual route. Clin Exp Allergy 2008;38:1819–29.

73. Marsland BJ, Gollwitzer ES. Host–microorganism interactions in lung diseases. Nat Rev Immunol 2014;14:827–35.

74. Moussu H, Van Overtvelt L, Horiot S, et al. Bifidobacterium bifidum NCC 453 promotes tolerance induction in murine models of sublingual immunotherapy. Int Arch Allergy Immunol 2012;158:35–42.

75. Schwarzer M, Srutkova D, Schabussova I, et al. Neonatal colonization of germfree mice with Bifidobacterium longum prevents allergic sensitization to major birch pollen allergen Bet v 1. Vaccine 2013;31:5405–12.

76. Fiocchi A. World Allergy Organization-McMaster University Guidelines for Allergic Disease Prevention (GLAD-P): probiotics. World Allergy Organ J 2015;8:4.

77. Costa DJ, Marteau P, Amouyal M, et al. Efficacy and safety of the probiotic Lactobacillus paracasei LP-33in allergic rhinitis: a double-blind, randomized, placebo-controlledtrial (GA2LEN Study). Eur J Clin Nutr 2014;68:602–7.

78. Rask C, Holmgren J, Fredriksson M, et al. Prolonged oral treatment with low doses of allergen conjugated to cholera toxin B subunit suppresses immunoglobulin E antibody responses in sensitized mice. Clin Exp Allergy 2000;30: 1024–32.

79. Gloudemans AK, Plantinga M, Guilliams M, et al. The mucosal adjuvant cholera toxin B instructs non-mucosal dendritic cells to promote IgA production via retinoic acid and TGF-β. PLoS One 2013;8:e59822.

80. Zuany-Amorim C, Manlius C, Trifilieff A, et al. Long-term protective and antigen-specific effect of heat-killed Mycobacterium vaccae in a murine model of allergic pulmonary inflammation. J Immunol 2002;169:1492–9.

81. Bakdash G, Schneider LP, van Capel TMM, et al. Intradermal application of vitamin D3 increases migration of CD14+ dermal dendritic cells and promotes the development of Foxp3+ regulatory T cells. Hum Vaccin Immunother 2013;9:250–8.

82. Heine G, Tabeling C, Hartmann B, et al. 25-hydroxvitamin D3 promotes the long-term effect of specific immunotherapy in a murine allergy model. J Immunol 2014;193:1017–23.
83. Majak P, Rychlik B, Stelmach I. The effect of oral steroids with and without vitamin D3 on early efficacy of immunotherapy in asthmatic children. Clin Exp Allergy 2009;39:1830–41.
84. Baris S, Kiykim A, Ozen A, et al. Vitamin D as an adjunct to subcutaneous allergen immunotherapy in asthmatic children sensitized to house dust mite. Allergy 2014;69:246–53.
85. Gregory AE, Titball R, Williamson D. Vaccine delivery using nanoparticles. Front Cell Infect Microbiol 2013;3:13.
86. Kawakita A, Shirasaki H, Yasutomi M, et al. Immunotherapy with oligomannose-coated liposomes ameliorates allergic symptoms in a murine food allergy model. Allergy 2012;67:371–9.
87. Ishii M, Koyama A, Iseki H, et al. Anti-allergic potential of oligomannose-coated liposome-entrapped Cry j 1 as immunotherapy for Japanese cedar pollinosis in mice. Int Immunopharmacol 2010;10:1041–6.
88. Erikçi E, Gursel M, Gürsel İ. Differential immune activation following encapsulation of immunostimulatory CpG oligodeoxynucleotide in nanoliposomes. Biomaterials 2011;32:1715–23.
89. Basomba A, Tabar AI, de Rojas DHF, et al. Allergen vaccination with a liposome-encapsulated extract of Dermatophagoides pteronyssinus: a randomized, double-blind, placebo-controlled trial in asthmatic patients. J Allergy Clin Immunol 2002;109:943–8.
90. De Souza Rebouças J, Esparza I, Ferrer M, et al. Nanoparticulate adjuvants and delivery systems for allergen immunotherapy. J Biomed Biotechnol 2012;2012: 474605.
91. Fadok VA, Bratton DL, Henson PM. Phagocyte receptors for apoptotic cells: recognition, uptake, and consequences. J Clin Invest 2001;108:957–62.
92. Kündig TM, Klimek L, Schendzielorz P, et al. Is the allergen really needed in allergy immunotherapy? Curr Treat Options Allergy 2015;2:72–82.
93. Kündig TM, Senti G, Schnetzler G, et al. Der p 1 peptide on virus-like particles is safe and highly immunogenic in healthy adults. J Allergy Clin Immunol 2006; 117:1470–6.
94. Senti G, Johansen P, Haug S, et al. Use of A-type CpG oligodeoxynucleotides as an adjuvant in allergen-specific immunotherapy in humans: a phase I/IIa clinical trial. Clin Exp Allergy 2009;39:562–70.
95. Klimek L, Willers J, Hammann-Haenni A, et al. Assessment of clinical efficacy of CYT003-QbG10 in patients with allergic rhinoconjunctivitis: a phase IIb study. Clin Exp Allergy 2011;41:1305–12.
96. Edlmayr J, Niespodziana K, Linhart B, et al. A combination vaccine for allergy and rhinovirus infections based on rhinovirus-derived surface protein VP1 and a nonallergenic peptide of the major timothy grass pollen allergen Phl p 1. J Immunol 2009;182:6298–306.
97. Sanders MT, Brown LE, Deliyannis G, et al. ISCOM-based vaccines: the second decade. Immunol Cell Biol 2005;83:119–28.
98. Beacock-Sharp H, Donachie AM, Robson NC, et al. A role for dendritic cells in the priming of antigen-specific CD4+ and CD8+ T lymphocytes by immune-stimulating complexes in vivo. Int Immunol 2003;15:711–20.
99. Craparo EF, Bondì ML. Application of polymeric nanoparticles in immunotherapy. Curr Opin Allergy Clin Immunol 2012;12:658–64.

100. Liu Z, Guo H, Wu Y, et al. Local nasal immunotherapy: efficacy of dermatophagoides farinae-chitosan vaccine in murine asthma. Int Arch Allergy Immunol 2009;150:221–8.
101. Razafindratsita A, Saint-Lu N, Mascarell L, et al. Improvement of sublingual immunotherapy efficacy with a mucoadhesive allergen formulation. J Allergy Clin Immunol 2007;120:278–85.
102. Saint-Lu N, Tourdot S, Razafindratsita A, et al. Targeting the allergen to oral dendritic cells with mucoadhesive chitosan particles enhances tolerance induction. Allergy 2009;64:1003–13.
103. Li GP, Liu Z-G, Liao B, et al. Induction of Th1-type immune response by chitosan nanoparticles containing plasmid DNA encoding house dust mite allergen Der p 2 for oral vaccination in mice. Cell Mol Immunol 2009;6:45–50.
104. Chew JL, Wolfowicz CB, Mao H-Q, et al. Chitosan nanoparticles containing plasmid DNA encoding house dust mite allergen, Der p 1 for oral vaccination in mice. Vaccine 2003;21:2720–9.
105. Roy K, Mao HQ, Huang SK, et al. Oral gene delivery with chitosan–DNA nanoparticles generates immunologic protection in a murine model of peanut allergy. Nat Med 1999;5:387–91.
106. Goldmann K, Ensminger SM, Spriewald BM. Oral gene application using chitosan-DNA nanoparticles induces transferable tolerance. Clin Vaccine Immunol 2012;19:1758–64.
107. Schöll I, Kopp T, Bohle B, et al. Biodegradable PLGA particles for improved systemic and mucosal treatment of Type I allergy. Immunol Allergy Clin North Am 2006;26:349–64, ix.
108. Schöll I, Weissenböck A, Förster-Waldl E, et al. Allergen-loaded biodegradable poly(D,L-lactic-co-glycolic) acid nanoparticles down-regulate an ongoing Th2 response in the BALB/c mouse model. Clin Exp Allergy 2004; 34:315–21.
109. Xiao X, Zeng X, Zhang X, et al. Effects of Caryota mitis profilin-loaded PLGA nanoparticles in a murine model of allergic asthma. Int J Nanomedicine 2013; 8:4553–62.
110. Salem AK. A promising CpG adjuvant-loaded nanoparticle-based vaccine for treatment of dust mite allergies. Immunotherapy 2014;6:1161–3.
111. Joshi VB, Adamcakova-Dodd A, Jing X, et al. Development of a poly (lactic-co-glycolic acid) particle vaccine to protect against house dust mite induced allergy. AAPS J 2014;16:975–85.
112. Maldonado RA, LaMothe RA, Ferrari JD, et al. Polymeric synthetic nanoparticles for the induction of antigen-specific immunological tolerance. Proc Natl Acad Sci U S A 2015;112:E156–65.
113. Singh A, Peppas NA. Hydrogels and scaffolds for immunomodulation. Adv Mater 2014;26:6530–41.
114. Gómez S, Gamazo C, Roman BS, et al. AN nanoparticles as an adjuvant for oral immunotherapy with allergens. Vaccine 2007;25:5263–71.
115. De S Reboucas J, Irache JM, Camacho AI, et al. Immunogenicity of peanut proteins containing poly(anhydride) nanoparticles. Clin Vaccine Immunol 2014;21: 1106–12.
116. Licciardi M, Montana G, Bondì ML, et al. International Journal of Pharmaceutics. Int J Pharm 2014;465:275–83.
117. De Boever EH, Ashman C, Cahn AP, et al. Efficacy and safety of an anti-IL-13 mAb in patients with severe asthma: a randomized trial. J Allergy Clin Immunol 2014;133:989–96.e4.

118. Ortega HG, Liu MC, Pavord ID, et al. Mepolizumab treatment in patients with severe eosinophilic asthma. N Engl J Med 2014;371:1198–207.
119. Lambert N, Guiddir T, Amat F, et al. Pre-treatment by omalizumab allows allergen immunotherapy in children and young adults with severe allergic asthma. Pediatr Allergy Immunol 2014;25:829–32.

Baked Milk and Egg Diets for Milk and Egg Allergy Management

Stephanie A. Leonard, MD[a],*, Anna H. Nowak-Węgrzyn, MD[b]

KEYWORDS

- Cow's milk allergy • Hen's egg allergy • Baked milk • Baked egg
- Extensively heated milk • Extensively heated egg • Milk allergy • Egg allergy

KEY POINTS

- Baked milk and egg are well tolerated in the diets of a majority of milk- and egg-allergic children.
- Inclusion of baked milk and egg in the diet of children who are tolerant of these baked forms may accelerate the resolution of milk and egg allergy.
- Clinical factors and biomarkers for predicting baked milk and egg tolerability or reactivity are lacking, and further research is needed.
- Tolerance to baked milk and egg may be a marker of a milder and transient milk and egg allergy.
- Anaphylaxis to baked milk and egg can occur, thus physician-supervised introduction is recommended.

INTRODUCTION

Cow's milk (CM) and egg allergies are some of the most common food allergies in young children. It is estimated that up to 3.8% and 2% of children less than 5 years of age have CM and egg allergy, respectively.[1] CM and egg are a large part of diets in many cultures. These allergens are commonly found in baked goods and are an important source of protein and calories, particularly in young children. Strict elimination of all CM and egg products may put children at risk for nutritional deficiencies as well as have a psychosocial impact. Studies show that the baked form of CM and egg is less allergenic and tolerated by a majority of CM- and egg-allergic children. The

The authors have nothing to disclose.
a Division of Pediatric Allergy & Immunology, Department of Pediatrics, Rady Children's Hospital San Diego, University of California, San Diego, 3020 Children's Way, MC 5114, San Diego, CA 92123, USA; b Division of Pediatric Allergy, Department of Pediatrics, Jaffe Food Allergy Institute, Icahn School of Medicine at Mount Sinai, Box 1198, One Gustave L. Levy Place, New York, NY 10029, USA
* Corresponding author.
E-mail address: saleonard@ucsd.edu

ability to add baked CM and egg products to the diets of CM- and egg-allergic children can improve the nutritional content of their diet and increase quality of life. In addition, data suggest that including baked CM and egg in the diet may accelerate resolution of CM and egg allergy. The goal of this review is to examine our current understanding of the effects of baked CM and egg in the management of CM and egg allergy.

PREVALENCE OF BAKED MILK AND EGG TOLERANCE

A CM allergy natural history study in a multi-site US population by Wood and colleagues,[2] which followed 293 infants, found that 21% (32 of 155) of subjects with CM allergy at the 5-year time point tolerated some baked milk products. An egg allergy natural history study in the same population by Sicherer and colleagues,[3] which followed 213 infants, found that 38% (43 of 113) of subjects with egg allergy at the 6-year time point tolerated some baked egg products. Percentages are typically higher in studies in which baked CM and egg tolerance are proactively evaluated with oral food challenges. For example, in a large population study in Australia by Peters and colleagues[4] in which baked egg challenges were offered at age 1 and 2 years of age to challenge-proven raw egg–reactive children, 80% (n = 126 of 157) of subjects tolerated baked egg at baseline.

Overall, studies show that between 69% and 83% of CM-allergic children can tolerate baked CM, and between 63% and 83% of egg-allergic children can tolerated baked egg, as detailed in **Tables 1** and **2, Box 1**. The studies that were reviewed used similar methods for baking CM and egg. In baked CM studies, a serving size was the equivalent of 0.5 to 2.6 g of CM protein in a muffin or cupcake baked at 350°F (180°C) for 20 to 30 minutes.[5–8] In baked egg studies, a serving size was the equivalent of 1 to 3 g egg protein in a muffin or cupcake baked at 350°F to 375°F (180°C–190°C) for 20 to 30 minutes.[9–16]

Not many studies have examined the tolerance of baked milk or egg in patients with eosinophilic esophagitis (EoE). One study examined 15 patients with EoE who were electively ingesting baked milk. Eleven patients (73%) showed tolerance of baked CM ingestion, and 4 patients showed a relapse of EoE disease on esophageal biopsy ($\geq$10 eosinophils per high-power field).[17] This small study suggests that baked milk and egg proteins may be tolerated most patients with EoE and warrant further investigation.

FOOD PROCESSING

Proteins possess both sequential and conformational epitopes that immunoglobulin E (IgE) antibodies may recognize and bind to. Heating alters conformational epitopes and induces other protein structural changes so that IgE antibodies may no longer bind.[18] Interaction of food proteins with one another (such as CM and egg with a wheat matrix) may also alter allergenicity.[19]

Casein makes up 80% of CM protein and is immunodominant, whereas whey makes up 20% and consists primarily of α-lactalbumin and β-lactoglobulin.[20] Casein and α-lactalbumin are more heat stable than β-lactoglobulin.[18] In one study, most children older than 9 years with persistent CM allergy had IgE binding to sequential (linear) casein epitopes as compared with patients younger than 3 years who are likely to outgrow CM allergy.[21]

Ovalbumin makes up 54% of egg white (EW) protein, however, ovomucoid (OM), which makes up 11%, is considered the immunodominant protein.[22] Compared with ovalbumin, OM is stable to both heat and digestive enzymes.[23] Children with persistent egg allergy have had higher levels of OM-specific IgE, specifically to sequential (linear) OM epitopes.[22,24]

Table 1
Prevalence of baked milk tolerance in studies using baked milk challenges

	Number of Subjects	Median Age (y) (Unless Indicated)	Unbaked Milk OFC?	Median CM IgE (kU$_A$/L) of BM Tolerant	Median CM IgE (kU$_A$/L) of BM Reactive	Median CM SPT Wheal (mm) of BM Tolerant	Median CM SPT Wheal (mm) of BM Reactive	Proportion Tolerant to BM (%)
Nowak-Wegrzyn et al,[5] 2008	91	Mean 7.5 (range, 2.1–17.3)	Yes; unless >95% PPV testing[a]	2.43 (range, 0–79.1)	11.6 (range, 0.69–101.0)	7 (range, 2.5–19.0)	9.5 (range, 5–24)	75
Caubet et al,[6] 2013[b]	121	BM tolerant: 7.5 (range, 4–11); BM reactive: 8.0 (range, 4.4–10.9)	Yes; unless >95% PPV testing[a]	4.0 (range, 0.2–42.3)	11.9 (range, 0.8–50.5)	—	—	69
Bartnikas et al,[7] 2012	35	BM tolerant: 8.9 (range, 3.9–18.1); BM reactive: 3.7 (range, 3.1–11.0)	No	1.93 (range, <0.35–20.6)	2.39 (range, <0.35–31.0)	10 (range, 0–20)	15 (range, 7–20)	83
Mehr et al,[8] 2014	70	BM tolerant: 4.5 (IQR, 2.5–8.0); BM reactive: 7.3 (IQR, 4.9–9.6)	No	—	—	8 (IQR, 7–10)	8.5 (IQR, 7.5–10)	73

Abbreviations: BM, baked milk; IgE, immunoglobulin E; IQR, interquartile range; OFC, oral food challenge; PPV, positive predictive value; SPT, skin prick test.
[a] Greater than 95% positive predictive value CM immunoglobulin E for milk allergy: greater than 5 kU$_A$/L in children 2 years of age or younger or greater than 15 kU$_A$/L in children older than 2 years; greater than 95% positive predictive value CM skin prick test wheal diameter of 8 mm or greater.
[b] Second cohort only; first cohort is already described in Nowak-Wegrzyn and colleagues.[5]

Table 2
Prevalence of baked egg tolerance in studies using baked egg challenges

	Number of Subjects	Median Age (y) (Unless Indicated)	Unbaked Egg OFC?	Median EW IgE (kUA/L) of BE Tolerant	Median EW IgE (kUA/L) of BE Reactive	Median EW SPT Wheal (mm) of BE Tolerant	Median EW SPT Wheal (mm) of BE Reactive	Proportion Tolerant to BE (%)
Lemon-Mule et al,[9] 2008	91	Mean 6.9 (range, 1.6–18.6)	Yes; unless >95% PPV testing[a]	1.3 (25%–75% IQR, 0.6–4.3)	5.1 (25%–75% IQR, 1.9–11.1)	6 (IQR, 5–8)	8 (IQR, 6.3–9)	70
Clark et al,[10] 2011	95	4.6 (IQR, 2.7–7.3)	Yes	2.2 (IQR, 0.7–7.7)	5.1 (IQR, 2.6–16.6)	4 (IQR, 3–5)	6 (IQR, 4–7.5)	66 (by 6 y of age)
Lieberman et al,[11] 2012	100	5.9 (range, 1.2–19.8)	No	2.81	5.85	7	7	66
Cortot et al,[12] 2012	52	7.2 (range, 2.2–18); BE tolerant: 8.8; BE reactive: 7.0	No	2.02 (range, <0.35–13.00)	1.52 (range, 0.51–6.10)	12 (range, 0–35)	17 (range, 10–30)	83
Turner et al,[13] 2013	236	BE tolerant: 3.2 (IQR, 1.8–5.8); BE mild-moderate symptoms: 4.7 (IQR, 1.9–6.8); BE anaphylaxis: 4.8 (range, 3.0–5.9)	No	—	—	8 (IQR, 7–10)	Mild-moderate symptoms: 9 (range, 6–11); anaphylaxis: 9 (range, 8.0–11.5)	64

Tan et al,[14] 2013	143	3.8 (IQR, 1.8–6.7)	No	—	—	8 (IQR, 7–11)	9 (IQR, 8–11)	63
Bartnikas et al,[15] 2013	169	BE tolerant: 5.22 (range, 0.84–17.07); BE reactive: 6.18 (range, 2.02–12.93)	No	1.31 (range, <0.35–42.00)	6.00 (range, <0.35–17.10)	9 (range, 0–35)	13 (range, 3–20)	84
Turner et al,[16] 2014	186	BE tolerant: 5.1 (IQR, 3.8–8.8); BE reactive: 5.6 (IQR, 2.7–10.6)	No	—	—	5 (IQR, 4–7)	8 (IQR, 5–10)	66

Abbreviations: BE, baked egg; EW, egg white; IgE, immunoglobulin E; IQR, interquartile range; OFC, oral food challenge; PPV, positive predictive value; SPT, skin prick test.

[a] Greater than 95% positive predictive value egg white immunoglobulin E for egg allergy: greater than 2 kU$_A$/L in children 2 years of age or younger or greater than 7 kU$_A$/L in children older than 2 years.

Box 1
Baked milk and egg challenge protocol

Preparation

- Provide baked milk or egg recipe to family.

- For children older than 2 years: If using recipes published in Leonard and colleagues,[33] ask the family to bring in 1 muffin if the recipe made 6 muffins or 2 to 3 muffins if it made greater than 6.

- For younger children less than 2 years of age and picky eaters, the total serving size should be adjusted, for example, one-half muffin.

- Schedule the challenge when other atopic conditions are stable (eczema, asthma, allergic rhinitis, urticaria/angioedema, and so forth).

- Medications that may interfere with the challenge should be discontinued at the appropriate time before the challenge.[36]
  o Antihistamines: 5 half-lives
  o H2-blockers: 12 hours
  o Oral/IM/IV steroids: 3 days to 2 weeks
  o Leukotriene antagonist: 24 hours
  o Short- and long-acting bronchodilators: 8 hours

- Consider delaying the challenge if patients have had a significant clinical reaction to the challenge food within the past 6 to 12 months.

Challenge day

- Ensure medications have been discontinued for the appropriate length of time.

- Obtain baseline vitals, including weight for medication dosing. Consider the pulmonary function test or peak flow in patients older than 5 years with a history of asthma.

- Perform a thorough physical examination. Patients should be free of fever, significant rash, upper or lower respiratory symptoms, abdominal symptoms, or vomiting and diarrhea within the past 48 hours.

- Calculate doses of emergency medications.

Challenge procedure

- Administer doses 15 to 20 minutes apart. Perform a brief physical examination between each dose. If there is a suspicion that a reaction may be developing, consider delaying the next dose, repeating the last dose, or stopping the challenge.

- Divide 1 muffin (containing 1.3 g milk protein or 2.2 g of egg protein) into
  o Dose 1: one-eighth muffin
  o Dose 2: one-eighth muffin
  o Dose 3: one-quarter muffin
  o Dose 4: one-half muffin

- With a higher-risk challenge, muffins may be divided into more doses.

Treatment of reactions

- Antihistamines
  o Cetirizine 0.25 mg/kg by mouth (max 10 mg)
  o Diphenhydramine 1.0 to 1.5 mg/kg by mouth/IM/IV (max 50 mg)

- Epinephrine 1:1000 concentration
  o 0.01 mL/kg (maximum 0.5 mL) IM anterolateral thigh
  o Auto-injector 0.15 mg (<25 kg) or 0.3 mg (>25 kg) anterolateral IM thigh

- Steroids: prednisolone by mouth or methylprednisolone (Solumedrol) IM/IV 1 to 2 mg/kg (max 60 mg)

- H2-antagonists: ranitidine 2 mg/kg by mouth or IV (max 50 mg)

- Albuterol: nebulization 2.5 to 5.0 mg × 3 doses

- Oxygen: 8 to 10 L/min via face mask

- IV fluids: 10 to 15 mL/kg bolus normal saline/lactated ringer bolus (max 1000 mL per bolus)

Discharge instructions

- Passed challenge:
  ○ Starting the following day, offer 1 to 3 servings of the baked foods daily, at minimum 3 times per week, using home-baked muffins or equivalents (eg, bread rolls or cupcakes) or store-bought baked foods with milk or egg listed as third ingredient or further down on the ingredient list.[33]
  ○ Continue avoidance of not well-baked foods with milk or egg ingredients.
  ○ Provide an emergency plan and prescription for epinephrine auto-injector in case of reactions to unbaked milk/egg.
  ○ Consider scheduling pizza challenge for baked-milk, muffin-tolerant patients.
  ○ Reevaluate skin prick tests and serum CM/egg white–specific IgE levels in 6 to 12 months and consider challenges to regular unbaked milk or egg based on the declining immunologic parameters.

- Failed challenge:
  ○ Continue strict avoidance of all forms of milk or egg.
  ○ Provide an emergency plan and prescription for epinephrine auto-injector.
  ○ Milk: Consider repeating the baked milk challenge in 1 to 3 years, with longer time intervals for the patients who had anaphylaxis during the baked milk challenge.
  ○ Egg: Consider repeating the baked egg challenge in 1 year.

Abbreviations: IM, intramuscular; IV, intravenous; max, maximum; min, minimum.

A recent study by Bloom and colleagues[25] using gel electrophoresis showed that the casein bands persisted for up to 60 minutes of heating, whereas β-lactoglobulin and α-lactalbumin bands were undetectable after 15 to 20 minutes of heating.[25] Immunoblotting using pooled serum from baked milk–reactive subjects showed preserved IgE binding to casein even with extended heating time. Similarly, the OM band persisted after 25 minutes of heating, whereas the ovalbumin band gradually weakened in the same amount of time. Immunoblotting using pooled serum from baked egg–reactive subjects showed stronger binding to scrambled EW, hardboiled EW, waffles and muffins containing egg, compared with baked egg or regular egg–tolerant subjects.

Previously it was shown that heating OM in a wheat matrix makes OM insoluble, likely from polymerization of wheat with OM via disulfide bonds.[19,26] Bloom and colleagues[25] also found that the presence of a wheat matrix during heating reduced IgE binding to CM proteins.

PREDICTIVE BIOMARKERS

As compared with evaluation of regular egg allergy, skin prick test (SPT) or specific IgE levels to CM or EW proteins have not been reliable in predicting baked milk or egg tolerance. Different patient populations and variability in methods of baking or heating CM and EW have resulted in varied proposed cutoffs.

Nowak-Wegrzyn and colleagues[5] found that only very high CM IgE levels had substantial positive predictive values (PPVs). A CM IgE level of 35 kU_A/L or greater only had a greater than 50% PPV, whereas CM IgE less than 0.35 kU_A/L had a 100% negative predictive value (NPV). A cutoff of CM IgE 5.0 kU_A/L was suggested for performing baked milk oral food challenge (OFC). Caubet and colleagues[6] evaluated data from 225 prospective baked milk OFCs, including 100 from Nowak-Wegrzyn and colleagues[5] and suggested cutoffs of casein IgE 4.95 kU$_A$/L (89% NPV, 54% PPV) and CM IgE 9.97 kU$_A$/L (86% NPV, 60% PPV). Bartnikas and colleagues[7] retrospectively studied physician-diagnosed milk-allergic children and found that a casein IgE of 0.9 kU$_A$/L and CM IgE of 1.0 kU$_A$/L had a greater than 90% NPV, while all subjects with casein IgE of greater than 10.3 kU$_A$/L and CM IgE greater than 20.6 kU$_A$/L had were baked milk reactive.

In regards to skin testing, Nowak-Wegrzyn and colleagues[5] found that a CM SPT of 14 mm had a greater than 50% PPV and a CM SPT less than 5 mm had a 100% NPV, with high sensitivity but poor specificity. Bartnikas and colleagues[7] found that all subjects with a CM SPT of less than 7 mm were baked milk tolerance, and all subjects with a casein SPT mm of greater than 15 mm were baked milk reactive. Conversely, Mehr and colleagues[8] found that CM or muffin SPT wheal was not predictive of baked milk tolerance.

In the natural history study by Sicherer and colleagues,[3] the baseline egg-specific IgE level did not predict who would go on to tolerate baked egg. Similarly, Cortot and colleagues[12] found no difference in EW-specific IgE levels between baked egg–tolerant and baked egg–reactive patients. Lemon-Mule and colleagues[9] found that only very high levels of OM-specific and EW-specific IgE had substantial PPVs. OM-specific IgE of 50 kU$_A$/L had a 90% PPV, and EW-specific IgE of 75 kU$_A$/L had greater than 50% PPV. An undetectable OM-specific IgE still had 10% PPV for baked egg reactivity. In the same population, Lieberman and colleagues[11] retrospectively studied baked egg tolerance in a clinical setting and found that an EW-specific IgE of 10 kU$_A$/L had a 60% PPV with high specificity but low sensitivity. Bartnikas and colleagues[15] found that OM-specific IgE was not superior to EW-specific IgE in predicting baked egg reactivity and suggested the following cutoffs with greater than 90% NPV for performing a baked-egg challenge: OM-specific IgE 0.35 kU$_A$/L and EW-specific IgE 6.0 kU$_A$/L.

In a large Japanese study, 108 children (median age, 34.5 months) with suspected egg allergy underwent double-blind, placebo-controlled food challenges with raw and heated egg.[27] Heated egg was prepared by heating liquid EW at 194°F (90°C) for 60 minutes, then freeze drying and homogenizing into a powder. The outcomes of the challenges were compared with the serum concentration of specific IgE antibodies and total IgE by using ImmunoCAP (Phadia AB, Uppsala, Sweden). Reactions to heated EW were observed in 38 children, considered allergic to raw and heated egg; 29 children reacted only to raw EW, and 41 children were heated and raw egg tolerant. Receiver operating characteristic analysis showed that EW-IgE was most accurate in the diagnosis of allergy to raw EW. The positive decision point, based on 95% clinical specificity, was 7.4 kU$_A$/L; the negative decision point, based on 95% clinical sensitivity, was 0.6 kU$_A$/L. For reaction to heated EW, OM-IgE was superior. The positive decision point was 10.8 kU$_A$/L, and the negative decision point was 1.2 kU$_A$/L. Collectively, data from various studies suggest that egg-allergic children with low levels of OM-specific IgE antibodies have the best odds of tolerating baked egg. In a research setting, a model that included the interactions between IgE and IgG$_4$ to ovalbumin and OM had enhanced accuracy in predicting reactivity to baked egg.[28]

With regard to skin testing, Lemon-Mule et al[9] found that a large EW SPT wheal of 15 mm only had a 60% PPV for baked egg reactivity and a negative EW SPT wheal had less than 5% PPV. Bartnikas and colleagues[15] suggested an EW SPT cutoff of 11 mm with greater than 90% NPV. Tan and colleagues[14] studied baked egg tolerance in egg-allergic children less than 7 years old and found that a large OM SPT of 11 mm or greater had a 100% PPV and a muffin SPT of 2 mm or less had a 88% NPV. In the study by Lieberman and colleagues,[11] EW SPT was not found to be significant.

Similarly, Turner and colleagues[16] retrospectively studied the ability of egg extract and raw egg SPT to predict baked egg tolerance in physician-diagnosed, egg-allergic children. Neither SPT nor the ratio of egg extract/raw egg SPT was helpful in predicting baked egg challenge outcomes.

INFLUENCE ON REGULAR COW'S MILK AND EGG TOLERANCE

In the natural history study by Wood and colleagues,[2] CM allergy resolution was 4 times more likely in subjects who tolerated baked milk ($P<.0001$). In the natural history study by Sicherer and colleagues,[3] egg allergy resolution rate was 70.8% in those consuming baked egg at an early 6-month follow-up, compared with 45.2% in those not consuming baked egg and 57.1% in those who reported a reaction to baked egg. This finding gave an instantaneous risk ratio of 3.4 for egg allergy resolution in the baked egg–consuming group versus the nonconsumption group ($P<.001$). In the natural history study by Peters and colleagues,[4] subjects reactive to baked egg at 1 year of age compared with subjects who were tolerant were 5 times more likely to have persistent egg allergy at age 2 years (13% vs 56%, respectively; adjusted odds ratio 5.27; $P = .02$).

Shorter time to regular CM and egg tolerance in patients who tolerate baked milk and egg may indicate a milder allergy phenotype. However, in Sicherer and colleagues,[3] the type of regular egg reaction and baseline egg IgE level did not predict who would go on to tolerate baked egg. Alternatively, higher rates of regular CM and egg tolerance in baked milk– and egg-tolerant patients may reflect a more proactive approach to evaluation for CM and egg allergy resolution when baked milk or egg is already tolerated. Adding baked milk and egg to the diet was the protocol for subjects who were tolerant in the baked milk study by Nowak-Wegrzyn and colleagues[5] and in the baked egg study by Lemon-Mule and colleagues[9]; however, it was not mandated in the CM and egg allergy natural history studies by Sicherer and colleagues[3] and Wood and colleagues,[2] which reported lower baked milk and egg tolerance. In Peters and colleagues,[4] it was noted that baked egg–tolerant subjects who frequently ($\geq$5 times per month) ingested baked egg versus infrequently or not at all were 3 times more likely to develop regular egg tolerance (adjusted odds ratio 3.52; $P = .009$).

Lastly, there are data suggesting that ingestion of baked milk and egg results in immune modulation and may actively lead to earlier tolerance of regular CM and egg, in a sense acting as a form of immunotherapy. In Nowak-Wegrzyn and colleagues[5], Kim and colleagues[29] and Leonard and colleagues,[30] ingesting baked milk and egg was associated with a significant decrease in CM- and EW- specific SPT wheal diameter and EW- and OM- specific IgE levels, and an increase in specific IgG4 levels to casein and OM. This finding is commonly seen in allergen immunotherapy, such as subcutaneous immunotherapy for allergic rhinitis or oral immunotherapy for food allergy. In Kim and colleagues,[29] subjects ingesting baked milk were 16 times more likely than the comparison group to become regular milk tolerant ($P<.001$). In Leonard and colleagues,[30] subjects ingesting baked egg were 14.6 times more likely than the comparison group to develop regular egg tolerance, and they developed tolerance earlier ($P<.0001$).

SAFETY

Inclusion of baked milk and egg into the diets of milk- and egg-allergic children who are tolerant appears to be very safe and well tolerated. In Kim and colleagues[29] and Leonard and colleagues,[30] no acute allergic reactions to properly baked milk and egg were reported at home. In addition, there was no worsening of underlying eczema, asthma, or allergic rhinitis. One baked milk–tolerant subject continued to tolerate baked milk after developing EoE.[29] A baked milk–reactive subject and 5 subjects in the comparison group also developed EoE while strictly avoiding milk. One baked egg–tolerant subject developed atypical food protein–induced enterocolitis syndrome to egg and subsequently removed all forms of egg from the diet.[30] In two other studies, acute reactions to baked milk (n = 3) and egg (n = 1) were reported at home, one to baked milk that required epinephrine.[7,13]

Anaphylaxis to baked milk and egg does occur.[5,9,12,14,16,31] In Nowak-Wegrzyn and colleagues,[5] reactivity to baked milk was a marker of a more severe CM allergy as only the baked milk–reactive subjects experienced anaphylaxis during OFC, compared with none of the baked milk–tolerant subjects who reacted to unheated milk. The following were not found to be predictors of baked milk anaphylaxis: age, history of asthma, respiratory symptoms at first reaction to milk or CM-induced anaphylaxis, elapsed time since last anaphylaxis, SPT size, or lifetime peak CM-specific IgE levels. In Mehr and colleagues,[8] 4 out of 19 positive baked milk OFCs required adrenaline, including one subject after ingesting one-sixteenth of a muffin (approximately 3 mg of baked CM protein). Baked milk reactivity predictors were found to include a history of CM-induced anaphylaxis, food allergies to greater than 3 food groups, asthma, and requiring asthma preventive therapy. Age at OFC, time since the last clinical reaction, previous anaphylaxis to other foods, and/or other atopic condition (eczema) were not predictive. In Turner and colleagues,[13] of the 86 children who were baked egg reactive, 12 (14%) developed anaphylaxis, including 4 to less than 100 mg baked egg protein. Adrenaline was given in 5 children, and a second dose was used for persistent hypotension in one child. Food allergy to 3 or more food groups was found to be predictive of baked egg reactivity; but SPT, prior EW-induced anaphylaxis, asthma on preventer therapy, history of another atopic condition, or a history of anaphylaxis to foods other than egg were not.

Conversely, in Clark and colleagues,[10] adrenaline was not required for any of the 28 of 77 (37%) positive baked egg challenges, when included gastrointestinal symptoms in 68% OFCs. The investigators suggested that reintroduction of baked egg in children aged 2 to 3 years with a history of previous mild reaction to egg and no asthma could be done at home. In general, however, because of the risk of anaphylaxis, it is recommended that evaluation of baked milk and egg tolerance be done under physician supervision in children who do not have a reliable history of already regularly tolerating them in clinically relevant amounts.[32]

DIETARY GUIDELINES

Published recipes and dietary guidelines for baked milk and egg can be found in the recent Leonard and colleagues[33] review. Although the exact frequency of baked milk and egg ingestion to be the most beneficial is not yet known, ingestion a few times a week seems reasonable.[33] Baked egg and milk tolerance may develop over time and in older children; therefore, rechallenging should be considered in those children who are initially baked milk or egg reactive.[5,9,10,34]

Although baked milk and egg may accelerate the resolution the milk and egg allergy, data do not support the use of baked milk and egg in the prevention of food allergy. In a study investigating associations between egg allergy at 12 months of age and age of introducing different forms of egg, Koplin and colleagues[35] found that between 4 and 6 months of age, first exposure to cooked egg (boiled, scrambled, fried, or poached) reduced the risk of egg allergy compared with first exposure to egg in baked good. Thus, more intact egg protein may be necessary for the prevention of egg allergy as compared to the use of modified egg protein in the possible treatment of the established allergy.

SUMMARY

Baked milk and egg appears to be well tolerated by most milk- and egg-allergic children. There is evidence that inclusion of baked milk and egg in the diets of children who are tolerant may accelerate the resolution of milk and egg allergy. Although further research is needed on biomarkers that can predict baked milk or egg reactivity, in general, the higher the specific IgE level or SPT, the less likely that baked milk and egg will be tolerated. Some data suggest that casein- and ovomucoid-specific IgE levels may be useful in predicting reactivity. Physician-supervised introduction of baked milk and egg is recommended since anaphylaxis to baked milk and egg has occurred and is difficult to predict. Tolerance of baked milk is a marker of a mild and transient milk allergy, whereas tolerance to baked egg is not as predictive of a milder phenotype of egg allergy. Children reactive to baked milk and egg have a more persistent milk and egg allergy and are in need of treatments that accelerate tolerance development.

REFERENCES

1. Sicherer SH. Epidemiology of food allergy. J Allergy Clin Immunol 2011;127: 594–602.
2. Wood RA, Sicherer SH, Vickery BP, et al. The natural history of milk allergy in an observational cohort. J Allergy Clin Immunol 2013;131:805–12.
3. Sicherer SH, Wood RA, Vickery BP, et al. The natural history of egg allergy in an observational cohort. J Allergy Clin Immunol 2014;133:492–9.
4. Peters RL, Dharmage SC, Gurrin LC, et al. The natural history and clinical predictors of egg allergy in the first 2 years of life: a prospective, population-based cohort study. J Allergy Clin Immunol 2014;133:485–91.
5. Nowak-Wegrzyn A, Bloom KA, Sicherer SH, et al. Tolerance to extensively heated milk in children with cow's milk allergy. J Allergy Clin Immunol 2008;122:342–7, 347.e1–2.
6. Caubet JC, Nowak-Wegrzyn A, Moshier E, et al. Utility of casein-specific IgE levels in predicting reactivity to baked milk. J Allergy Clin Immunol 2013;131: 222–4.e1–4.
7. Bartnikas LM, Sheehan WJ, Hoffman EB, et al. Predicting food challenge outcomes for baked milk: role of specific IgE and skin prick testing. Ann Allergy Asthma Immunol 2012;109:309–13.e1.
8. Mehr S, Turner PJ, Joshi P, et al. Safety and clinical predictors of reacting to extensively heated cow's milk challenge in cow's milk-allergic children. Ann Allergy Asthma Immunol 2014;113:425–9.
9. Lemon-Mule H, Sampson HA, Sicherer SH, et al. Immunologic changes in children with egg allergy ingesting extensively heated egg. J Allergy Clin Immunol 2008;122:977–83.e1.
10. Clark A, Islam S, King Y, et al. A longitudinal study of resolution of allergy to well-cooked and uncooked egg. Clin Exp Allergy 2011;41:706–12.
11. Lieberman JA, Huang FR, Sampson HA, et al. Outcomes of 100 consecutive open, baked-egg oral food challenges in the allergy office. J Allergy Clin Immunol 2012;129:1682–4.e2.
12. Cortot CF, Sheehan WJ, Permaul P, et al. Role of specific IgE and skin-prick testing in predicting food challenge results to baked egg. Allergy Asthma Proc 2012;33:275–81.

13. Turner PJ, Mehr S, Joshi P, et al. Safety of food challenges to extensively heated egg in egg-allergic children: a prospective cohort study. Pediatr Allergy Immunol 2013;24:450–5.

14. Tan JW, Campbell DE, Turner PJ, et al. Baked egg food challenges - clinical utility of skin test to baked egg and ovomucoid in children with egg allergy. Clin Exp Allergy 2013;43:1189–95.

15. Bartnikas LM, Sheehan WJ, Larabee KS, et al. Ovomucoid is not superior to egg white testing in predicting tolerance to baked egg. J Allergy Clin Immunol Pract 2013;1:354–60.

16. Turner PJ, Kumar K, Fox AT. Skin testing with raw egg does not predict tolerance to baked egg in egg-allergic children. Pediatr Allergy Immunol 2014;25:657–61.

17. Leung J, Hundal NV, Katz AJ, et al. Tolerance of baked milk in patients with cow's milk-mediated eosinophilic esophagitis. J Allergy Clin Immunol 2013;132: 1215–6.e1.

18. Nowak-Wegrzyn A, Fiocchi A. Rare, medium, or well done? The effect of heating and food matrix on food protein allergenicity. Curr Opin Allergy Clin Immunol 2009;9:234–7.

19. Kato Y, Oozawa E, Matsuda T. Decrease in antigenic and allergenic potentials of ovomucoid by heating in the presence of wheat flour: dependence on wheat variety and intermolecular disulfide bridges. J Agric Food Chem 2001;49:3661–5.

20. Gjesing B, Osterballe O, Schwartz B, et al. Allergen-specific IgE antibodies against antigenic components in cow milk and milk substitutes. Allergy 1986; 41:51–6.

21. Chatchatee P, Jarvinen KM, Bardina L, et al. Identification of IgE- and IgG-binding epitopes on alpha(s1)-casein: differences in patients with persistent and transient cow's milk allergy. J Allergy Clin Immunol 2001;107:379–83.

22. Bernhisel-Broadbent J, Dintzis HM, Dintzis RZ, et al. Allergenicity and antigenicity of chicken egg ovomucoid (Gal d III) compared with ovalbumin (Gal d I) in children with egg allergy and in mice. J Allergy Clin Immunol 1994;93:1047–59.

23. Dang TD, Mills CE, Allen KJ. Determination of the clinical egg allergy phenotypes using component-resolved diagnostics. Pediatr Allergy Immunol 2014;25: 639–43.

24. Jarvinen KM, Beyer K, Vila L, et al. Specificity of IgE antibodies to sequential epitopes of hen's egg ovomucoid as a marker for persistence of egg allergy. Allergy 2007;62:758–65.

25. Bloom KA, Huang FR, Bencharitiwong R, et al. Effect of heat treatment on milk and egg proteins allergenicity. Pediatr Allergy Immunol 2014;25:740–6.

26. Kato Y, Watanabe H, Matsuda T. Ovomucoid rendered insoluble by heating with wheat gluten but not with milk casein. Biosci Biotechnol Biochem 2000;64: 198–201.

27. Ando H, Moverare R, Kondo Y, et al. Utility of ovomucoid-specific IgE concentrations in predicting symptomatic egg allergy. J Allergy Clin Immunol 2008;122: 583–8.

28. Caubet JC, Bencharitiwong R, Moshier E, et al. Significance of ovomucoid- and ovalbumin-specific IgE/IgG(4) ratios in egg allergy. J Allergy Clin Immunol 2012; 129:739–47.

29. Kim JS, Nowak-Wegrzyn A, Sicherer SH, et al. Dietary baked milk accelerates the resolution of cow's milk allergy in children. J Allergy Clin Immunol 2011;128: 125–31.e2.

30. Leonard SA, Sampson HA, Sicherer SH, et al. Dietary baked egg accelerates resolution of egg allergy in children. J Allergy Clin Immunol 2012;130:473–80.e1.

31. Konstantinou GN, Giavi S, Kalobatsou A, et al. Consumption of heat-treated egg by children allergic or sensitized to egg can affect the natural course of egg allergy: hypothesis-generating observations. J Allergy Clin Immunol 2008;122:414–5.
32. Leonard SA, Nowak-Wegrzyn A. Re-defining food allergy phenotypes and management paradigm: is it time for individualized egg allergy management? Clin Exp Allergy 2011;41:609–11.
33. Leonard SA, Caubet JC, Kim JS, et al. Baked milk- and egg-containing diet in the management of milk and egg allergy. J Allergy Clin Immunol Pract 2015;3:13–23 [quiz: 4].
34. Des Roches A, Nguyen M, Paradis L, et al. Tolerance to cooked egg in an egg allergic population. Allergy 2006;61:900–1.
35. Koplin JJ, Osborne NJ, Wake M, et al. Can early introduction of egg prevent egg allergy in infants? A population-based study. J Allergy Clin Immunol 2010;126:807–13.
36. Nowak-Wegrzyn A, Assa'ad AH, Bahna SL, et al. Work group report: oral food challenge testing. J Allergy Clin Immunol 2009;123:S365–83.

Biomarkers for Allergen Immunotherapy
A "Panoromic" View

Philippe Moingeon, PhD

KEYWORDS

- Allergen • Biomarker • Companion diagnostic • Efficacy • Immunotherapy
- Precision medicine • Safety

KEY POINTS

- Allergen immunotherapy would benefit from biomarkers (BMKs) that can stratify patients in terms of predicting treatment response and assessing efficacy.
- Although no such established BMKs are available, candidate biomarkers of efficacy include allergen-specific regulatory T lymphocytes, blocking antibodies (IgG4), as well as signatures associated with blood regulatory and proallergic (DC2) dendritic cells.
- The combined used of omics technologies allows application of nonhypothesis-driven approaches to the identification of novel candidate BMKs (the "panoromic" view).

INTRODUCTION

The National Institutes of Health Biomarkers Definitions Working Group defines a biomarker (BMK) as "a characteristic that is objectively measured and evaluated as an indicator of normal biological processes, pathogenic processes, or pharmacologic responses to a therapeutic intervention."[1] The quest for BMKs reflects a global trend in postmodern medicine toward stratification of patients into different categories based on their distinctive biological characteristics or the underlying molecular mechanisms involved in their disease.[2,3] Stratified medicine, also referred to as precision or targeted medicine, aims to implement therapies tailored to subsets or even individual patients, based on the use of such BMKs. This paradigm became the reference model after evidence in oncology that drugs such as trastuzumab (Herceptin) or imatinib (Gleevec) were remarkably efficacious in subsets of patients who have cancer.[2,3] Such a patient-centric approach contrasts with the previous 1-drug-fits-all belief

Disclosure: The author is an employee at Stallergenes SA.
Research and Development, Stallergenes SA, 6 Rue Alexis de Tocqueville, Antony Cedex 92183, France
E-mail address: pmoingeon@stallergenes.com

Immunol Allergy Clin N Am 36 (2016) 161–179
http://dx.doi.org/10.1016/j.iac.2015.08.004
0889-8561/16/$ – see front matter © 2016 Elsevier Inc. All rights reserved.

immunology.theclinics.com

that had been prevailing in traditional medicine. Practically, it implies that diagnostic and therapies should be better integrated, leading to the codevelopment of a targeted therapy with its companion diagnostic.[2–4]

In contrast to pharmacologic treatments, allergen immunotherapy (AIT) is the only treatment addressing the cause of the disease by reorienting inappropriate T-helper lymphocyte type 2 (Th2) immune responses to the allergens toward a Th1/regulatory T-cell profile.[5–7] AIT can act quickly (in a few hours or days) and also mediate a sustained and disease-modifying effect.[8] In this regard, whereas the subcutaneous route of immunization has been historically considered as a reference for AIT, sublingual immunotherapy (SLIT) is established as a noninvasive alternative to treat type I allergic rhinoconjunctivitis, with or without mild asthma.[9–11] New routes of immunization (eg, epicutaneous, intradermal, intralymphatic, oral) are being considered for AIT, together with new indications, such as food allergy or atopic dermatitis.[12,13]

In this context, distinct types of candidate BMKs can theoretically support AIT, in relationship with efficacy or safety (**Table 1**).[14–16] BMKs can benefit numerous stakeholders, including the patients themselves (improving compliance to treatment), physicians (supporting decision making before, during, and after AIT), regulators and payers (creating more value for money), and allergy vaccine manufacturers (increasing chances of success and decreasing time lines during development). BMKs will likely emerge as algorithms combining information on the patient (both in terms of his/her disease, immune status, and environmental interactions), as well as on protective mechanisms elicited by AIT (**Fig. 1**). To this aim, knowledge networks should be created to generate and assemble complex sets of data into algorithms that can be used to inform decisions (**Fig. 1**). The search for BMKs of efficacy has been focusing on immunologic parameters, from our current understanding of AIT mechanisms of action.[5–7] As developed later, new omics technologies provide the opportunity to move from inductive (ie, hypothesis-driven) to nonhypothesis-driven approaches (**Fig. 1**) in the context of more comprehensive "panoromic" strategies.[4]

THE IDEAL BIOMARKER

A molecular signature specific of either the allergic condition or of a protective biological mechanism elicited by AIT can be used as a valid BMK.[14–16] Sources of BMKs can

Table 1	
Applications of BMKs supporting allergen immunotherapy	
Types of Marker	**Applications**
BMK for diagnosis	Stratify patients to predict disease severity or progression
BMK predicting AIT safety or efficacy	Improve efficacy by selecting patients more likely to benefit from AIT
	Reduce cohort size needed for clinical development
	Reduce risk or severity of side effects
BMK of early onset of AIT efficacy	Confirm or not treatment efficacy after a few weeks
	Adjust treatment modalities (eg, dosing, immunization scheme)
	Improve patient compliance
BMK of long-term AIT efficacy	Document whether immune protection has been reached (support decision to pursue or stop AIT)
	Confirm lasting protection after stopping AIT (support decision to resume or not AIT)
	Improve patient compliance

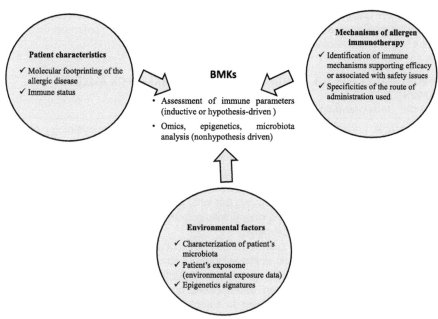

Fig. 1. Knowledge networks supporting the search for BMKs. To identify BMKs, information is assembled from various sources, including the comprehensive molecular fingerprinting of the patient (disease characteristics, immune status), the known immune mechanisms of AIT (with potential specificities of the route of administration), as well as environmental data specific to the patient (microbiota analysis, exposome, epigenetic signatures). As a consequence, cross-disciplinary knowledge networks are necessary to integrate complex data sets produced using both inductive (hypothesis-driven) and nonhypothesis-driven approaches.

be cells, DNA variants or mutants, RNAs (including messenger, micro, long noncoding RNAs), proteins (secreted, intracellular, membrane-associated), metabolites, etc. In any case, BMKs should be objectively measured in easily accessible body fluids, for example, in the blood, and reflect physiologic or pathologic changes induced in target organs during AIT. Supporting this assumption, a recent study[17] confirmed that a nasal allergen challenge in individuals allergic to grass pollen results in molecular changes at the level of basophil, dendritic, and T cells detectable in peripheral blood several hours after challenge. Well-standardized analytical methods, such as enzyme-linked immunosorbent assays or polymerase chain (PCR) assays, should be developed to quantify the BMK and a cutoff value for positivity should be established. BMKs should persist in biological fluids for several days or weeks to be used as a smoking gun of residual allergic inflammation or treatment efficacy.

Some information on the function of the BMK might be useful (ie, does it play a role in allergic inflammation? Is it linked with either a protective or a deleterious immune response?) to provide some mechanistic insights beyond its predictive value. Nonetheless, the relevance of a BMK does not require any causal association with disease severity or treatment efficacy. The performance of a BMK is classically evaluated, in terms of specificity and sensitivity, by its ability to distinguish treatment responders from nonresponders. Classically, those parameters are analyzed using a receiver operating curve representation to identify algorithms combining, as appropriate, multiple BMKs to increase the overall predictive value. In addition, because the development and implementation of a companion diagnostic are costly, the ideal BMK should be assessed as well in terms of health economics, with confirmed evidence that it has a positive cost-benefit value.

OPPORTUNITIES FOR THE IDENTIFICATION OF BIOMARKERS FOR ALLERGEN IMMUNOTHERAPY
A Better Understanding of Allergic Diseases

Considerable knowledge has accumulated regarding the pathophysiology of IgE-mediated allergic diseases. Standard models have been established, which integrate innate and adaptive immune mechanisms involved in allergic inflammation, with a central role played by allergen-specific CD4[+] T-helper cells through the production of cytokines such as interleukin 4 (IL-4), IL-5, IL-9, IL-13, and IL-17.[5–7] Cellular and molecular mechanisms of airway, skin, and gut inflammation are also better understood, with emerging insights on the role of epithelial cells in the initiation of effector immune responses after exposure to allergens.[18]

Advances have also been made in the diagnosis of allergic diseases. For example, component-resolved diagnostic is increasingly used to characterize patterns of IgE sensitization in allergic patients using batteries of purified natural or recombinant allergens displayed on commercial (eg, immunosolid-phase allergen chip) or customized miniaturized arrays.[19] Beyond helping to select the right allergen extract(s) for AIT based on evidence for real sensitization as opposed to IgE cross-reactivity, such detailed profiling of IgE sensitization provides an opportunity to stratify patients, with ongoing attempts to link some of those patterns to disease progression or severity.[20–22] The application of component-resolved diagnosis to the selection of patients more likely to respond to AIT has been suggested, with the hypothesis that multisensitized patients with broad patterns of IgE reactivity to multiple minor allergens, or cross-reactive panallergens such as profilins or polcalcins, may show poor responses to AIT.[16] In our experience, grass pollen immunotherapy was found to be efficacious irrespective of the patients' IgE sensitization profiles.[23]

Progress has also been made in the characterization of immune responses developed by nonallergic individuals when exposed to allergens. For example, many nonallergics have circulating allergen-specific CD4[+] T cells producing interferon γ (IFN-γ) (Th1 cells) or IL-10 (regulatory T cells), often associated with the secretion of allergen-specific IgGs as opposed to IgEs.[24,25] Those responses can be considered as being potentially naturally protective and may provide clues for the identification of candidate BMKs of AIT efficacy.

A Better Understanding of Allergen Immunotherapy Mechanisms

Changes in the polarization of allergen-specific CD4[+] T cells are considered to be critical for the efficacy of immunotherapy.[5–7] Many studies have documented that successful AIT is associated with a downregulation of allergen-specific CD4[+] Th2 cells in parallel with the induction of IFN-γ-secreting Th1 and IL-10-producing regulatory CD4[+] T'cells.[26–33] Given the dramatic differences in patterns of cytokines produced by these distinct subsets of CD4[+] T cells, such changes explain as well in large part the impact of AIT on allergen-specific antibody responses and on the recruitment and activation of proinflammatory innate cells in target organs.[5–7] Those general mechanisms of action are believed to be elicited regardless of the route of administration used for AIT (ie, epicutaneous, intradermal, oral, subcutaneous, sublingual). However, it cannot be excluded that some differences could be observed in the balance of induced systemic versus local immune responses, with the notion that mucosal routes are more likely to induce immunologic changes at mucosal surfaces.[6]

Harnessing the Power of Omics Technologies

Many powerful technologies are now available to perform nonhypotesis-driven and comprehensive genome-wide, transcriptome-wide, and proteome-wide analyses.[4] In this regard, the capacity of omics (ie, genomics, epigenetics, transcriptomics and RNA sequencing, proteomics, metabolomics) technologies to perform comprehensive molecular characterizations makes it easier to perform comparative analyses between biological samples from clinical responders and nonresponders or between pretreatment and posttreatment samples for a given patient, thus focusing exclusively on the molecular differences observed.

CHALLENGES FOR THE IDENTIFICATION OF BIOMARKERS FOR ALLERGEN IMMUNOTHERAPY
Heterogeneity of Allergic Diseases

The pathophysiology of allergic diseases is influenced by exposure conditions to the allergens (eg, seasonal vs perennial, dose, route), monosensitization versus polysensitization, intercurrent infections, genetic susceptibilities. In addition, tremendous variability is observed regarding the patients' immune status, beyond the fact that they are atopic. For example, most patients with pollinosis or food allergy have pure Th2 responses to the allergen(s).[25,34] However, in contrast, patients allergic to house dust mites develop mixed Th2/Th1, Th2/Th17, or even Th1/Th17 immune responses to mite allergens, likely as a consequence of chronic exposure.[35] It is undocumented whether AIT is equally efficacious in all those patient subsets. It is not known either whether BMKs of efficacy differ between AIT approaches, when conducted in patients allergic to grass pollen, food, or house dust mite.

Clinical Development Issues

Clinical trials documenting biological changes during AIT commonly include small studies often lacking a placebo group, which as a consequence do not allow such changes to be correlated with clinical improvement. Objective quantification of allergy symptoms, for example, in association with respiratory allergies, is difficult, because it consists classically of an autoevaluation by the patient of their symptoms associated with the nose and the eye, using a grading system for each individual symptom to build up a global symptom score.[36,37] Efficacy is also measured by considering the impact of AIT on the use of symptomatic treatments (medication score).[36,37] Combining the symptom and medication scores is recommended by health authorities, although no broadly accepted algorithm is available. Nasal, conjunctival, and bronchial provocation tests, as well as oral food challenges or skin prick tests, can be used to provide clinical readouts, although both the allergens and the procedures should be well standardized. Another specificity of AIT as it applies to the treatment of type I allergies is that it is associated with a significant placebo effect.[38] BMKs should relate to protective biological responses supporting clinical benefit induced by the active treatment, beyond such a placebo effect.

The search for BMKs of efficacy should be conducted in sufficiently powered double-blind placebo-controlled clinical studies. In addition, all biological analyses should be performed on samples coded to the operator. To be used as a tool to guide physicians' decision making during AIT, a correlation between a biological change and clinical benefit has to be established at an individual patient level. Even if correlations at a cohort level may provide interesting mechanistic insights, they cannot support the identification of candidate BMKs. In this context, for the purpose of identifying candidate BMKs, it is interesting to consider allergen challenge chambers.[39] Although such a setting allows enrolling only small cohorts of patients, 1 advantage is that challenge chambers provide standardized conditions for allergen exposure, as well as for measurement of clinical symptoms. A baseline evaluation of allergic symptoms can easily be performed during a pretreatment challenge, making it possible to document clinical improvement after AIT for each individual patient.[39] Candidate BMKs identified in this setting should be validated in the context of larger efficacy studies conducted under natural exposure conditions.

Handling of Biological Samples

Biological analyses are most often conducted in blood samples (eg, total blood, serum, plasma, isolated peripheral blood mononuclear cells [PBMCs]). Attention must be paid in handling, shipping, and storing biological samples, using standardized procedures to avoid introducing any bias in the conservation of potentially fragile molecules, most particularly when a clinical study involves multiple geographically dispersed recruiting centers. In this regard, 1 interesting approach is to perform blood sampling using syringes prefilled with compounds to lyse cells and stabilize RNAs from total blood until shipment to the laboratory. Other measurements can be performed on nasal secretions or saliva, although it remains difficult to standardize both sampling and biological analyses in those mucosal fluids.[40] Tissue biopsies are a highly relevant source of material to identify or validate BMKs, but they are not convenient for routine testing. As an alternative, biological analyses can be conducted in bronchoalveolar lavages, sputum, or exhaled air condensates believed to be relevant to document inflammatory mechanisms locally at play in the airways.[41–44] It is important to constitute biobanks, collected from patients after informed consent and approval by ethics committees. In this regard, clinical study protocols should contain as a provision the possibility to use such collected biological samples for retrospective analyses of emerging candidate BMKs, as novel mechanistic hypotheses arise.

Big Data Management

As summarized in **Fig. 1**, convergence has to be made between many sources of information to extract smart data from noise, and further, to draw information supporting decision making. Data mining among molecular signatures allows clustering molecules or genes into biological pathways (referred as functional genomics), thereby providing information regarding mechanisms underlying a disease or supporting a positive or negative outcome during AIT. The management of such big data is considered by many as the most critical bottleneck to transform multiomics data into decision algorithms combining up to hundreds of molecular signatures.[2–4] In the near future of e-health, data exchange and management should be facilitated by the use of connected devices transmitting in real-time biological and clinical measurements from patients to their physicians. However, the need to guarantee the confidentiality of such personal big data will likely raise significant ethical issues.

Regulatory Issues

As stated earlier, it is interesting to consider a coordinated development of BMKs together with a specific AIT.[2,3] In this regard, phase 3 efficacy studies should be used to validate candidate BMKs identified earlier during clinical development. However, 1 common practical issue is that when such large-scale efficacy studies are initiated, the potential value of candidate BMKs as a companion diagnostic is not sufficiently established to justify the cost and complexity of such a joint development.

Thus, the search for BMKs supporting AIT in a specific indication should ideally be initiated early on during clinical development.

DIAGNOSTIC BIOMARKERS IN SUPPORT OF ALLERGEN IMMUNOTHERAPY

Diagnostic BMKs help stratify patients based on objective biological readouts linked to a specific risk for disease severity or progression in patient subpopulations. Consequently, such markers could pave the ground for primary or secondary prophylactic approaches. The most common diagnostic test used in allergy (ie, allergen-specific IgE reactivity testing) is associated with sensitization, not disease. Using the expanding set of data available on patterns of IgE sensitization generated by using component-resolved diagnostic testing, some inferences regarding subsets of patients are already emerging. For example, patients allergic to peanuts with high serum IgE levels to Ara h 2 are reported to have an earlier onset of peanut allergy and a higher risk of systemic reactions to peanut allergens.[45] Similarly, IgE sensitization to plant food nonspecific lipid transfer proteins is associated with a higher risk of systemic reactions after allergen exposure.[46] The MeDALL (Mechanisms of the Development of Allergy) consortium has been assembled to better understand the links between comorbidities of allergic diseases (eg, asthma, rhinitis, atopic dermatitis) with patterns of IgE sensitization.[20,21] Young children with specific profiles of IgE sensitization (eg, high titers to pathogenesis-related class 10 allergens) are more likely to develop subsequently allergic rhinoconjunctivitis or asthma in their adolescence or young adulthood.[22]

Diagnostic markers allowing stratification of disease phenotypes into endotypes have also been identified for allergic asthma.[42,47] For example, genome-wide gene–environment interaction studies show that IL-9 induction after stimulation of patients' PBMCs with mite allergens predicts a higher risk for severe asthma exacerbation in children.[48] Nuclear magnetic resonance, as well as mass spectrometry–based metabolomic analyses applied to exhaled breath condensates might also be of interest to categorize asthmatic children, based on their individualized metabolite profiles.[41,43] Patterns of DNA methylation observed in blood mononuclear cells predict the clinical reactivity to oral food challenges in allergic children.[49]

PREDICTIVE BIOMARKERS OF ALLERGEN IMMUNOTHERAPY EFFICACY

BMKs useful to predict responsiveness to pharmacologic or biological treatments have been identified for allergic asthma. For example, patients with high serum levels of periostin, increased eosinophil counts in sputum, or high values of inflammatory BMKs such as FeNO (fraction of exhaled nitric oxide) have Th2-mediated asthmas showing positive responses to anti-IL-13 antibodies or corticosteroids.[42,47] Transcriptomic analyses comparing peripheral blood leukocytes from children with either therapy-resistant or controlled asthma show distinct gene expression profiles.[50] Similarly, measurement of the expression and methylation of the Vanin-1 gene in nasal epithelial cells can be used to discriminate asthmatic children who will not respond to systemic corticosteroids.[51]

No such BMKs are available to predict AIT efficacy in patients with respiratory or food allergies. Nonetheless, in line with the observation that patients with severe rhinoconjunctivitis react positively to AIT,[52] both high titers of specific IgEs (relative to total IgEs)[31,53] and high basophil responsiveness to the allergen[54] before treatment have been documented in patients showing subsequent benefit from AIT (**Table 2**). In addition, we recently identified a sialylated variant of the Fetuin A (Fet A) molecule expressed at high levels in pretreatment sera from patients allergic to grass pollen

Table 2
Relevance of immune parameters as biomarkers of allergen immunotherapy efficacy

Parameters	Predictive Value Before AIT	Changes Documented During Short-Term AIT (hours to <1 wk)	Changes Documented During Middle-Term AIT (1 wk to 6 mo)	Changes Documented During Long-Term AIT (6 mo to Several years)	References
Allergen-specific CD4+ T-cell responses	Not applicable	Not significantly affected in such a short time frame	Induction of Th1 or regulatory T cells producing IL-10 or TGF-β in peripheral blood and in mucosae Th2 CD4+ T cells: not significantly decreased in peripheral blood, but potential decrease in Th2 cytokine production	Induction of Th1 or regulatory T cells producing IL-10 or TGF-β in peripheral blood and in mucosae Induction of Foxp3 expression in memory regulatory T cells in association with epigenetic modifications Decrease in Th2 cytokines (IL-5, IL-9, IL-13) in serum or in PBMC cultures	26–33,62
			Changes in the polarization of CD4+ T-cell responses in peripheral blood have not been correlated with clinical benefit at an individual patient level Several AIT studies failed to document significant changes in allergen-specific CD4+ T-cell responses in peripheral blood despite evidence for clinical benefit	Such changes in the polarization of CD4+ T-cell responses in peripheral blood have not been correlated with clinical benefit at an individual patient level	63–66
Allergen-specific antibody responses	High specific IgE/total IgE ratio (unconfirmed)	Not significantly affected in such a short time frame	Boosting of existing specific IgE levels in serum, but not in nasal secretions Induction of allergen-specific IgG1s, IgG4s, and IgAs in serum and mucosae, in association with an IgE-blocking activity In a SLIT study conducted in a pollen chamber, patients with strong allergen-specific humoral responses show clinical responses. However, evidence for clinical responders without any detectable antibody response	Progressive decline in specific IgE titers in serum Induction of allergen-specific IgG1s, IgG4s, and IgAs in serum and mucosae, in association with an IgE-blocking activity Persistence of the IgE- blocking activity (whereas specific IgG4s decline to baseline levels) 1 y after AIT cessation	31,53,57,67–76

| Innate immune paramets | High basophil responsiveness | • During rush venom immunotherapy:
  ○ Downregulation of basophil activation (↘FcεRI, ↘c-Syk)
  ○ Induction of ILT3, ILT4, cyclic adenosine monophosphate, as well as IL-10 production by monocytes | Several studies (SCIT and SLIT in respiratory allergies, OIT in peanut allergy), but not all, documented a decrease in blood basophil activation. Association with clinical benefit is proposed at a cohort level in some, but not all studies | Decrease in blood basophil activation concomitantly with the decrease in serum IgE levels | 33,54,78,79 |
| | A sialylated variant of Fetuin A is highly expressed in sera from patients allergic to grass pollen responding to SLIT | | Markers associated with regulatory DCs are upregulated whereas markers associated with proallergic DC2 are rather downregulated in peripheral blood of patients showing clinical benefit during SLIT | After 1 y of SLIT, evidence for monocyte-derived DCs in the blood with low expression of CD86, reduced production of IL-12 and increased IL-10 secretion | 80–82 |

Abbreviations: DC, dendritic cell; DC2, DCs supporting the differentiation of Th2 cells; TGF-β, transforming growth factor β.

benefiting from SLIT, when compared with nonresponders. Fet A has previously been reported as a molecule involved in controlling inflammation associated with metabolic and infectious, as well as cardiovascular diseases and cancer.[55] Although no link between Fet A and allergy had been established, we confirmed that this molecule can either amplify or downregulate allergic inflammation depending on its posttranslational modifications (our unpublished results).

FOLLOW-UP BIOMARKERS OF ALLERGEN IMMUNOTHERAPY EFFICACY
Changes in the Polarization of Allergen-Specific CD4$^+$ T Cells

Subcutaneous immunotherapy (SCIT), SLIT, oral immunotherapy (OIT), and epicutaneous immunotherapy with pollen, mite, or food allergens have been reported to elicit Foxp3$^+$ regulatory T cells and IL-10-producing Foxp3$^-$ Tr1 cells, as well as transforming growth factor β–secreting Th3 cells (**Table 2**).[26–33] Whereas these regulatory T cells are commonly detected in the patients' blood, the presence of Foxp3$^+$ and IL-10$^+$ CD4$^+$ T cells has also been documented within the oral and nasal mucosae after SCIT or SLIT.[56,57] Mechanistically, such Tregs differentiate from naive T cells in the periphery, and their induction has been linked to epigenetic modifications (such as hypomethylation of Foxp3 CpG sites) occurring during AIT.[33,58] AIT has been shown as well to elicit allergen-specific IFN-γ-producing Th1 cells, in parallel with a decline in Th2 CD4$^+$ T lymphocytes involving both apoptosis and anergy induction (**Table 2**).[5–7,26,59–61]

Those changes in the polarization of allergen-specific T cells occur in an epitope-specific manner, and they are considered as central to AIT efficacy.[5–7,61] Nonetheless, it remains difficult to summarize in a simple picture the kinetics of those changes, likely as a consequence of differences in dosing regimens and immunization schemes between studies. For example, SLIT in patients allergic to grass pollen was shown to downregulate specifc Th2 responses within 4 months, before the induction of regulatory T cells.[61] In contrast, other studies document an upregulation of regulatory T cells in the first few months of AIT.[6,62] However, AIT for respiratory allergies starts decreasing symptoms within 1 week and venom immunotherapy within hours, whereas no major modulation of T cell responses is observed in such a time frame.[63] Modifications in the balance between regulatory T lymphocytes and Th2 cells are more consistently documented in long-lasting (>6 months) AIT regimens.[29]

Several clinical studies have failed to document any induction of regulatory T lymphocytes, or even alterations in peripheral CD4$^+$ T cell responses, during AIT.[63–66] For example, in our SLIT study conducted in an allergen challenge chamber over 4 months,[63] changes in phenotype and cytokine secretion in grass pollen–specific CD4$^+$ T cells were limited, with no differences between clinical responders and non-responders detected in peripheral blood. Similarly, ragweed pollen immunotherapy did not affect numbers of allergen-specific T cells, although intracellular staining showed a potential lower secretion of IL-5 by those cells.[66] Such discrepancies with the aforementioned studies may be first explained by the tremendous capacity of CD4$^+$ T cells to circulate throughout the body, making the analysis of in transit T cells in the blood unreliable to document pathophysiologic mechanisms occurring in target organs. Furthermore, standardization of quantitative T cell assays is difficult, most particularly in longitudinal studies requiring the use of frozen cell samples. For those reasons combined, it is unlikely that quantification of allergen-specific Treg or Th2 cells can be used as a BMK of AIT efficacy. Not surprisingly, no firm correlation between changes in patterns of allergen-specific CD4$^+$ T cells in the blood and clinical improvement has yet been established at an individual patient level (**Table 2**).

Changes in Allergen-Specific Antibody Responses

During AIT, an initial boosting of allergen-specific IgE serum levels is commonly observed in the first few months in most patients, including those with documented clinical benefit. This observed recall of existing IgEs is well tolerated because it occurs in peripheral blood but not in the airways.[23] A progressive decline in specific IgEs is observed after 6 months to 1 year of AIT (**Table 2**), consistent with a decrease of long-lived bone marrow–resident IgE-secreting plasma cells. In parallel, AIT induces allergen-specific IgG4 secretion by IL-10-producing regulatory B cells as early as after 2 weeks, and such IgGs are still detected in serum for more than a year after treatment cessation.[67–70] Serum IgG4 titers do not represent an absolute marker of clinical efficacy, because there is now strong evidence that functional properties (such as IgE-blocking activity) reflecting the induction of IgG4 antibodies with a high affinity for the allergen are more relevant to AIT efficacy.[71] In murine asthma models, the efficacy of SLIT conducted with allergens formulated in vector systems is consistently associated with a strong induction of IgAs in respiratory mucosae.[72] Thus, allergen-specific IgAs produced during AIT may provide as well a source of highly relevant blocking antibodies at mucosal surfaces.[73] Such blocking antibodies inhibit IgE binding to the allergen, leading as a consequence to a decrease in histamine release by basophils, as well as in CD23-dependent allergen presentation to T cells.[74] IgGs can also engage FcγRIIB (CD32) inhibitory receptors, thereby downregulating B-cell, mast cell, and basophil activation.[67,74] In this context, it has been proposed to measure allergen-specific IgE reactivity as a readout for AIT efficacy, using low allergen concentrations immobilized on a solid phase, to document residual IgE binding in presence of blocking IgGs.[75]

The induction of specific IgG4s and, even more convincingly, of blocking antibodies after AIT have been correlated with clinical improvement at a cohort level.[70,71] For example, 2 years of SCIT in patients allergic to mites or grass pollen elicits high levels of allergen-specific IgG4s, which revert back to pretreatment levels within a year after treatment cessation, despite preserved clinical benefit. An IgE-blocking activity persists in posttreatment sera, which better correlates with clinical responses than IgG4 levels.[70,71] In our SLIT study conducted in a challenge pollen chamber,[23] clinical responders were found to encompass both immunoreactive patients with strong grass pollen–specific IgE, IgG, and IgG4 responses and blocking antibodies, as well as non-immunoreactive patients without any detectable antibody responses distinguishing them from patients receiving placebo. We observed similarly in a large cohort of patients allergic to mites that a 1-year course of SLIT induces specific IgG4 antibodies only in a subset (ie, 15%) of patients, irrespective of clinical benefit.[76] It seems that allergen-specific IgG4 responses likely contribute to tolerance induction in some, but not all, patients in large part through their IgE-blocking activity. Nonetheless, such antibody responses cannot be used as a marker of efficacy for AIT at an individual patient level (**Table 2**).

Changes at the Level of the Innate Immune System

As a consequence of changes in the cytokine milieu elicited during AIT, the recruitment and activation of proinflammatory innate cells (ie, mast cells, basophils, eosinophils, neutrophils) is significantly reduced in the skin, nose, and eye, as well as in bronchial and oral mucosae after provocation or natural exposure to the allergens.[5–7] Detailed studies evaluating changes in innate immunity parameters have been conducted in the context of venom immunotherapy performed via the subcutaneous route. In such a setting, several alterations of immune parameters are seen within hours, which include a decrease in basophil activation (associated with a downregulation of FcεRI and c-Syk and the upregulation of the H2R histamine receptor), the induction of immunoglobulin-like transcript ILT3 and ILT4 expression, as well as IL-10 and intracellular cyclic adenosine monophosphate production in monocytes.[77–79]

Many studies have specifically documented a decrease in basophil responsiveness to in vitro restimulation with the allergen, after 6 months or less of SCIT or SLIT for respiratory allergies or OIT for peanut allergy (**Table 2**).[5–7] In contrast, we failed to detect any impact of a 4-month course of SLIT on basophil activation despite evidence for clinical benefit in patients.[54] Those discrepancies might be explained in part by differences of duration of AIT in those various studies, and possibly by the use of CD63 as opposed to CD203c as readouts of basophil activation. Long-term (>6 months) AIT has been more consistently associated with a decrease in basophil activation, in parallel with a decrease in specific IgE levels. However, an OIT study in patients allergic to peanuts failed to correlate tolerance induction with such changes in basophil responsiveness.[33]

We have as well recently observed a significant impact of AIT on blood dendritic cells, with evidence for induction by SLIT in patients allergic to grass pollen of regulatory dendritic cells (DCs) (DCregs) expressing high levels of C1Q and Stabilin.[80] The C1Q molecule itself was subsequently shown to have a powerful inhibitory activity against Th2 responses in a murine asthma model, suggesting that DCregs can not only support the differentiation of regulatory T cells but also mediate a direct antiinflammatory activity by themselves (our unpublished results). Furthermore, this induction of blood DCregs is paralleled by a decrease in the blood of markers such as CD141 and OX40 L associated with proallergic DC2s (ie, DCs supporting the differentiation of Th2 cells). This change in the DCreg/DC2 balance was detectable in peripheral blood by quantitative PCR only in those patients showing clinical responses, further corroborating at the level of the innate immune system the central paradigm that a reorientation of immune responses from a Th2 to a regulatory profile is critical to the success of AIT. In agreement with these findings, SLIT for 1 year in children allergic to house dust mite resulted in a decrease of the capacity of monocyte-derived DCs to mature and produce IL-12 and upregulated IL-10 secretion, consistent with their acquisition of a tolerogenic phenotype.[81] Also, DCs isolated from the blood of patients allergic to peanuts after 2 years of OIT significantly downregulate Foxp3 CpG methylation when cultured with T lymphocytes.[33] Another study reported an increase in PD-L1 (programmed cell death-ligand 1)–expressing antigen-presenting cells and IL-10-producing CD14+ monocytes during AIT.[82] These studies confirm a significant and persisting impact of AIT on innate immunity, with evidence that the induction of DCreg signatures are correlated with clinical improvement in patients allergic to grass pollen .

BIOMARKERS FOR ALLERGEN IMMUNOTHERAPY SAFETY

No BMK is available to predict and prevent severe or systemic reactions to AIT. The rate and type of side effects associated with AIT are anticipated based on the route of immunization used. For example, SCIT carries a risk of unfrequent, but potentially life-threatening anaphylactic reaction, whereas SLIT mostly causes local reactions, with severe systemic reactions being rare.[83,84] As stated earlier, specific patterns of IgE sensitization may help identify those patients prone to developing systemic reactions when exposed to the allergen(s).[45,46] Also, measurement of serum mast cell tryptase is proposed to help in the diagnosis of anaphylaxis.[85] Further research is clearly needed in this area, with the encouraging result that an increase of a prostaglandin D_2 metabolite in serum could be used to predict systemic reactions to AIT.[86]

FUTURE CONSIDERATIONS
Characterization of Patients' Microbiota

The presence of commensal or pathogenic bacteria in mucosae can promote either tolerogenic or proinflammatory mechanisms, after engagement of pattern-recognition receptors at the surface of resident immune cells. Bacteria can significantly influence the maturation of the immune system, most particularly at mucosal surfaces.[87] Thus, differences between individuals in terms of flora composition could possibly influence both the susceptibility to allergic diseases[87] and AIT efficacy. Comprehensive studies of human microbiota are conducted at various body sites, including the oral, intestinal, nasal, and respiratory mucosae, both in healthy individuals and in allergic patients.[88,89] Using 16S ribosomal RNA sequencing, the characterization of commensal bacteria has already shed light on both the uniqueness of each individual's microbiota, as well as the considerable variation found between individuals with respect to patterns of bacterial genes expressed in their tissues.[88,89] As we better understand the role of microbiota in shaping local immune responses, patterns associated with positive or negative AIT outcomes may be identified.

New Players in the Regulation of Allergen-Specific Immune Responses

The recent identification of new players involved in the modulation of regulatory or proinflammatory responses to allergens provides potential new sources of candidate BMKs of efficacy. The latter include for example, microRNAs (miRNAs)[90] and innate lymphoid cells (ILCs).[91] miRNAs are small noncoding RNAs involved in the posttranscriptional regulation of gene expression in mammalian cells. Selected miRNAs have been shown to regulate T-cell polarization and activation (eg, miRNA-21 and miRNA-146) or eosinophil development (miRNA-21 and miRNA-223).[90,92] MiRNA-21, miRNA-126, miRNA-145, and let-7b are significantly induced in the airways of mice exposed to allergens.[91] The existence of extracellular forms of those miRNAs that can be easily measured in body fluids have been shown. In addition, specific long noncoding RNAs are expressed during Th2 differentiation of CD4$^+$ T cells.[93] Although the use of such RNAs as BMKs of AIT efficacy remains largely unexplored, we recently observed in a pilot study that miRNA-132 (expressed in monocyte-derived DC1 and DC2 cells) is upregulated during SLIT in relationship with clinical benefit (our unpublished results).

A major interest has been raised as well by the recent identification of ILCs as a new family of lymphocyte-like cells lacking specific antigen receptors and producing large amounts of proinflammatory cytokines such as IFN-γ, IL-5, IL-13, IL-17, and IL-22. These cells encompass 3 distinct subsets (ILC1s, ILC2, ILC3) based on their patterns of cytokine production, which match those of polarized CD4$^+$ T lymphocytes.[91] ILCs play a role in the initiation and persistence of allergic inflammation, with evidence that numbers of circulating ILC2 cells are increased in the blood of asthmatic patients and that ILC3s can contribute to asthma associated with obesity.[94,95] Recently, a study conducted in a small cohort of patients allergic to grass pollen[96] showed that SCIT blunts the upregulation of ILC2 cells observed in the blood during the pollen season. In our hands, a 4-month regimen of SLIT in a pollen chamber had no detectable effect on circulating ILC2s. The potential heterogeneity of ILCs and their role in allergic diseases as well as the impact of long-term AIT on ILC2 frequencies and activation need to be further investigated.

REFERENCES

1. Biomarkers Definitions Working Group. Biomarkers and surrogate end points: preferred definitions and conceptual framework. Clin Pharmacol Ther 2001;69: 89–95.
2. Trusheim MR, Burgess B, Xinghua Hu S, et al. Quantifying factors for the success of stratified medicine. Nat Rev Drug Discov 2011;10:817–33.
3. Willis JC, Lord GM. Immune biomarkers: the promises and pitfalls of personalized medicine. Nat Rev Immunol 2015;15:323–9.
4. Topol EJ. Individualized medicine from prewomb to tomb. Cell 2014;157: 241–53.
5. Shamji MH, Durham SR. Mechanisms of immunotherapy to aeroallergens. Clin Exp Allergy 2011;41:1235–46.
6. Moingeon P. Update on immune mechanisms associated with sublingual immunotherapy: practical implications for the clinician. J Allergy Clin Immunol Pract 2013;1:228–41.
7. Akdis M, Akdis C. Mechanisms of allergen-specific immunotherapy: multiple suppressor factors at work in immune tolerance to allergens. J Allergy Clin Immunol 2014;133:621–31.
8. Marogna M, Spadolini I, Massolo A, et al. Long lasting effects of sublingual immunotherapy according to its duration: a 15 year prospective study. J Allergy Clin Immunol 2010;126:969–75.
9. Canonica GW, Bousquet J, Casale T, et al. Sublingual immunotherapy: World Allergy Organization Position Paper. Allergy 2009;64(Suppl 91):1–59.
10. Cox L, Nelson H, Lockey R, et al. Allergen immunotherapy: a practice parameter third update. J Allergy Clin Immunol 2011;127(Suppl):S1–55.
11. Burks AW, Calderon MA, Casale T, et al. Update on allergen immunotherapy: American Academy of Allergy, Asthma and Immunology/European Academy of Allergy and Clinical Immunology. PRACTALL consensus report. J Allergy Clin Immunol 2013;131:1288–96.
12. Moingeon P, Mascarell L. Novel routes of allergen specific immunotherapy: safety, efficacy and modes of action. Immunotherapy 2012;4:1–12.
13. Passalacqua G, Compalati E, Canonica GW. Sublingual immunotherapy: other indications. Immunol Allergy Clin North Am 2011;31(2):279–87.
14. Alam R. Biomarkers in asthma and allergy. Immunol Allergy Clin North Am 2012; 32:11–2.
15. Shamji MH, Ljørring C, Würtzen PA. Predictive biomarkers of clinical efficacy of allergen-specific immunotherapy: how to proceed. Immunotherapy 2013;5: 203–6.
16. Popescu FD. Molecular biomarkers for grass pollen immunotherapy. World J Methodol 2014;4:26–45.
17. Shamji MH, Bellido V, Scadding GW, et al. Effector cell signature in peripheral blood following nasal allergen challenge in grass pollen allergic individuals. Allergy 2015;70:171–9.
18. Lloyd CM, Saglani S. T cells in asthma: influences of genetics, environment, and T-cell plasticity. J Allergy Clin Immunol 2013;131:1267–74.
19. Harwanegg C, Laffer S, Hiller R, et al. Microarrayed recombinant allergens for diagnosis of allergy. Clin Exp Allergy 2003;33:7–13.
20. Bousquet J, Antó JM, Auffray C, et al. MeDALL (Mechanisms of the Development of ALLergy): an integrated approach from phenotypes to systems medicine. Allergy 2011;66:596–604.

21. Antó JM, Pinart M, Akdis M, et al. Understanding the complexity of IgE-related phenotypes from childhood to young adulthood: a Mechanisms of the Development of Allergy (MeDALL) seminar. J Allergy Clin Immunol 2012;129:943–54.

22. Westman M, Lupinek C, Bousquet J, et al. Early childhood IgE reactivity to pathogenesis-related class 10 proteins predicts allergic rhinitis in adolescence. J Allergy Clin Immunol 2015;135:1199–206.

23. Baron-Bodo V, Horiot S, Lautrette A, et al. Heterogeneity of antibody responses among clinical responders during grass pollen sublingual immunotherapy. Clin Exp Allergy 2013;43:1362–73.

24. Akdis M, Verhagen A, Taylor F, et al. Immune responses in healthy and allergic individuals are characterized by a fine balance between allergen-specific T regulatory 1 and T helper 2 cells. J Exp Med 2004;199:1567–75.

25. Van Overtvelt L, Wambre E, Maillere B, et al. Assessment of Bet v 1-specific CD4[+] T cell responses in allergic and nonallergic individuals using MHC class II peptide tetramers. J Immunol 2008;180:4514–22.

26. Jutel M, Pichler WJ, Skrbic D, et al. Bee venom immunotherapy results in decrease of IL4 and IL5 and increase in IFNγ secretion in specific allergen stimulated T cell cultures. J Immunol 1995;154:4178–94.

27. Francis JN, Till SJ, Durham SR. Induction of IL10+ CD4+ CD25+ T cells by grass pollen immunotherapy. J Allergy Clin Immunol 2003;111:1255–61.

28. Bohle B, Kinaciyan T, Gerstmayr M, et al. Sublingual immunotherapy induces IL-10-producing T regulatory cells, allergen-specific T-cell tolerance, and immune deviation. J Allergy Clin Immunol 2007;120:707–13.

29. Eifan AO, Akkoc T, Yildiz A, et al. Clinical efficacy and immunological mechanisms of sublingual and subcutaneous immunotherapy in asthmatic/rhinitis children sensitized to house dust mite: and open randomized controlled trial. Clin Exp Allergy 2010;40:922–32.

30. Mondoulet L, Dioszeghy V, Puteaux E, et al. Specific epicutaneous immunotherapy prevents sensitization to new allergens in a murine model. J Allergy Clin Immunol 2015;135(6):1546–57.e4.

31. Fujimura T, Yonekura S, Horiguchi S, et al. Increase of regulatory T cells and the ratio of specific IgE to total IgE are candidates for response monitoring or prognostic biomarkers in 2-year sublingual immunotherapy (SLIT) for Japanese cedar pollinosis. Clin Immunol 2011;139:65–74.

32. O'Hehir RE, Gardner LM, de Leon MP, et al. House dust mite sublingual immunotherapy. The role for transforming growth factor B and functional regulatory T cells. Am J Respir Crit Care Med 2009;180:936–47.

33. Syed A, Garcia MA, Lyu SC, et al. Peanut oral immunotherapy results in increased antigen-induced regulatory T-cell function and hypomethylation of forkhead box protein 3 (FOXP3). J Allergy Clin Immunol 2014;133:500–10.

34. Nowak-Wegrzyn A, Albin S. Oral immunotherapy for food allergy: mechanisms and role in management. Clin Exp Allergy 2014;45:368–83.

35. Wambre E, Bonvalet M, Bodo V, et al. Seasonal (Bet v 1) and perennial (Der p 1/Der p 2) allergens elicit distinct memory CD4[+] T cell responses. Clin Exp Allergy 2011;41:192–203.

36. European Medicines Agency. Guideline on the clinical development of products for specific immunotherapy for the treatment of allergic diseases. CHMP/EWP/18504/2006. 2008.

37. Devilliers P, Chassany O, Vicaut E, et al. The minimally important difference in the rhinoconjunctivitis total symptom score in grass pollen-induced allergic rhinoconjunctivitis. Allergy 2014;69:1689–95.

38. Narkus A, Lehnigk U, Haefner D, et al. The placebo effect in allergen-specific immunotherapy trials. Clin Transl Allergy 2013;3:42.
39. Horak F, Zieglmayer P, Zieglmayer R, et al. Early onset of action of a 5-grass-pollen 300-IR sublingual immunotherapy tablet evaluated in an allergen challenge chamber. J Allergy Clin Immunol 2009;124:471–7.
40. Scadding G, Hellings P, Iobid I, et al. Diagnostic tools in rhinology EAACI position paper. Clin Transl Allergy 2011;1:2.
41. Carraro S, Rezzi S, Reniero F, et al. Metabolomics applied to exhaled breath condensate in childhood asthma. Am J Respir Crit Care Med 2007;175:986–90.
42. Fajt ML, Wenzel SE. Asthma phenotypes and the use of biologic medications in asthma and allergic disease: the next steps toward personalized care. J Allergy Clin Immunol 2015;135:299–310.
43. Martinez-Lozano Sinues P, Kohler M, Zenobi R. Human breath analysis may support the existence of individual metabolic phenotypes. PLoS One 2013;8:e59909.
44. Peters MC, Mekonnen ZK, Yuan S, et al. Measures of gene expression in sputum cells can identify Th2-high and Th2-low subtypes of asthma. J Allergy Clin Immunol 2014;133:388–94.
45. Ballmer-Weber BK, Lidholm J, Fernandez-Rivas M, et al. IgE recognition patterns in peanut allergy are age dependent: perspectives of the EuroPrevall study. Allergy 2015;70:391–407.
46. Romano A, Scala E, Rumi G, et al. Lipid transfer proteins: the most frequent sensitizer in Italian subjects with food-dependent exercise-induced anaphylaxis. Clin Exp Allergy 2012;42:1643–53.
47. Cowan DC, Taylor DR, Peterson LE, et al. Biomarker-based asthma phenotypes of corticosteroid response. J Allergy Clin Immunol 2015;135:877–83.
48. Sordillo JE, Kelly R, Bunyavanich S, et al. Genome-wide expression profiles identify potential targets for gene-environment interactions in asthma severity. J Allergy Clin Immunol 2015. [Epub ahead of print].
49. Martino D, Dang T, Sexton-Oates A, et al. Blood DNA methylation biomarkers predict clinical reactivity in food-sensitized infants. J Allergy Clin Immunol 2015;135: 1319–28.
50. Persson H, Kwon AT, Ramilowski JA, et al. Transcriptome analysis of controlled and therapy-resistant childhood asthma reveals distinct gene expression profiles. J Allergy Clin Immunol 2015;136(3):638–48.
51. Xiao C, Biagini Myers JM, Ji H, et al. Vanin-1 expression and methylation discriminate pediatric asthma corticosteroid treatment response. J Allergy Clin Immunol 2015. [Epub ahead of print].
52. Howarth P, Malling HJ, Molimard M, et al. Analysis of allergen immunotherapy studies shows increased clinical efficacy in highly symptomatic patients. Allergy 2012;67:321–7.
53. Di Lorenzo G, Mansueto P, Pacor ML, et al. Evaluation of serum s-IgE/total IgE ratio in predicting clinical response to allergen-specific immunotherapy. J Allergy Clin Immunol 2009;123:1103–10.
54. Van Overtvelt L, Baron-Bodo V, Horiot S, et al. Changes in basophil activation during grass-pollen sublingual immunotherapy do not correlate with clinical efficacy. Allergy 2011;66:1530–7.
55. Mori K, Emoto M, Inaba M. Fetuin-A: a multifunctional protein. Recent Pat Endocr Metab Immune Drug Discov 2011;5:124–46.
56. Nouri-Aria KT, Wachholz PA, Francis JN, et al. Grass pollen immunotherapy induces mucosal and peripheral IL10 responses and blocking IgG responses. J Immunol 2004;172:3252–9.

57. Scadding GW, Shamji MH, Jacobson MR, et al. Sublingual grass pollen immunotherapy is associated with increases in sublingual Foxp3-expressing cells and elevated allergen-specific immunoglobulin G4, immunoglobulin A and serum inhibitory activity for immunoglobulin E-facilitated allergen binding to B cells. Clin Exp Allergy 2010;40:598–606.

58. Swamy RS, Reshamwala N, Hunter T, et al. Epigenetic modifications and improved regulatory T-cell function in subjects undergoing dual sublingual immunotherapy. J Allergy Clin Immunol 2012;130:215–24.

59. Wambre E, DeLong JH, James EA, et al. Differentiation stage determines pathologic and protective allergen-specific CD4+ T-cell outcomes during specific immunotherapy. J Allergy Clin Immunol 2012;129:544–51.

60. Wambre E, DeLong JH, James EA, et al. Specific immunotherapy modifies allergen-specific CD4+ T cell responses in an epitope-dependent manner. J Allergy Clin Immunol 2014;133:872–9.

61. Suárez-Fueyo A, Ramos T, Galán A, et al. Grass tablet sublingual immunotherapy downregulates the Th2 cytokine response followed by regulatory T-cell generation. J Allergy Clin Immunol 2014;133:130–8.

62. Francis JN, James LK, Paraskevopoulos G, et al. Grass pollen immunotherapy: IL-10 induction and suppression of late responses precedes IgG4 inhibitory antibody activity. J Allergy Clin Immunol 2008;121:1120–5.

63. Bonvalet M, Moussu H, Wambre E, et al. Allergen-specific CD4+ T cell responses in peripheral blood do not predict the early onset of clinical efficacy during grass pollen sublingual immunotherapy. Clin Exp Allergy 2012;42:1745–55.

64. Rolinck-Werninghaus CKM, Liebke C, Lange J, et al. Lack of detectable alterations in immune responses during sublingual immunotherapy in children with seasonal allergic rhinoconjunctivitis to grass pollen. Int Arch Allergy Immunol 2005;136:134–41.

65. Dehlink E, Eiwegger T, Gerstmayr M, et al. Absence of systemic immunologic changes during dose build-up phase and early maintenance period in effective specific sublingual immunotherapy in children. Clin Exp Allergy 2006;36:32–9.

66. Campbell JD, Buchmann P, Kesting S, et al. Allergen-specific T cell responses to immunotherapy monitored by CD154 and intracellular cytokine expression. Clin Exp Allergy 2010;40:1025–35.

67. Wachholz PA, Durham SR. Mechanisms of immunotherapy: IgG revisited. Curr Opin Allergy Clin Immunol 2004;4:313–8.

68. Bahceciler NN, Arikan C, Taylor A, et al. Impact of sublingual immunotherapy on specific antibody levels in asthmatic children allergic to house dust mites. Int Arch Allergy Immunol 2005;136:287–94.

69. Van de Veen W, Stanic B, Yaman G, et al. IgG4 production is confined to human IL-10-producing regulatory B cells that suppress antigen-specific immune responses. J Allergy Clin Immunol 2013;131:1204–12.

70. James LK, Shamji MH, Walker SM, et al. Long term tolerance after allergen immunotherapy is accompanied by selective persistence of blocking antibodies. J Allergy Clin Immunol 2011;127:509–16.

71. Shamji MH, Ljorring C, Francis JN, et al. Functional rather than immunoreactive levels of IgG4 correlate closely with clinical response to grass pollen immunotherapy. Allergy 2012;67:217–26.

72. Razafindratsita A, Saint-Lu N, Mascarell L, et al. Improvement of sublingual immunotherapy efficacy with a mucoadhesive allergen formulation. J Allergy Clin Immunol 2007;120:278–85.

73. Pilette C, Nouri-Aria KT, Jacobson MR, et al. Grass pollen immunotherapy induces an allergen-specific IgA2 antibody response associated with mucosal TGF-beta expression. J Immunol 2007;178:4658–66.

74. Flicker S, Valenta R. Renaissance of the blocking antibody concept in type I allergy. Int Arch Allergy Immunol 2003;132:13–24.

75. Wollmann E, Lupinek C, Kundi M, et al. Reduction in allergen-specific IgE binding as measured by microarray: a possible surrogate marker for effects of specific immunotherapy. J Allergy Clin Immunol 2015;136(3):806–9.e7.

76. Baron-Bodo V, Batard T, Nguyen H, et al. Absence of IgE neosensitization in house dust mite allergic patients following sublingual immunotherapy. Clin Exp Allergy 2012;42:1510–8.

77. Michils A, Baldassare S, Ledent C, et al. Early effect of ultrarush venom immunotherapy on the IgG antibody response. Allergy 2000;55:455–62.

78. Bussmann C, Xia J, Allam JP, et al. Early markers for protective mechanisms during rush venom immunotherapy. Allergy 2010;65:1558–65.

79. Čelesnik N, Vesel T, Rijavec M, et al. Short-term venom immunotherapy induces desensitization of FcεRI-mediated basophil response. Allergy 2012;67:1594–600.

80. Zimmer A, Bouley J, Le Mignon M, et al. A regulatory dendritic cell signature correlates with the clinical efficacy of allergen immunotherapy. J Allergy Clin Immunol 2012;129:1020–30.

81. Angelini F, Pacciani V, Corrente S, et al. Dendritic cells modification during sublingual immunotherapy in children with allergic symptoms to house dust mites. World J Pediatr 2011;7:24–30.

82. Piconi S, Trabattoni D, Rainone V, et al. Immunological effects of sublingual immunotherapy: clinical efficacy is associated with modulation of programmed cell death ligand 1, IL-10, and IgG4. J Immunol 2010;185:7723–30.

83. Bernstein DI, Epstein T, Murphy-Berendts K, et al. Surveillance of systemic reactions to subcutaneous immunotherapy injections: year 1 outcomes of the ACAAI and AAAAI collaborative study. Ann Allergy Asthma Immunol 2010;104:530–5.

84. Calderon MA, Simons FE, Malling HJ, et al. Sublingual allergen immunotherapy: mode of action and its relationship with the safety profile. Allergy 2012;67:302–11.

85. Brown SG, Blackman KE, Heddle RJ. Can serum mast cell tryptase help diagnose anaphylaxis? Emerg Med Australas 2004;16:120–4.

86. Rank MA, Kita H, Li JT, et al. Systemic reactions to allergen immunotherapy: a role for measuring a PGD2 metabolite? Ann Allergy Asthma Immunol 2013;110:57–8.

87. Ohnmacht C, Park JH, Cording S, et al. The microbiota regulates type 2 immunity through RORγt+ T cells. Science 2015;349(6251):989–93.

88. Human Microbiome Project Consortium. Structure, function and diversity of the healthy human microbiome. Nature 2012;486:207–14.

89. Mika M, Mack I, Korten I, et al. Dynamics of the nasal microbiota in infancy: a prospective cohort study. J Allergy Clin Immunol 2015;135:905–12.

90. Lu TX, Rothenberg ME. Diagnostic, functional, and therapeutic roles of microRNA in allergic diseases. J Allergy Clin Immunol 2013;132:3–13.

91. Spits H, Di Santo JD. The expanding family of innate lymphoid cells: regulators and effectors of immunity and tissue remodelling. Nat Immunol 2010;12:21–7.

92. Plant K, Maltby S, Mattes J, et al. Targeting translational control as a novel way to treat inflammatory disease: the emerging role of microRNAs. Clin Exp Allergy 2013;43:981–99.

93. Hu G, Tang Q, Sharma S, et al. Expression and regulation of intergenic long noncoding RNAs during T cell development and differentiation. Nat Immunol 2013; 14:1190–8.

94. Bartemes KR, Kephart GM, Fox SJ, et al. Enhanced innate type 2 immune response in peripheral blood from patients with asthma. J Allergy Clin Immunol 2014;134:671–8.

95. Barlow JL, McKenzie AN. Type-2 innate lymphoid cells in human allergic disease. Curr Opin Allergy Clin Immunol 2014;14:397–403.

96. Lao-Araya M, Steveling E, Scadding GW, et al. Seasonal increases in peripheral innate lymphoid type 2 cells are inhibited by subcutaneous grass pollen immunotherapy. J Allergy Clin Immunol 2014;134:1193–5.

Allergen Immunotherapy Outcomes and Unmet Needs: A Critical Review

Davide Caimmi, MD[a,b], Moises A. Calderon, MD, PhD[c],
Jean Bousquet, MD, PhD[b], Pascal Demoly, MD, PhD[a,d],*

KEYWORDS

- Allergen immunotherapy (AIT) • Allergic rhinitis • Clinical outcomes
- Primary end point • Unmet needs

KEY POINTS

- Allergen immunotherapy (AIT) is a disease-modifying treatment of allergic patients.
- AIT trials do not use a uniformed primary outcome.
- There is a lack of consensus on how to properly evaluate AIT efficacy for all allergic diseases.
- Total combined symptom score could be a standardized tool to evaluate the primary outcome in AIT trials for allergic rhinitis.

INTRODUCTION

Allergen immunotherapy (AIT) is an effective treatment for both adults and children, mainly prescribed for allergic rhinitis, allergic conjunctivitis, and allergic asthma.[1] Although, on one hand, pharmacologic therapies are capable of providing temporary symptoms relief, on the other hand, AIT is the only treatment that can actually modify the atopic march and induce long-term disappearance of the allergic symptoms. For allergic rhinitis, medications (relief therapies) include mast cell stabilizers, antihistamines, glucocorticoids, leukotriene receptor antagonists, and nasal decongestants.[2,3]

Disclosure: See last page of article.
[a] Division of Allergy, Department of Pulmonology, Hôpital Arnaud de Villeneuve, University Hospital of Montpellier, 371, av. du Doyen Gaston Giraud – 34295, Montpellier cedex 5, France; [b] MACVIA-LR, European Innovation Partnership on Active and Healthy Ageing Reference Site, University Hospital of Montpellier, 371, av. du Doyen Gaston Giraud – 34295, Montpellier cedex 5, France; [c] Section of Allergy and Clinical Immunology, Imperial College London, National Heart & Lung Institute, Royal Brompton Hospital, Sydney Street, London SW3 6NP, UK; [d] Sorbonne Universités, UPMC Paris 06, UMR-S 1136, IPLESP, Equipe EPAR, F-75013, 4, Place Jussieu – 75005 Paris, France
* Corresponding author. Division of Allergy, Department of Pulmonology, Hôpital Arnaud de Villeneuve, 371, Av du Doyen Gaston Giraud, Montpellier 34090, France.
E-mail address: pascal.demoly@inserm.fr

Immunol Allergy Clin N Am 36 (2016) 181–189
http://dx.doi.org/10.1016/j.iac.2015.08.011   immunology.theclinics.com
0889-8561/16/$ – see front matter © 2016 Elsevier Inc. All rights reserved.

Intranasal steroids are considered as the most effective treatment to control symptoms and are prescribed as a first-line therapy, very often in association with antihistamines.[2] Their effects quickly disappear when the treatment is stopped. AIT has, therefore, to be considered as the only real possible disease-modifying treatment of allergic patients.[4]

The two most commonly prescribed routes for aeroallergen AIT are subcutaneous (subcutaneous allergen immunotherapy [SCIT]) and sublingual (sublingual allergen immunotherapy [SLIT]).[5] The type of prescribed route and the more interest of one over the other is different worldwide, depending on different variables, such as the availability of a regulatory-approved extract, geography, patient preferences, reimbursement policies, and cost both for the local health care system and for patients.[5]

Besides the primary indications mentioned, AIT may be effective in some patients with atopic dermatitis, food allergy, and other allergic conditions[6,7] (**Table 1**). Nevertheless, it has to be underlined that, as for food immunotherapy, many issues still need to be clarified in terms of long-term tolerance after discontinuation.[8,9]

When evaluating the effectiveness of AIT, both statistically significant and clinically relevant outcomes need to be taken into account.[1] Therefore, both clinical trials and daily effectiveness should be considered, even though it is difficult to separate them in research articles. Several issues still need to be addressed in order to properly identify a specific tool capable of predicting the real efficacy of such a treatment. A clinical trial outcome should be a measure allowing one to decide whether the null hypothesis should be accepted or rejected.[10] Classically, there is a differentiation between the *primary outcome*, which usually includes the measurement of symptoms and the use of rescue drugs, and the *secondary outcomes*, which may include the patients' quality-of-life improvement, and several other markers that change from one study to the other.[3,11] Also, more cost-effectiveness studies are urgently needed.

PRIMARY OUTCOMES

The European Medicines Agency (EMA) guidance on statistical principles for clinical trials defines the primary variable as the one "capable of providing the most clinically relevant and convincing evidence directly related to the primary objective of the trial."[10] In 2008, the EMA stated that, so far, no validated symptom and medication scoring method for clinical trials could be clearly used in evaluating AIT effectiveness.[3] Nevertheless, the agency pointed out a possible preferred primary outcome measure for AIT clinical trials, the total combined score (TCS), which is the sum of the total symptom score (TSS) and total medication score (TMS).[3] The Allergy-Control-SCORE has been actually validated to assess patients' allergy disease severity by recording both symptoms and the concomitant use of symptomatic treatments.[12]

Table 1	
AIT indications and other possible uses	
Primary Indications of AIT	**Other Possible Uses of AIT**
Allergic rhinitis	Atopic dermatitis
Allergic conjunctivitis	Large local venom allergic reaction
Allergic asthma	Food allergy
Hymenoptera venom allergy	Oral allergy syndrome
—	Latex allergy
—	Allergic urticaria/angioedema

Such a score considers the severity of the disease, and the need to consult for the allergic condition and the validated Rhinoconjunctivitis Quality of Life Questionnaire[13] and is a good method to evaluate respiratory allergy severity in clinical trials.[12] However, very few trials have used this tool.

Regardless, it is important to combine the TSS and the TMS, because the severity of the symptoms and the use of relief medications are 2 interdependent variables that should both be considered when evaluating patients' benefits from such treatment.[1] The use of the TCS has to be considered as the best approach to evaluate the primary outcome of AIT, being able to highlight both the largest effect size and the most efficient (clinically relevant) treatment.[14] Nevertheless, there is no agreed scoring system for TCS yet.[1]

In general, to evaluate the TSS, several double-blind placebo-controlled trials have used the patient self-rated Total Nasal Symptom Score (TNSS), assessed over the whole pollen season (with variable definition of the season) or the peak of the pollen season (with variable definition but around 2 weeks in general) for seasonal allergic rhinitis (SAR) and over a 4- to 8-week period for persistent allergic rhinitis (PAR).[15] The TNSS is generally based on 4 symptoms: sneezing, rhinorrhea, nasal congestion, nasal pruritus.[1] The other score that is usually assessed is the total ocular symptom score (TOSS), which is based on the following symptoms: ocular pruritus and watery eyes.[1] Patients record a diary and score their symptoms usually daily, by using a 4-point rating scale ranging between 0 (no symptoms) and 3 (severe symptoms) (**Fig. 1**).[16]

The symptoms may be recorded in the evening in trials for SAR and in the morning in PAR trials.[3] A task force by the World Allergy Organization (WAO) has suggested including in the symptoms score lower respiratory symptoms as well (chest tightness, shortness of breath, cough, and wheezing).[11]

The EMA guidelines recommend that the "*efficacy for the nasal and eye-symptoms should be proven separately*" and "*the overall-effect should be balanced.*"[3] Nevertheless, clinical trials are different in considering what kind of TSS is used: They may vary from simply TNSS including 4 nasal symptoms,[17–21] 4 nasal and 3 eye symptoms,[21] 4 nasal and 2 eye symptoms,[20] 4 nasal and one eye symptom,[21–24] or 3 nasal and one eye symptom.[25] Some other trials only consider the TOSS as a primary end

Score		0 No symptoms	1 Mild, not bothersome, easily tolerated	2 Moderate, bothersome, but tolerable	3 Severe symptoms
Nasal symptoms	Sneezing				
	Rhinorrhea				
	Nasal congestion				
	Nasal pruritus				
Oular symptoms	Ocular pruritus				
	Watery eyes				

Fig. 1. Possible daily symptoms score sheets for patients in AIT trials.

point.[26,27] On the whole, there is a deep lack of homogeneity in the different AIT trials because of what symptom they focus on.

One major issue is the recording of the allergen season. In AIT trials, allergen exposure is typically assessed by pollen counts; but these may misrepresent exposure if performed remotely from multiple study centers, because pollen counts vary widely across centers and do not represent the real allergen exposure for individual patients. Moreover, pollen counts may vary daily even during the season. A novel placebo score-based method, which may better reflect the variations in pollen counts, was proposed.[28] Electronic-health (e-health) technologies may be used in the future to include a clinical decision support system coupled to cell phones and visual analog scales (VASs) comparing placebo and AIT-treated patients.[29]

SECONDARY OUTCOMES

Secondary outcome parameters may also be evaluated in AIT trials. These parameters may include several different assessments, as summarized in **Table 2**.

Evaluations of AIT efficacy may, therefore, include different responder analyses. Only a few studies have used the VAS to estimate the severity and/or control of symptoms.[30–32] Quality of life has been assessed through a specific questionnaire in several studies in adults[23,24,33,34] and in children.[17]

COST-EFFECTIVENESS OF ALLERGEN IMMUNOTHERAPY

Allergic rhinitis and asthma are among the most common and costliest chronic conditions worldwide.[5] Data from the Medical Expenditure Panel Survey run in the United States estimated the direct costs of allergic rhinitis to be $11.5 billion in 2005, with prescription medications (59%).[35] When considering the cost associated with over-the-counter (OTC) drugs, another $1.2 to $1.7 billion was to be added in a 2008 survey[36]; this cost is likely to increase in the future, when more medications will become OTC. Moreover, these total costs do not consider lost work productivity due to patients' absence at work.[5] As for asthma, the total direct and indirect medical care cost in the United States was estimated at $56 billion in 2007.[37] The financial burden of allergic diseases to both society and patients is, therefore, considerable; AIT seems to be associated with a significant cost savings (as high as 80%),[7] even though these results are based on SCIT studies only and there are only a limited number of studies that have included cost comparisons between AIT and other treatments.[5] One systematic review highlighted that both SCIT and SLIT are cost-effective compared with other therapies, but this outcome is proven only 6 years after AIT is started.[38,39]

| Table 2 | | |
Possible way to assess secondary outcomes in AIT trials		
Rhinoconjunctivitis quality of life	Well and hell days	Allergen challenge chambers
Allergen-specific immunoglobulin G antibodies	Inflammatory parameters	Score in individual symptoms
VASs	Nasal provocation tests	Skin reactivity
Conjunctival provocation tests	Bronchial provocation tests	Functional measures
Generic questionnaires	Disease-specific questionnaires	Others

Once again, there is no homogeneity in the way the economic outcomes are expressed and/or measured.[5] However, a health technology assessment study funded by the UK National Institute for Health Research Health Technology Assessment program concluded:

A benefit from both SCIT and SLIT compared with placebo has been consistently demonstrated, but the extent of this effectiveness in terms of clinical benefit is unclear. Both SCIT and SLIT may be cost-effective compared with AIT from around 6 years (threshold of £20,000–30,000 per [quality-adjusted life-year] QALY). Further research is needed to establish the comparative effectiveness of SCIT compared with SLIT and to provide more robust cost-effectiveness estimates.[38]

UNMET NEEDS

Several articles evaluated the efficacy of AIT in patients with allergic rhinitis (AR), but it seems clear that there is no method/end point that is actually universally accepted. In fact, heterogeneous end points have been used in different published trials with a lack of standardization for primary and secondary outcomes. In 2014, the European Academy of Allergy and Clinical Immunology (EAACI) Immunotherapy Interest Group has conducted a task force on "recommendations for the standardization of clinical outcomes used in AIT trials for allergic rhino-conjunctivitis."[29] The position paper is based on EMA guidelines, the American recommendation of the Food and Drug Administration (FDA), already published phase III trials, and expert discussion. The aim of the article was both to highlight and evaluate the current clinical outcomes used in AIT clinical trials and to recommend a consensus position for the best clinical outcomes to consider for future AIT products for allergic rhino-conjunctivitis.[29] The EAACI position paper confirms that the TCS should be used as a primary outcome in allergic rhino-conjunctivitis trials, associated nose and eyes symptoms, and the need for concomitant symptomatic therapies. Nevertheless, the TCS is still not validated; there is no strict consensus/direction from the EAACI or regulatory authorities for clinical AIT trials.[29] As for AIT trials in asthmatic patients, the position paper does not give recommendations for clinical end points.

One unmet need that requires clarification in AIT trials is how to measure the magnitude of clinical efficacy using, for example, effect sizes or a minimal clinically important difference (MCID). MCID is the smallest change in an outcome identified as important by patients. Glacy and colleagues,[40] from the US Agency for Healthcare Research and Quality, detail the different ways to calculate the MCID. Here as well, there is no consensus regarding the optimal methodology. In contrast to pharmacotherapy trials, AIT field trials allow patients to use rescue drugs, making it impossible to consider the placebo group as "medications free."[5] The only setting where patients do not use rescue medications is the environmental exposure chambers,[29] but these studies are not accepted as phase III trials.[3] The WAO task force has underlined that the effect size of AIT efficacy should exceed 20% of the one recorded in the placebo group,[11] without clear justifications for this number. In AIT trials, the placebo group is equivalent to a symptomatic-therapy-alone group.[5] Even considering this aspect, AIT trials have all demonstrated a significant clinical efficacy of the treatment when compared with placebo both in allergic rhino-conjunctivitis and asthma studies.[4] The FDA seems to request an effect size of 15% with a lower 95% confidence interval band no smaller than 10% for pollen allergic rhinitis. These numbers are by far greater than what has always been requested for allergic rhinitis pharmacotherapy.

Another interesting point that needs to be clarified is that symptoms, in pollen allergic patients, are obviously more severe during the pollen season. Trials should, therefore, be run during the relevant season; but a standard definition of pollen season and peak pollen season does not really exist and varies from one phase III trial to another. EAACI is currently running a task force to address this issue. As for perennial allergens, such as mites, a higher exposure is highlighted during the fall; choosing the period when the outcomes are measured is crucial. AIT trials take into account this aspect, whereas pharmacologic trials usually do not consider such an increase in allergen exposure, patients being included when they are very symptomatic, meaning very exposed. Also, mite allergic patients are not usually evaluated for ocular symptoms, which might underestimate the presence of allergic conjunctivitis if compared with pollen allergic patients. In mite studies, therefore, eye symptoms often appear as secondary end points, which does not line up with the new recommendations of the EAACI task force.[29]

However, the future of AIT will be in patient stratification and novel health systems. There is a need to define the patient population that will need AIT and the population that will benefit. This aspect will be the critical issue of AIT in the next 5 years. To help stratifying patients, e-health technology and biomarkers should be combined.[29] Biomarkers should define the patients who need to receive AIT (patient stratification), assess the early benefits of AIT after a few months (ie, after the first season for pollens and after a few months for indoor allergens) to decide whether AIT should be stopped or discontinued, determine the long-term benefits of AIT (after 3 years) to decide whether AIT should be continued or can be discontinued, and determine the efficacy of AIT when it is stopped.

Health systems in most countries are based on acute care and severe diseases (eg, cancer). They are often successful in the small proportion of the population needing this type of care. However, chronic diseases and their comorbidities represent the new paradigm of medicine.[41,42] More than 100 million patients have allergic rhinitis in Europe, and self-management support interventions should be implemented[43]; integrated care pathways should be developed at the national or regional levels.[44] The importance of e-health is undisputable. This approach will lead to novel health care models in which AIT should be considered.

All these issues still need to be clarified, validated, and standardized for future AIT trials.

SUMMARY

Several articles have been published over the years on AIT treatments and efficacy. Prevention of both asthma and the appearance of new sensitizations in patients with allergic rhinitis are crucial objectives of AIT[45] and not yet demonstrated for the newly developed products. However, registration is a stepwise process, starting with the demonstration of short-term (1 year) efficacy and safety. Primary end points are not homogeneous throughout publications, and secondary end points vary from one article to the other.[46] The main unmet need for all AIT trials is to find a validated and uniform primary end point for all studies. This consistency would allow clinicians to decide in a standardized manner whether AIT is an appropriate therapy for their patients[1] and indirectly compare products. Nevertheless, even if the total combined symptoms score seems to be a proper tool for a primary end point evaluation, and it would make trials as close as possible to real-life circumstances, its validation is still missing.[46] Also, international guidelines should identify both at what time, in relation with the pollen season or the allergen peak, the clinical significance of AIT should be evaluated and what exact magnitude of treatment efficacy should be considered over the placebo group. Once these issues are solved, AIT trials will be uniform and a real comparison between results and treatment efficacy will be possible.

DISCLOSURE

D. Caimmi has nothing to disclose. M.A. Calderon has received consulting fees, honoraria for lectures, and/or research funding from ALK, Stallergenes, Merck, Allergopharma, and HAL. J. Bousquet has received honoraria for scientific and advisory boards: Almirall, Meda, Merck, MSD, Novartis, Sanofi-Aventis, Takeda, Teva, and Uriach; lectures during meetings: Almirall, AstraZeneca, Chiesi, GSK, Meda, Menarini, Merck, MSD, Novartis, Sanofi-Aventis, Takeda, Teva, and Uriach; and board of directors: Stallergènes. P. Demoly is a consultant (and a speaker) for Stallergenes, Circassia, ALK, DBV, and Chiesi and was a speaker for Merck, Astra Zeneca, Pierre Fabre Médicaments, Menarini, Allergopharma, Allergy Therapeutics Ltd, ThermoFischer Scientific, and GlaxoSmithKline.

REFERENCES

1. Makatsori M, Pfaar O, Calderon MA. J Allergen immunotherapy: clinical outcomes assessment. J Allergy Clin Immunol Pract 2014;2:123–9.
2. Bousquet J, Khaltaev N, Cruz AA, et al. Allergic Rhinitis and its Impact on Asthma (ARIA) 2008 update (in collaboration with the World Health Organization, GA(2) LEN and AllerGen). Allergy 2008;63:S8–160.
3. European Medicines Agency (EMA). Committee for medicinal products for human use (CHMP). Guideline on the clinical development of medicinal products for the treatment of allergic rhinoconjunctivitis (CHMP/EWP/2455/02). Available at: http://www.ema.europa.eu/docs/en_GB/document_library/Scientific_guideline/2009/09/WC500003554.pdf. Accessed June 7, 2015.
4. Burks AW, Calderon MA, Casale T, et al. Update on allergy immunotherapy: American Academy of Allergy, Asthma & Immunology/European Academy of Allergy and Clinical Immunology/PRACTALL consensus report. J Allergy Clin Immunol 2013;131:1288–96.
5. Cox L. Allergy immunotherapy in reducing healthcare cost. Curr Opin Otolaryngol Head Neck Surg 2015;23:247–54.
6. Schneider L, Tilles S, Lio P, et al. Atopic dermatitis: a practice parameter update 2012. J Allergy Clin Immunol 2013;131:295–9.
7. Cox L, Calderon M, Pfaar O. Subcutaneous allergen immunotherapy for allergic disease: examining efficacy, safety and cost-effectiveness of current and novel formulations. Immunotherapy 2012;6:1–16.
8. Pajno GB, Cox L, Caminiti L, et al. Oral immunotherapy for treatment of immunoglobulin E-mediated food allergy: the transition to clinical practice. Pediatr Allergy Immunol Pulmonol 2014;27:42–50.
9. Wood RA, Sampson HA. Oral immunotherapy for the treatment of peanut allergy: is it ready for prime time? J Allergy Clin Immunol Pract 2014;2:97–8.
10. European Medicines Agency (EMA). Committee for medicinal products for human use (CHMP): ICH topic E 9. Statistical principles for clinical trials. Note for guidance on statistical principles for clinical trials (CPMP/ICH/363/96). Available at: http://www.ema.europa.eu/docs/en_GB/document_library/Scientific_guideline/2009/09/WC500002928.pdf 1998. Accessed June 7, 2015.

11. Canonica GW, Baena-Cagnani CE, Bousquet J, et al. Recommendations for standardization of clinical trials with allergen specific immunotherapy for respiratory allergy. A statement of a World Allergy Organization (WAO) task force. Allergy 2007;62:317–24.

12. Hafner D, Reich K, Matricardi PM, et al. Prospective validation of 'Allergy-Control Score™': a novel symptom-medication score for clinical trials. Allergy 2011;66: 629–36.

13. Juniper EF, Guyatt GH. Development and testing of a new measure of health status for clinical trials in rhinoconjunctivitis. Clin Exp Allergy 1991;21:77–83.

14. Clark J, Schall R. Assessment of combined symptom and medication scores for rhinoconjunctivitis immunotherapy clinical trials. Allergy 2007;62:1023–8.

15. US Department of Health and Human Services. Food and Drug Administration (FDA). Center for Drug Evaluation and Research (CDER): guidance for industry. Allergic rhinitis: clinical development programs for drug products. Available at: http://www.fda.gov/downloads/Drugs/.GuidanceComplianceRegulatoryInformation/Guidances/ucm071293.pdf. Accessed 2000.

16. Pfaar O, Kleine-Tebbe J, Hörmann K, et al. Allergen-specific immunotherapy: which outcome measures are useful in monitoring clinical trials? Immunol Allergy Clin North Am 2011;31:289–309.

17. Potter P, Maspero JF, Vermeulen J, et al. Rupatadine oral solution in children with persistent allergic rhinitis: a randomized, double-blind, placebo-controlled study. Pediatr Allergy Immunol 2013;24:144–50.

18. Ciebiada M, Gorska-Ciebiada M, Barylski M, et al. Use of montelukast alone or in combination with desloratadine or levocetirizine in patients with persistent allergic rhinitis. Am J Rhinol Allergy 2011;25:e1–6.

19. Meltzer EO, Lee J, Tripathy I, et al. Efficacy and safety of once-daily fluticasone furoate nasal spray in children with seasonal allergic rhinitis treated for 2 wk. Pediatr Allergy Immunol 2009;20:279–86.

20. Sastre J, Mullol J, Valero A, et al. Efficacy and safety of bilastine 20 mg compared with cetirizine 10 mg and placebo in the treatment of perennial allergic rhinitis. Curr Med Res Opin 2012;28:121–30.

21. Meltzer E, Ratner P, Bachert C, et al. Clinically relevant effect of a new intranasal therapy (MP29-02) in allergic rhinitis assessed by responder analysis. Int Arch Allergy Immunol 2013;161:369–77.

22. Marmouz F, Giralt J, Izquierdo I. Morning and evening efficacy evaluation of rupatadine (10 and 20 mg), compared with cetirizine 10 mg in perennial allergic rhinitis: a randomized, double-blind, placebo-controlled trial. J Asthma Allergy 2011;4:27–35.

23. Rogkakou A, Villa E, Garelli V, et al. Persistent allergic rhinitis and the XPERT study. World Allergy Organ J 2011;4:S32–6.

24. Hashemi SM, Okhovat A, Amini S, et al. Comparing the effects of botulinum toxin-A and cetirizine on the treatment of allergic rhinitis. Allergol Int 2013;62:245–9.

25. Guilemany JM, Garcia-Pinero A, Alobid I, et al. The loss of smell in persistent allergic rhinitis is improved by levocetirizine due to reduction of nasal inflammation but not nasal congestion (the CIRANO study). Int Arch Allergy Immunol 2012;158:184–90.

26. Keith P, Lee LA. Fluticasone furoate nasal spray is the only intranasal corticosteroid to reduce the ocular symptoms of seasonal allergic rhinitis consistently. J Allergy Clin Immunol 2011;127:288–9.

27. Prenner BM, Lanier BQ, Bernstein DI, et al. Mometasone furoate nasal spray reduces the ocular symptoms of seasonal allergic rhinitis. J Allergy Clin Immunol 2010;125:1247–53.

28. Frew AJ, Dubuske L, Keith PK, et al. Assessment of specific immunotherapy efficacy using a novel placebo score-based method. Ann Allergy Asthma Immunol 2012;109:342–7.

29. Pfaar O, Demoly P, Gerth van Wijk R, et al. Recommendations for the standardization of clinical outcomes used in allergen immunotherapy trials for allergic rhinoconjunctivitis: an EAACI position paper. Allergy 2014;69:854–67.

30. Demoly P, Bousquet PJ, Mesbah K, et al. Visual analogue scale in patients treated for allergic rhinitis: an observational prospective study in primary care: asthma and rhinitis. Clin Exp Allergy 2013;43:881–8.

31. Wu KG, Li TH, Wang TY, et al. A comparative study of loratadine syrup and cyproheptadine HCL solution for treating perennial allergic rhinitis in Taiwanese children aged 2-12 years. Int J Immunopathol Pharmacol 2012;25:231–7.

32. Mehuys E, Gevaert P, Brusselle G, et al. Self-medication in persistent rhinitis: overuse of decongestants in half of the patients. J Allergy Clin Immunol Pract 2014;2:313–9.

33. Bautista AP, Eisenlohr CP, Lanz MJ. Nasal nitric oxide and nasal eosinophils decrease with levocetirizine in subjects with perennial allergic rhinitis. Am J Rhinol Allergy 2011;25:383–7.

34. Bousquet J, Zuberbier T, Canonica GW, et al. Randomized controlled trial of desloratadine for persistent allergic rhinitis: correlations between symptom improvement and quality of life. Allergy Asthma Proc 2013;34:274–82.

35. Soni A. Allergic rhinitis: trends in use and expenditures, 2000 to 2005. Statistical brief #204. Bethesda (MD): Agency for Healthcare Research and Quality; 2008.

36. Blaiss MS. Allergic rhinitis: direct and indirect costs. Allergy Asthma Proc 2010; 31:375–80.

37. Barnett SB, Nurmagambetov TA. Costs of asthma in the United States: 2002–2007. J Allergy Clin Immunol 2011;127:145–52.

38. Meadows A, Kaambwa B, Novielli N, et al. A systematic review and economic evaluation of subcutaneous and sublingual allergen immunotherapy in adults and children with seasonal allergic rhinitis. Health Technol Assess 2013;17:vi, xi-xiv, 1–322.

39. Hankin CS, Cox L. Allergy immunotherapy: what is the evidence for cost saving? Curr Opin Allergy Clin Immunol 2014;14:363–70.

40. Glacy J, Putnam K, Godfrey S, et al. Treatments for seasonal allergic rhinitis. Rockville (MD): Agency for Healthcare Research and Quality (US); 2013. Available at: http://effectivehealthcare.ahrq.gov/ehc/products/376/1588/allergy-seasonal-report-130711.pdf.

41. Bousquet J, Jorgensen C, Dauzat M, et al. Systems medicine approaches for the definition of complex phenotypes in chronic diseases and ageing. From concept to implementation and policies. Curr Pharm Des 2014;20:5928–44.

42. Grover A, Joshi A. An overview of chronic disease models: a systematic literature review. Glob J Health Sci 2015;7:210–27.

43. Franek J. Self-management support interventions for persons with chronic disease: an evidence-based analysis. Ont Health Technol Assess Ser 2013;13:1–60.

44. Bousquet J, Addis A, Adcock I, et al. Integrated care pathways for airway diseases (AIRWAYS-ICPs). Eur Respir J 2014;44:304–23.

45. Verheggen BG, Westerhout KY, Schreder CH, et al. Health economic comparison of SLIT allergen and SCIT allergoid immunotherapy in patients with seasonal grass-allergic rhinoconjunctivitis in Germany. Clin Transl Allergy 2015;5:1.

46. Calderon MA, Eichel A, Makatsori M, et al. Comparability of subcutaneous and sublingual immunotherapy outcomes in allergic rhinitis clinical trials. Curr Opin Allergy Clin Immunol 2012;12:249–56.

Allergy Work-Up Including Component-Resolved Diagnosis

How to Make Allergen-Specific Immunotherapy More Specific

Jörg Kleine-Tebbe, MD[a],*, Paolo M. Matricardi, MD[b],
Robert G. Hamilton, PhD, D.ABMLI[c]

KEYWORDS

- Allergen-specific immunotherapy • Allergy diagnosis
- Component-resolved diagnosis • Pollen pan-allergen • Profilin • Polcalcin
- Major allergen

KEY POINTS

- Identification of clinically relevant inhalant allergen sources, that is, tree, grass, or weed pollen, is required before allergen-specific immunotherapy.
- In the case of IgE sensitizations to plant pan-allergens (minor allergens profilin and/or polcalcin) diagnostic pollen extracts lack analytical specificity and show all-over positive and thus misleading results.
- Molecular marker allergens for allergen-specific IgE detection help to separate specific sensitizations to tree and/or grass and/or weed pollen from IgE sensitizations to pollen pan-allergens.
- Candidates for molecular allergy diagnostics to identify specific allergen sensitivities (ie, major allergen markers) are Bet v 1 (birch, hazel, alder, beech, and oak) Ole e 1 (olive and ash), Jun a 1 (cedar), Phl p 1/5 (Pooideae grasses), Amb a 1 (ragweed), Art v 1 (mugwort), and Par j 2 (pellitory).
- Allergen extract compositions based on confirmed IgE sensitizations to major allergen markers might facilitate more targeted allergen-specific immunotherapy.

[a] Allergy & Asthma Center Westend, Outpatient Clinic Hanf, Ackermann & Kleine-Tebbe, Spandauer Damm 130, Haus 9, Berlin D-14050, Germany; [b] AG Molecular Allergology and Immuno-modulation, Department of Pediatric Pneumology and Immunology, Charité Medical University, Augustenburger Platz 1, Berlin D-13353, Germany; [c] Johns Hopkins Dermatology, Allergy and Clinical Immunology Reference Laboratory, Johns Hopkins Asthma and Allergy Center, Johns Hopkins University School of Medicine, 5501 Hopkins Bayview Circle, Room 1A20, Baltimore, MD 21224, USA
* Corresponding author.
E-mail address: kleine-tebbe@allergie-experten.de

Immunol Allergy Clin N Am 36 (2016) 191–203
http://dx.doi.org/10.1016/j.iac.2015.08.012   immunology.theclinics.com
0889-8561/16/$ – see front matter © 2016 Elsevier Inc. All rights reserved.

INTRODUCTION

Allergy diagnosis is based on the recording of characteristic symptoms after a known allergen exposure and demonstrating immunoglobulin E(IgE) sensitizations (**Fig. 1**) to the underlying (protein) allergen or allergen source (ie, plant, animal, or fungal species). A positive history corresponding to positive sensitization test results indicates a clinically relevant allergy. Allergylike symptoms without corresponding IgE sensitizations indicate a "localized allergy"[1] or a nonallergic cause (ie, nonspecific, nonallergic rhinoconjunctivitis).[2] Isolated positive diagnostic IgE antibody test results without corresponding symptoms are considered "silent IgE sensitizations." Their clinical relevance might have been apparent in the past or might develop in the future. The following overview discusses diagnostic tools for successful implementation of allergen-specific immunotherapy (AIT). Judicious use of allergen molecules in the diagnostic evaluation permits a more targeted selection of allergen sources for subsequent use in AIT.[3-6]

CLINICAL INFORMATION WHEN ALLERGY IS SUSPECTED

The patient's allergy history provides the clinician with the individual's symptoms and the onset, course, and trend of the disease. Seasonal allergic symptoms may be linked to exposure to a number of allergen sources (ie, tree, grass, and weed pollen). The relevant allergen sources are more readily identified in both the northern and southern hemispheres, at temperate latitudes where moderate climate zones provide more definitive separation of pollen seasons among the dominant pollen species (**Fig. 2**, upper panel).

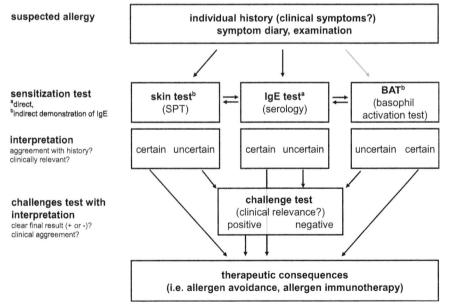

Fig. 1. Diagnostic algorithm. A rational allergy work-up considers the benefits and risks to the individual. These can involve suitability of a particular allergen source and test method and the suitability of the patient for skin or blood testing (ie, interfering drug intake, dermographisms, or comorbidities).

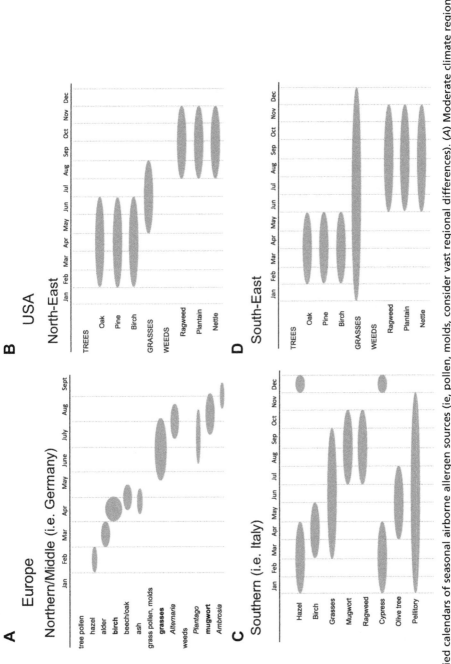

Fig. 2. Simplified calendars of seasonal airborne allergen sources (ie, pollen, molds, consider vast regional differences). (*A*) Moderate climate regions (northern/middle Europe, ie, Germany). (*B*) Northern parts of America (ie, Canada, northern parts of the United States). (*C*) Mild climate regions (southern Europe, ie, Italy). (*D*) Regions of America with hot or subtropical climates (ie, southern parts of the United States).

Other areas within the subtropical or tropical climate zones show overlapping pollen seasons, which may hamper conclusions based on history-derived symptom data from the allergic individual (see **Fig. 2**, lower panel).

Valuable information can be collected in the case of a clear temporal or local manifestation of characteristic allergy symptoms after allergen exposure. This information is often far from clear. Therefore, the data collected in a complete allergy-related history might be supplemented by

- Additional (parent's) atopic history (ie, in infants and children)
- Allergy symptom diary (ie, prospective in the upcoming season)
- Software or mobile phone-based symptom calendars (ie, AllergyMonitor,[7] Pollen-App 3.0 (http://www.pollenstiftung.de), National Allergy Bureau of the AAAAI (http://www.aaaai.org/global/nab-pollen-counts.aspx)

The time spent in obtaining a thorough allergy history along with additional tools, such as symptom diaries, is well invested as this clinical information serves as the basis for the selection of the allergen to be included in the subsequent AIT formulation. In contrast, selections of therapeutic allergens for AIT based on vague patient information carries the risk of unsuitable prescriptions, resulting in failed AIT responses.[8]

PRINCIPLES FOR THE DEMONSTRATION OF IMMUNOGLOBULIN E SENSITIZATION
Skin Prick Test Reagents Are Considered Drugs in European Law

In the case of immediate-type hypersensitivity (type I allergy), sensitization tests are based on the demonstration of allergen-specific IgE antibody. A positive skin prick test (SPT) with allergens provides indirect evidence of allergen-specific IgE on cutaneous mast cells. SPTs are robust and easy to use screening instruments for common allergen sources. Allergen extracts for in vivo diagnostic use are classified as drugs according to a European Directive and must fulfil the criteria for market authorization by the competent authorities (ie, Paul-Ehrlich-Institute, Langen, Germany: http://www.pei.de/DE/arzneimittel/allergene/test-allergene/pricktest/pricktest-node.html). At present, certain extracts are no longer available on the market in certain European countries (ie, Germany) because of a number of quality control requirements and the increased costs of maintaining mandatory pharmacovigilance data input in Europe. Switching to another SPT solution from a different allergen manufacturer carries the risk that the composition, total potency, and the size of the SPT reaction can vary, despite being from the same allergen source. In the United States, extracts are treated as biologics. A biologic is defined as a "biological product" (meaning an allergenic product or analogous product) applicable to the prevention, treatment, or cure of a disease or condition of human beings. Only 19 of the more than 1000 diagnostic and therapeutic extracts have a standardized potency.[9]

Serologic Immunoglobulin E Diagnostics with Aeroallergens

In the case of missing skin test reagents, serologic in vitro diagnostic tests (see **Fig. 1**) are an alternative option. They provide a direct assessment of circulating allergen-specific IgE. The results of specific IgE concentrations can vary considerably depending on the test method used. Their performance is compared in proficiency trials in Germany and other European countries, whereas in North America their performance is compared by the College of American Pathologists depending on the type of diagnostic assay that is provided by each manufacturer.

For optimal interpretation, allergen-specific IgE antibody results should be viewed in the context of the individual's total serum IgE level (to define the relative specific IgE to total IgE ratio).[10,11] This approach is particularly important in the case of extremely low (<20 kU/L) or very high (>1000 kU/L) total IgE concentrations.

Recently, commercially available allergen extract reagents for specific IgE detection have been complemented by the addition of single allergens. The use of allergenic molecule-based allergosorbents are able to improve the analytical working range of the assay (eg, lower limit of quantitation), particularly in the case of allergens that are missing or in low abundance in an extract. An additional indication for the use of single allergens includes the assessment of cross-reactivity, which can interfere with the analytical specificity of IgE antibody analyses that use allergen extracts (see later).

Basophil Activation Test for Sera with Extremely Low Total Immunoglobulin E Levels

In the case of extremely low total serum IgE levels, the basophil activation test (BAT) allows a highly sensitive indirect demonstration of allergen-specific IgE on the surface of human effector cells from fresh blood.[12,13] This approach is used in the diagnostic work-up of patients with negative specific IgE results and convincing clinical history (ie, to insect venoms) and may be due to extremely low total IgE concentrations. In patients with typical allergylike symptoms but negative SPT and allergen-specific IgE serology ("localized allergy"), a positive allergen-specific BAT has been demonstrated in 50% of cases, which suggests a weak systemic IgE sensitization.[14]

Concordance and Interpretation of Sensitization Tests

In general, the results of in vivo and in vitro IgE sensitization tests are in good qualitative concordance, providing either a positive or a negative result. Because additional variables add to their complexity,[15,16] indirect sensitization tests (SPT, BAT) do not necessarily demonstrate quantitative concordance with the direct demonstration of specific IgE in serum.[17] Proper interpretation requires taking into account that a negative test result would ideally rule out an IgE sensitization. However, a positive test result indicates IgE sensitization and is only clinically relevant when the individual has corresponding allergic symptoms. Subsequently, all diagnostic sensitization test results require clinical information derived from the patient's history to allow a definitive interpretation by the physician.

ALLERGEN SOURCES FOR DEMONSTRATING SENSITIZATION BEFORE ALLERGEN-SPECIFIC IMMUNOTHERAPY

Because of the structural similarity and close taxonomical relationship of some major allergens, selected common allergen sources are classified as homologs by the European Medicines Agency.[18,19] On this basis, diagnostic tests that demonstrate IgE sensitization to these specificities can be simplified. The use of 1 dominant and representative allergen specificity is frequently sufficient to represent a whole group of allergen sources in its "taxonomic family" due to its content of homologous major allergen(s). Examples of these taxonomic families are

- Birch pollen (with cross-sensitization to pollen allergens from alder, hazel and to a lesser extent to oak, beech, chestnut and hornbeam)
- Olive tree pollen (with cross-sensitization to pollen allergens of other Oleaceae, ie, ash tree, privet, elder)
- Cedar pollen (with cross-sensitization to other pollen allergens, ie, cypress)
- Timothy grass pollen or pollen from Poaceae (also applied as a mix with extensive cross-sensitization among all members of the Poaceae)
- *Dermatophagoides pteronyssinus* or *farinae* (members of the genus *Dermatophagoides* with extensive cross-reactivity between species)

Other inhalant allergen sources including pollen from various weeds, mold spores, and allergens from furry animals are commonly tested separately from species to species (**Table 1**).

DIAGNOSTIC HURDLES AS A RESULT OF MULTISENSITIZATION TO UNRELATED POLLEN SPECIES
Sensitization to Pollen Pan-allergens

A minority of pollen-allergic individuals produce positive sensitization tests (ie, SPT, IgE serology) to numerous or occasionally many pollen plants, independent of their taxonomic relationship. Approximately 15% to 30% of pollen-allergic individuals exhibit sensitization to highly conserved and extensively cross-reactive pan-allergens. Members of the pan-allergen families include profilins (ubiquitous proteins in all pollens and numerous plant foods) and polcalcins (Ca^{2+}-binding proteins in all pollens).

Diagnostic Approach in the Case of Pollen Pan-allergen Sensitization

Suspected sensitizations to pollen pan-allergens can be effectively confirmed by measuring specific IgE antibody to 1 of the members of the profilin family (ie, Phl p 12 or Bet v 2) and of the polcalcin family (ie, Phl p 7 or Bet v 4). Alternatively, sensitization can be excluded in the case of a negative IgE antibody result to these allergens. If a positive result occurs to 1 of the pollen pan-allergens, an allergen-specific diagnosis cannot be established any further using pollen extracts. The analytical specificity is lost because it is impossible to differentiate between tree, grass, or weed pollen sensitizations in the case of detectable IgE anti-pollen pan-allergen positivity. Considering this diagnostic dilemma, sensitizations to unrelated pollen species can only be differentiated by detecting IgE antibody to the corresponding immunodominant major allergen that is unique for each of the important allergen sources (**Fig. 3**): Examples of unique allergen specificities that permit differentiation in the case of pan-allergen cross-reactivity include

a. Bet v 1 (representative for hazel, alder, birch, oak, beech, chestnut and hornbeam)
b. Ole e 1 (representative for Oleaceae, ie, olive tree, ash tree, privet, elder)
d. Cup a 1 (cypress)

Table 1
Modified standard skin prick test for aeroallergens (European standard adapted for northern and middle European countries)

Pollen Species	Other Aeroallergens
Birch, hazel, alder, oak, beech	**Alternaria**, Cladosporium
Ash (olive tree)	Aspergillus, Penicillium
Cypress (cedar)	**Cat**
Plantane	**Dog**
Grass(es)	Horse
Mugwort	*D. pteronyssinus*
Ambrosia, Parietaria	*D. farinae*
Goose foot, nettle, plane	Cockroach

Dominant allergen sources for SPT (bold type) with potential indication for AIT (italic type). Because of cross-reactivity of some major allergens, selected allergen sources (bold type) are sufficient to demonstrate IgE sensitizations. Exceptions: some weeds beyond mugwort, *Ambrosia*, and *Parietaria*.
Adapted from Heinzerling L, Mari A, Bergmann KC, et al. The skin prick test – European standards. Clin Transl Allergy 2013;3:3.

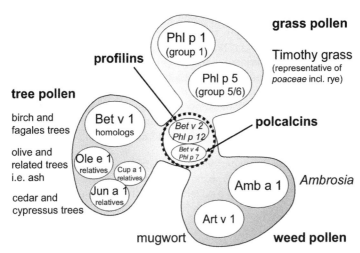

Fig. 3. Propeller model for molecular diagnostics with pollen allergens. Highly cross-reactive pollen pan-allergens (profilins, polcalcins, center of the propeller) and specific indicators of family or species-specific sensitizations (blades). In the case of IgE sensitization to pollen pan-allergens the analytical specificity of extracts is not sufficient to differentiate tree from grass or weed pollen sensitizations. Thus, major pollen allergens (blades) for allergen-specific IgE determinations are suitable to demonstrate sensitizations to important pollen sources.

e. Phl p 1 and Phl p 5 (representative for all grasses from Poaceae)
f. Art v 1 (major allergen of mugwort pollen)
g. Amb a 1 (major allergen of ragweed pollen)
h. Par j 2 (pellitory)

Among 651 Italian children with moderate-to-severe pollen-related allergic rhinitis, no IgE antibodies to major allergens were detected in a significant proportion of patients who presented with a clinical history consistent with a specific seasonal allergen, for example, mugwort (45 of 65, 69%), Betulaceae (146 of 252, 60%), pellitory (78 of 257, 30%), olive (111 of 390, 28%), cypress (28 of 184, 15%), and grass (56 of 568, 10%).

IgE to profilins or polcalcins, or both could identify 173 (37%) of 464 of these SPT reactions. After component-resolved diagnosis (CRD), the SPT-based decision on specific immunotherapy prescription or composition was changed in 277 (42%) of 651 or 315 (48%) of 651 children according to the European or American approach, respectively, and in 305 (47%) of 651 children according to the opinion of 14 local pediatric allergists.[4] This study therefore shows that, in a complex area, the effect of CRD on the composition of prescriptions used in AIT is high. Similar conclusions were reached in a study that investigated sensitization patterns to major grass and olive pollen allergens in 1263 Spanish patients with seasonal allergic rhinitis, and positive SPTs to grass and olive pollens. Based on a traditional diagnostic approach, 922 (73%) patients would have received an AIT prescription with both grass and olive pollens; however, the investigators changed the composition of AIT based on additional CRD IgE antibody data in 56.8% of the patients.[5]

The Evolution of the Immunoglobulin E Response to Grass Pollen and its Impact on Allergen-Specific Immunotherapy

The IgE response to grass pollen (eg, *Phleum pratense*) usually evolves from a simple, monomolecular stage to an oligomolecular stage and eventually to a polymolecular sensitization stage.[20] This phenomenon has been defined as "molecular spreading," which is "the sequential development of an antibody (IgE) response to distinct non-cross-reacting molecules from the same antigenic (allergenic) source, starting with an 'initiator' (allergenic) molecule" (**Fig. 4**).[21] Phl p 1 is the probable initiator molecule in most patients,[20] and the immune response progressively evolves to Phl p 4 or Phl p 5, then Phl p 2 and Phl p 11, and, finally, Phl p 12 or Phl p 7. The practical consequence of this phenomenon is that the longer the duration of disease, the broader the repertoire of IgE specificities against the different molecules within a single pollen. The sequence of IgE responses described in a German birth cohort (a multicenter allergy study), and the molecular spreading phenomenon in general, has been recently confirmed in a second birth cohort study.[22]

The observation that the IgE repertoire is expanding progressively before and during the expression of seasonal allergic rhinitis symptoms has also led to the consideration that AIT should be started earlier in a patient's clinical care, possibly even immediately

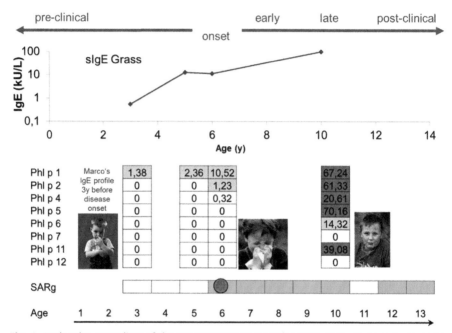

Fig. 4. Molecular spreading of the IgE response to Timothy grass. Potential implications for allergen-specific immunologic intervention in a child with seasonal allergic rhinitis to grass pollen (SARg) (a case from the multicenter allergy study birth cohort). This child started experiencing hay fever symptoms at the age of 6 years. The IgE response against *Phleum pratense* started 3 years previously with a weak, monomolecular sensitization to Phl p 1. This IgE response became stronger and also directed to Phl p 2 and Phl p 4 at disease onset. After disease onset, the IgE response became progressively stronger and directed to Phl p 5, Phl p 6, and Phl p 11. In clinical practice, allergen-specific immunotherapy (AIT) would be "normally" prescribed at this advanced stage, after some years of symptoms (age 10 years). An interesting hypothesis is that AIT would be more efficient if started much earlier, ideally at disease onset (age 6 years) (early AIT). Moreover, the question of whether an immune intervention at the earliest, preclinical stages (age 3 years) of disease could more effectively change the natural history of the sensitization and prevent or delay disease onset (allergen-specific immunoprophylaxis, SIP) could be investigated. The use of recombinant allergens would be easier at this stage as less molecules would be used (component-resolved immune-prophylaxis, CRP).

after the first season in which the allergic respiratory symptoms are observed ("early AIT").[21] The molecular spreading process follows different pathways in different children. Some patients remain sensitized only to the initiator molecule, whereas others become sensitized to most or all allergenic molecules. Consequently, a population of patients allergic to grass pollen apparently homogeneous if examined with an allergen extract, can be remarkably heterogeneous when examined with allergenic molecules (**Fig. 5**).[23]

Clinical Consequences of Pollen Pan-allergen Sensitizations

Approximately 15% to 30% of pollen-allergic individuals are sensitized to profilin and approximately 5% are sensitized to polcalcins. It is thus rare (approximately <2%) that sensitization occurs to both pan-allergens in the same individual. Sensitization to profilin and polcalcin typically occurs in regions with high grass pollen exposure, and this leads to the induction of a broad IgE antibody repertoire specific for grass pollen allergens with their numerous cross-reactive major and minor allergens.[20,23] In addition, profilin sensitized allergic individuals can develop oropharyngeal and, rarely, systemic symptoms after the ingestion of melon, Rosacea fruits, citrus fruits, avocado, banana, cucumber, or other plant foods.[24]

The question of whether sensitization to these minor profilin and/or polcalcin allergens should preclude subsequent AIT has never been addressed prospectively. Retrospectively, less successful courses of AIT have been associated with pan-allergen sensitization to profilin and/or polcalcin.[25] In the case of pollen pan-allergen sensitization, major allergen-specific diagnosis should be established before AIT is initiated (see **Fig. 4**). Monosensitization to these pollen pan-allergens is considered to be uncommon and is presumed to be less suitable for AIT, because the content of profilin and polcalcin in pollen extracts used for AIT and their subsequent therapeutic effect following AIT is far from clear.

INTERPRETATION OF SENSITIZATION TESTS

The detection of allergen-specific IgE in the skin with SPT using commercially available inhalant allergen extracts[26,27] and serum using state-of-the-art singleplex auto-analyzers[28,29] are both considered equivalently sensitive diagnostic methods to detect IgE sensitization to aeroallergens.

A negative IgE antibody result can largely exclude IgE sensitization. When the total IgE level is high enough, and the allergens are intact and in sufficient abundance, the analytical sensitivity is optimized (low threshold level of 0.1 kU_A/L).

A positive result is only clinically relevant and supportive of a decision for subsequent treatment when the individual manifests corresponding allergy symptoms. Therefore, interpretation of the sensitization test results requires plausible historical information from the patient. In the case of a vague clinical history or an underlying allergen source that is in question, or when an allergen exposure cannot be confirmed, subsequent interpretation of a positive sensitization test remains inconclusive.

CHALLENGE TESTS IN THE CASE OF UNRESOLVED CLINICAL RELEVANCE

Particularly in Europe, allergen application to mucosal surfaces (nasal, conjunctival) is considered to be a tool[30] that provides more objective evidence for the clinical relevance of questionable IgE sensitization (examples given in **Table 2**). Nasal and ocular challenges are less commonly used in general practice in the United States. In the event of a negative challenge test result, the evaluated allergen source should not be included in the AIT treatment extract. A clearly positive challenge result verifies

Profile APCS code	profile's binary code (8 molecules): cut-off 0.35 kU/L	rPhl p 1	rPhl p 2	rPhl p 4	rPhl p 5	rPhl p 6	rPhl p 7	rPhl p 11	rPhl p 12	n pos. mol.	n	%	cum. %
128	10000000	●								1	36	20,8	21
248	11111000	●	●	●	●	●				5	21	12,1	33
160	10100000	●		●						2	10	5,8	39
184	10111000	●		●	●	●				4	8	4,6	43
186	10111010	●		●	●	●		●		5	8	4,6	48
251	11111011	●	●	●	●	●		●	●	7	8	4,6	53
192	11000000	●	●							2	7	4,0	57
216	11011000	●	●		●	●				4	7	4,0	61
249	11111001	●	●	●	●	●			●	6	7	4,0	65
250	11111010	●	●	●	●	●		●		6	7	4,0	69
32	100000			●						1	5	2,9	72
224	11100000	●	●	●						3	5	2,9	75
152	10011000	●			●	●				3	4	2,3	77
185	10111001	●		●	●	●			●	5	4	2,3	79
208	11010000	●	●		●					3	3	1,7	81
218	11011010	●	●		●	●		●		5	3	1,7	83
48	110000			●	●					2	2	1,2	84
64	1000000		●							1	2	1,2	85
144	10010000	●			●					2	2	1,2	86
162	10100010	●		●				●		3	2	1,2	87
187	10111011	●		●	●	●		●	●	6	2	1,2	88
193	11000001	●	●						●	3	2	1,2	90
217	11011001	●	●		●	●			●	5	2	1,2	91
225	11100001	●	●	●					●	4	2	1,2	92
16	10000				●					1	1	0,6	92
34	100010			●				●		2	1	0,6	93
58	111010			●	●	●		●		4	1	0,6	94
96	1100000		●	●						2	1	0,6	94
129	10000001	●							●	2	1	0,6	95
130	10000010	●						●		2	1	0,6	95
132	10000100	●					●			2	1	0,6	96
156	10011100	●			●	●	●			4	1	0,6	97
188	10111100	●		●	●	●	●			5	1	0,6	97
194	11000010	●	●					●		3	1	0,6	98
232	11101000	●	●	●		●				4	1	0,6	98
240	11110000	●	●	●	●					4	1	0,6	99
254	11111110	●	●	●	●	●	●	●		7	1	0,6	99
255	11111111	●	●	●	●	●	●	●	●	8	1	0,6	100
0	0									0	3	1,7	

Fig. 5. Highly variable IgE repertoires to single grass pollen allergens. Profiles of IgE sensitization to 8 Phleum pratense molecules in 176 sensitized children with allergen-specific IgE to Phleum pratense and complete dataset. The Allergen Profile Codification System (APCS) code and the absolute and cumulative frequency are shown. (*From* Tripodi S, Frediani T, Lucarelli S, et al. Molecular profiles of IgE to Phleum pratense in children with grass pollen allergy: implications for specific immunotherapy. J Allergy Clin Immunol 2012;129:837.e8; with permission.)

Table 2	
Allergen sources for challenge testing	
Aeroallergen Sources (Examples)	**Rational to Apply Challenge Tests**
Birch pollen	Diagnosis not clear, ie, positive case history and negative sensitization test (rare)
Ash pollen	Checking for present clinical relevance (symptoms on exposure?)
Grass pollen	Diagnosis not clear, ie, positive case history and negative sensitization test (rare)
Mugwort pollen	Checking for present clinical relevance
Other weeds: plane, goose foot, nettle	Checking for present clinical relevance
Alternaria	Checking for present clinical relevance (frequently positive in the case of positive sensitization)
House dust mites (*D. pteronyssinus* or *D. farinae*)	Checking for present clinical relevance
Animal dander (cat, dog)	Demonstration of present clinical relevance

Challenge tests (nasal and conjunctival provocation) indicate clinical relevance by demonstrating mucosal reactivity.[30] Generally, challenges are only useful and applied in the routine setting if potential consequences (ie, decision on extract composition for AIT) can be drawn from the results (positive or negative).

an allergic reaction with mucosal exposure and supports the clinical relevance of the tested inhalant allergen, providing the clinical history indicates that the patient has symptoms with natural exposure to the allergen.

Physicians may be hesitant to perform nasal or ocular allergen challenges because of the requirement for extra instrument-based tools (ie, nasal challenge with rhinomanometry), the subjective nature of its interpretation (ie, conjunctival challenge), or lack of appropriate training in the technique. However, from a practical point of view, a simple score-based "clinical mucosal challenge" based entirely on symptoms may provide valuable information if the extract being used has a known potency. Therefore, some European state allergy organizations are promoting these diagnostic tools to identify the suitable allergen sources for subsequent AIT. However, proper reimbursement or validated challenge procedures are lacking.

SUMMARY

Allergists and other specialists in Europe and the United States have well-suited test instruments for proper allergy diagnosis. In the moderate climate of the northern hemisphere, a carefully obtained allergy clinical history is generally sufficient to identify the underlying, dominant outdoor grass, tree, and weed allergen sources if there are clearly separated periods of seasonal airborne allergen exposures. Considering subtropical or tropical areas, the clinical history becomes less informative because of potentially overlapping pollen and/or mold spore exposures. Available sensitization tests (skin tests, in vitro allergen-specific IgE assays, and, in a few cases, BATs) allow a more comprehensive diagnostic work-up to identify or rule out the most important allergen sources that elicit a given individual's allergy symptoms. Additional serology testing with individual major allergenic molecules facilitates an allergen-specific diagnosis, especially in the case of questionably multisensitized individuals, even with an underlying pan-allergen (profilin and/or polcalcin) sensitization. For proper interpretation of sensitization tests, plausible clinical data from previous anamnesis and/or symptom diaries of the patients are absolutely essential. AIT with principal or dominant allergens is only useful when there are corresponding airway symptoms and clearly demonstrated clinical relevance of allergen exposure leading to an individual's allergic disease symptoms.

REFERENCES

1. Rondon C, Campo P, Togias A, et al. Local allergic rhinitis: concept, pathophysiology, and management. J Allergy Clin Immunol 2012;129:1460–7.
2. Van Gerven L, Boeckxstaens G, Hellings P. Up-date on neuro-immune mechanisms involved in allergic and non-allergic rhinitis. Rhinology 2012;50:227–35.
3. Sastre J, Landivar ME, Ruiz-Garcia M, et al. How molecular diagnosis can change allergen-specific immunotherapy prescription in a complex pollen area. Allergy 2012;67:709–11.
4. Stringari G, Tripodi S, Caffarelli C, et al. The effect of component-resolved diagnosis on specific immunotherapy prescription in children with hay fever. J Allergy Clin Immunol 2014;134:75–81.
5. Moreno C, Justicia JL, Quiralte J, et al. Olive, grass or both? Molecular diagnosis for the allergen immunotherapy selection in polysensitized pollinic patients. Allergy 2014;69:1357–63.
6. Sastre J, Rodriguez F, Campo P, et al. Adverse reactions to immunotherapy are associated with different patterns of sensitization to grass allergens. Allergy 2015;70:598–600.
7. Costa C, Menesatti P, Brighetti MA, et al. Pilot study on the short-term prediction of symptoms in children with hay fever monitored with e-Health technology. Eur Ann Allergy Clin Immunol 2014;46:216–25.
8. Murphy K, Gawchik S, Bernstein D, et al. A phase 3 trial assessing the efficacy and safety of grass allergy immunotherapy tablet in subjects with grass pollen-induced allergic rhinitis with or without conjunctivitis, with or without asthma. J Negat Results Biomed 2013;12:10.
9. Slater JE, Menzies SL, Bridgewater J, et al. The US food and drug administration review of the safety and effectiveness of nonstandardized allergen extracts. J Allergy Clin Immunol 2012;129:1014–9.
10. Hamilton RG, MacGlashan DW Jr, Saini SS. IgE antibody-specific activity in human allergic disease. Immunol Res 2010;47:273–84.
11. Gupta RS, Lau CH, Hamilton RG, et al. Predicting outcomes of oral food challenges by using the allergen-specific IgE-total IgE ratio. J Allergy Clin Immunol Pract 2014;2:300–5.
12. MacGlashan DW Jr. Basophil activation testing. J Allergy Clin Immunol 2013;132:777–87.
13. Van Gasse AL, Mangodt EA, Faber M, et al. Molecular allergy diagnosis: status anno 2015. Clin Chim Acta 2015;444:54–61.
14. Gomez E, Campo P, Rondon C, et al. Role of the basophil activation test in the diagnosis of local allergic rhinitis. J Allergy Clin Immunol 2013;132:975–6.e1–5.
15. Kleine-Tebbe J. Old questions and novel clues: complexity of IgE repertoires. Clin Exp Allergy 2012;42:1142–5.
16. Kleine-Tebbe J, Erdmann S, Knol EF, et al. Diagnostic tests based on human basophils: potentials, pitfalls and perspectives. Int Arch Allergy Immunol 2006;141:79–90.
17. Purohit A, Laffer S, Metz-Favre C, et al. Poor association between allergen-specific serum immunoglobulin E levels, skin sensitivity and basophil degranulation: a study with recombinant birch pollen allergen Bet v 1 and an immunoglobulin E detection

system measuring immunoglobulin E capable of binding to Fc epsilon RI. Clin Exp Allergy 2005;35:186–92.

18. Lorenz AR, Luttkopf D, May S, et al. The principle of homologous groups in regulatory affairs of allergen products–a proposal. Int Arch Allergy Immunol 2009; 148:1–17.

19. EMA guideline on allergen products: production and quality issues. 2009. Available at: http://www.ema.europa.eu/docs/en_GB/document_library/Scientific_guideline/2009/09/WC500003333.pdf. Accessed October 5, 2015.

20. Hatzler L, Panetta V, Lau S, et al. Molecular spreading and predictive value of preclinical IgE response to Phleum pratense in children with hay fever. J Allergy Clin Immunol 2012;130:894–901.e5.

21. Matricardi PM. Allergen-specific immunoprophylaxis: toward secondary prevention of allergic rhinitis? Pediatr Allergy Immunol 2014;25:15–8.

22. Custovic A, Sonntag HJ, Buchan IE, et al. Evolution pathways of IgE responses to grass and mite allergens throughout childhood. J Allergy Clin Immunol 2015. [Epub ahead of print].

23. Tripodi S, Frediani T, Lucarelli S, et al. Molecular profiles of IgE to *Phleum pratense* in children with grass pollen allergy: implications for specific immunotherapy. J Allergy Clin Immunol 2012;129:834–9.e8.

24. Hauser M, Roulias A, Ferreira F, et al. Panallergens and their impact on the allergic patient. Allergy Asthma Clin Immunol 2010;6:1.

25. Schmid-Grendelmeier P. Rekombinante Allergene – Routinediagnostik oder Wissenschaft? Hautarzt 2010;61:946–53.

26. Makatsori M, Pfaar O, Lleonart R, et al. Recombinant allergen immunotherapy: clinical evidence of efficacy–a review. Curr Allergy Asthma Rep 2013;13:371–80.

27. Heinzerling L, Mari A, Bergmann KC, et al. The skin prick test – European standards. Clin Transl Allergy 2013;3:3.

28. Hamilton RG, Matsson PN, Chan S, et al. Analytical performance characteristics, quality assurance and clinical utility of immunological assays for human immunoglobulin E (IgE) antibodies of defined allergen specificities. 3rd edition. P. I/LA20–A3. International CLSI-Guideline 2015, in press.

29. Hamilton RG, Williams PB, Specific IgE Testing Task Force of the American Academy of Allergy Asthma & Immunology, American College of Allergy Asthma & Immunology. Human IgE antibody serology: a primer for the practicing North American allergist/immunologist. J Allergy Clin Immunol 2010;126:33–8.

30. Agache I, Bilo M, Braunstahl GJ, et al. In vivo diagnosis of allergic diseases–allergen provocation tests. Allergy 2015;70:355–65.

Solving the Problem of Nonadherence to Immunotherapy

Bruce G. Bender, PhD[a],*, Richard F. Lockey, MD[b]

KEYWORDS

- Allergen immunotherapy • Adherence • Patient-centered care
- Shared decision making • Motivational interviewing

KEY POINTS

- Fewer than one-half of patients compete a course of allergen immunotherapy.
- Very little research has been conducted to address nonadherence to immunotherapy.
- Communication models including patient-centered care, shared decision making, and motivation interviewing can be used to help improve immunotherapy adherence.
- Sensitivity to health literacy, language, and cultural differences are also important to improved immunotherapy adherence.

INTRODUCTION

Allergen immunotherapy (AIT) is an effective form of therapy to treat subjects with allergic rhinoconjunctivitis, allergic asthma, stinging insect hypersensitivity, and atopic eczema. It involves the gradual administration of increasing doses of the causative allergens, for example, inhalant allergens for allergic rhinoconjunctivitis, asthma, and atopic eczema and stinging insect venom allergens for individuals allergic to Hymenoptera or stinging insects. Whereas conventional vaccination, for example, tetanus or diphtheria, initiate and boost the immunologic memory and thereby protect against these diseases, AIT decreases established immune responses mediated by immunoglobulin (Ig)E and allergen-specific memory T cells through a gradual and controlled exposure to the offending allergens.[1]

Subcutaneous immunotherapy (SCIT) has been used to treat allergic diseases for over a century; however, it was not a universally accepted form of therapy until the end of the 20th century when the World Health Organization (WHO) sponsored a

[a] Center for Health Promotion, National Jewish Health, 1400 Jackson Street, Denver, CO 80206, USA; [b] Division of Allergy and Immunology, Department of Internal Medicine, University of South Florida Morsani College of Medicine, 12901 Bruce B. Downs Boulevard, Tampa, FL 33612, USA
* Corresponding authors.
E-mail address: bender@njhealth.org

Immunol Allergy Clin N Am 36 (2016) 205–213
http://dx.doi.org/10.1016/j.iac.2015.08.014   immunology.theclinics.com
0889-8561/16/$ – see front matter © 2016 Elsevier Inc. All rights reserved.

treatise on AIT entitled "WHO Position Paper, Allergen Immunotherapy: Therapeutic Vaccines for Allergic Diseases." This treatise summarized the scientific evidence for such therapy and broadened its appeal to physicians and subjects who suffer from these diseases throughout the world.[2]

New forms of AIT, particularly sublingual immunotherapy (SLIT), now complement SCIT. However, as with any form of therapy, efficacy depends on appropriate diagnosis, selection, and education of patients who suffer from these diseases. Many subjects who begin a course of either SCIT or SLIT for a variety of different reasons do not complete or continue these forms of therapy.

ADHERENCE TO ALLERGEN IMMUNOTHERAPY

Despite the clinical value of AIT, patient adherence is often very low. Reports of AIT adherence rates have varied greatly. For example, a review of 12 studies (6 SCIT, 5 SLIT, and 1 nasal immunotherapy) reported adherence rates ranging from 27% to 97%.[3] Variance in reported adherence likely reflects differing methodologies used to measure adherence. AIT clinical trials that rely on self-report data record unrealistically high adherence rates for reasons that include the implied obligation of patients to use their medication in the trial setting and inaccuracy of diary card data. Further, the adherence of clinical trial dropouts is frequently omitted from the reported data, thus further inflating an artificially high adherence rate. The consequence of these factors creates a distorted picture of actual adherence in clinical settings. For example, diary card trials have reported mean SLIT adherence rates of 87%,[3] 99%,[4] 90%[5] and 80%.[6] Self-report by means other than diary card is similarly subject to exaggeration. Of 71 families of SLIT-treated children interviewed by telephone, 84% reported adherence of greater than 75% at 6 months, again with no objective confirmation.[7] Despite seeming to be more objective, chart review studies fare only slightly better because they still rely on patient self-report.[5,6] Objective, methodologically sound measurement of adherence has often been absent from AIT trials. However, informative data emerge in asthma trials that have clearly demonstrated the inaccuracy of patient self-report when compared with objective adherence measures. In the final year of the 4-year Childhood Asthma Management Program clinical trial, patients on average took only 52% of their controller medication (as measured by returned medication), while reporting 91% adherence on diary cards (**Fig. 1**).[8] In a 4-month study of 104 children with asthma, inhaled corticosteroid adherence measured by an electronic

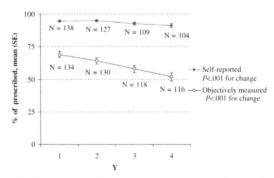

Fig. 1. Objective and self-reported adherence to asthma controller medication. SE, standard error. (*From* Krishnan J, Bender B, Wamboldt F, et al. Adherence to inhaled corticosteroids: an ancillary study of the childhood asthma management program clinical trial. J Allergy Clin Immunol 2012;129:112–8; with permission.)

device attached to their inhaler was contrasted with 1 of 3 forms of self-report: diary card, in-person interview, or computer interview. Adherence was significantly overreported in all self-report conditions; one-half of families exaggerated their adherence by more than 25% and one-third reported perfect adherence when no medication was taken.[9]

Pharmacy database studies reporting on AIT refill rates provide more objective data that do not rely on patient self-reports or estimates from physicians and other health care professional (PHCP). When a patient stops filling their medication, they have clearly abandoned that treatment. Although refill data are not reliable in short-term intervals, when used to evaluate adherence over a year or more, they provide insightful information. Adherence measurements by refill data correlate well with electronic tracking devices.[10–13] A large pharmacy refill database has shown that 53% to 56% of SLIT and SCIT patients discontinued treatment in year 1 and 84% to 87% by years 3 to 4 (**Fig. 2**).[14] In a side-by-side comparison of 6486 immunotherapy patients, 77% of those on SCIT and 93% of those on SLIT discontinued treatment before reaching 3 years.[15] Another study of SCIT and SLIT treatment termination revealed that attrition from SCIT was markedly higher in the first 2 months of treatment and SLIT attrition increased after 2 months; over 24 months, the overall rates of attrition approached 50% for both forms of AIT (**Fig. 3**).[16]

COST VERSUS BENEFIT

Most allergy treatments, such as intranasal corticosteroids and antihistamines, provide short-term benefit as long as they are used. Patterns of use often depend on current symptoms, and discussions of nonadherence are less relevant because these medications are largely dictated by the patient's perceived need for relief. In contrast, AIT is intended to modify the underlying immune system response and hence benefit follows only from persistent long-term use. Modest symptom relief may be received with a year of treatment, but maximum, lasting benefit is obtained with at least 3 years of treatment.[17] Collective evidence indicates that persistence is equally problematic for both SCIT and SLIT. The assessment of cost versus benefit must, therefore, take into account the loss of any benefit resulting from early termination of therapy. A large retrospective analysis of pharmacy data in The Netherlands indicated that only 23% of SCIT patients and 7% of SLIT patients completed a full 3 years of

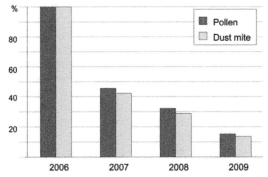

Fig. 2. Proportion of patients continuing sublingual immunotherapy. (*From* Senna G, Lombardi C, Canonica G, et al. How adherent to sublingual immunotherapy prescriptions are patients? the manufacturers' viewpoint. J Allergy Clin Immunol 2010;126:668–9; with permission.)

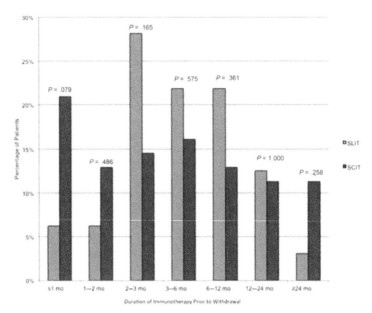

Fig. 3. Duration of sublingual immunotherapy (SLIT) and subcutaneous immunotherapy (SCIT). (*From* Hsu N, Reisacher W. A comparison of attrition rates in patients undergoing sublingual immunotherapy vs subcutaneous immunotherapy. Int Forum Allergy Rhinol 2012;2(4):280–4; with permission.)

treatment, representing a $4000 cost per nonpersistent patient that was "largely misspent."[15] To establish a satisfactory cost versus benefit balance with an effective treatment, it becomes particularly important that PHCPs be equipped to identify patients most likely to commit to and benefit from a full course of AIT and to engage communication tools to maximize adherence.

IDENTIFYING PATIENTS LIKELY TO BE NONADHERENT

Multiple studies have documented an association between AIT nonadherence and patient characteristics that include younger age,[18,19] lower socioeconomic status,[20] government insurance,[21,22] minority race,[23,24] and cost.[3] A primary reason for subjects discontinuing SCIT is the inconvenience of receiving injections,[3,25] because injections cannot be administered at home. A physician well-versed and competent in treating a systemic allergic reaction must be present because SCIT can induce a systemic allergic reaction and even cause death.[26] Other patient-reported reasons for SCIT and SLIT nonadherence summarized in a review of more than 25 studies included concurrent illness, perceived ineffectiveness, symptom improvement, change in residence or clinic, adverse reaction, systemic reaction, local reaction, inconvenience, and cost or lack of insurance (**Table 1**).[25] Somewhat unexpectedly, adherence to SLIT seems to be even more problematic than adherence with SCIT. Although SLIT maintains a strong safety profile and can be administered at home, the primary reason given by patients for SLIT discontinuation and/or nonadherence was an "inability to take medication according to schedule and/or non-compliance." Other reasons were "time-consuming and/or inconvenience, not effective, concurrent illness and/or medical condition, adverse effects, cost."[25]

Table 1	
Patient-reported reasons for discontinuation of allergen immunotherapy	
Subcutaneous Immunotherapy	**Sublingual Immunotherapy**
Inconvenience	Inability to take medication according to schedule and/or forgetting and/or noncompliance
Concurrent illness	Time consuming and/or inconvenient
Not effective	Not effective
Symptoms improved	Concurrent illness and/or medical condition
Changed residence or clinic	Adverse effects
Adverse reaction	Cost
Systemic reaction	—
Local reaction	—

From Cox L, Hankin C, Lockey R. Allergy immunotherapy adherence and delivery route: location does not matter. J Allergy Clin Immunol Pract 2014;2(2):156–60; with permission.

COMMUNICATION STRATEGIES TO MAXIMIZE ADHERENCE TO ALLERGEN IMMUNOTHERAPY

PHCPs can adopt brief, effective, evidence-based strategies to improve AIT adherence. Randomized trials of interventions to improve AIT adherence are in process; until these data are available, interventions directed at other health conditions including asthma can be applied to AIT. The key elements of an effective AIT adherence intervention plan come from studies of patient-centered care, shared decision making, and motivational interviewing.

Patient-Centered Care

Patient-centered care is a model for care in which PHCPs create partnerships with patients and their family members. The Institute of Medicine strongly endorses this model, emphasizing the importance of "providing care that is respectful of and responsive to individual patient preferences, needs, and values, and ensuring that patient values guide all clinical decisions."[27] Guided by the principles of patient-centered care, PHCPs focus on establishing a caring relationship from the first meeting with the patient. Trust is more likely to develop when the PHCP is warm and friendly, demonstrates genuine interest in the patient's problem, and does not seem to be rushed. In patient-centered care, the PHCP listens carefully to the patient, allows sufficient time for the patient to share their primary concerns and what they hope to accomplish in the visit, verifies to be sure that the PHCP has correctly understood the patient, and addresses the patient's concerns during the visit.[28] Clinic barriers that interfere with patient-centered care include time pressures that produce a need to move quickly through the encounter, and in turn an increasing tendency to speak rapidly and decrease listening time. When PHCPs listen carefully to patients and are supportive, understanding, and nonjudgmental, patients express greater satisfaction and are more likely to be adherent to treatment.[29–31]

Motivational Interviewing

In its original format, motivational interviewing, although effective, is impractical for most PHCPs. Programs to decrease alcohol consumption or improve physical activity[32] or medication adherence[33–35] have required 1 to 5 hours of motivational interviewing to accomplish changes in patient behavior. Few primary care PHCPs or specialists have the luxury of time to allow this degree of patient interaction. Nonetheless, recent work has developed time- and resource-efficient approaches to motivational interviewing that can enhance patient motivation and adherence.[36,37] Two specific motivational interviewing techniques that can be used to improve AIT adherence are (1) asking open-ended questions and (2) reflective listening. Open-ended questions cannot be answered "yes" or "no" and allow the patient to express their concerns and expectations regarding this visit. Reflective listening includes summarizing back to the patient what the PHCP has heard from the patient to ensure a correct understanding of the patient's perspective and preferences. Motivational interviewing strategies have proven effective in improving asthma adherence[38] and may be similarly applied to patients with allergic disorders.

Shared Decision Making

Strategies of patient-centered care and motivational interviewing integrate well with shared decision making. All 3 concepts embrace the importance of communicating effectively, listening closely, and respecting patient concerns and wishes. All 3 strategies avoid lecturing patients or imparting the expectation that PHCPs will be disappointed if the patient does not comply with the PHCP's recommendations. Shared decision making builds on strong listening skills by providing a guideline for choosing treatments. This communication strategy includes attempts to increase concordance about treatment choices and goals, leads to higher adherence in patients with asthma,[39] and is well-suited to PHCP–patient discussions regarding AIT. When using shared decision making, the PHCP is deferring some control over treatment decisions to the patient. Differences in patient and PHCP goals and patient expectations must be discussed and resolved before the treatment plan is finalized.[40] To reach this point, the PHCP must make sure that the patient has an adequate understanding of the illness and treatment options. Hence, patient education becomes an important step in creating a patient–PHCP partnership. Patients differ significantly in the degree to which they want or understand detailed information. Therefore, sensitivity to health literacy, language, cultural differences, and desire for choices are essential in PHCP–patient communication.[41] Information about health, illness, and treatment should be delivered in clear language and at a pace that seems to be comfortable to each patient. One-size-fits-all education often leaves many patients dissatisfied. The principles of adult learning, established decades ago[42] continue to be helpful guides and include (1) assessing the person's knowledge of a topic before teaching, (2) progressing from simple to complex, (3) encouraging questions and discussion, (4) repeating and reinforcing new information, and (5) practicing new skills (eg, the correct self-administration of a inhaler or tablet medication).

SUMMARY AND FUTURE CONSIDERATIONS

AIT is an effective therapy that can improve allergic response by modifying the underlying disease. However, many patients are nonadherent with AIT regardless of the mode of delivery, including SLIT. Medication refill studies reveal that barely 10% of patients complete a full 3-year course of AIT, and one-half of patients quit taking AIT in the first year. PHCP teams can improve AIT adherence by (1) appropriately diagnosing and selecting patients likely to benefit, (2) avoiding prescribing AIT prematurely to patients not yet ready to commit to treatment, (3) providing sufficient education about the treatment, and (4) using effective communication strategies to motivate and activate patients toward greater adherence. Evidence-based communication strategies are drawn from patient-centered care, motivational interviewing, and shared decision making. Collectively, the key strategies from these include (1) establishing trust, (2) working diligently to understand patient concerns and priorities, (3) taking sufficient time, and (4) involving the patient in decisions regarding whether and when to initiate AIT. Sensitivity to health literacy, language, cultural differences, and a desire for choices are essential to this PHCP–patient communication. Using these strategies, PHCP teams can enhance both AIT adherence and consequent benefit to patients.

REFERENCES

1. Shamji M, Till S, Durham S. Immunological responses to subcutaneous allergen immunotherapy. In: Lockey RF, Ledford DK, editors. Allergens and allergen immunotherapy: subcutaneous, sublingual and ora. New York: CRC Press/Taylor & Francis Group; 2014. p. 51–65.
2. Bousquet J, Lockey R, Malling H. WHO position paper. Allergen immunotherapy: therapeutic vaccines for allergic diseases. Allergy 1998;53(44):1–42.
3. Incorvaia C, Ariano R, Berto P, et al. Economic aspects of sublingual immunotherapy. Int J Immunopathol Pharmaco 2009;22(4 Suppl):27–30.
4. Roder E, Berger M, deGrott H, et al. Sublingual immunotherapy in youngsters: adherence in a randomized clinical trial. Clin Exp Allergy 2008;38:1659–67.
5. Park D, Daher N, Blaiss M. Adult and pediatric clinical trails of sublingual immunotherapy in the USA. Expert Rev Clin Immunol 2012;8:557–64.
6. Amar S, Harbeck R, Sills M, et al. Response to sublingual immunotherapay with grass pollen extract: monotherapy versus combination in a multiallergen extract. J Allergy Clin Immunol 2009;124(1):150–6.
7. Passalacqua G, Musarra A, Pecora S, et al. Qualitative assessment of the compliance with a once-daily sublingual immunotherapy regime in real life. J Allergy Clin Immunol 2006;117:946–8.
8. Krishnan J, Bender B, Wamboldt F, et al. Adherence to inhaled corticosteroids: an ancillary study of the childhood asthma management program clinical trial. J Allergy Clin Immunol 2012;129:112–8.
9. Bender B, Long A, Parasuraman B, et al. Factors influencing patient decisions about the use of asthma controller medication. Ann Allergy Asthma Immunol 2007;98:322–8.
10. Choo P, RAnd C, Inui T, et al. Validation of patient reports, automated pharmacy records, and pill counts with electronic monitoring of adherence to antihypertensive therapy. Med Care 1999;37(9):846–57.
11. Hansen R, Kim M, Song L, et al. Comparison of methods to assess medication adherence and classify nonadherence. Ann Pharmacother 2009;43:413–22.
12. Grymonpre R, Cheang M, Frase M, et al. Validity of a prescription claims database to estimate medication adherence in older persons. Med Care 2006; 44(5):471–7.
13. Ndubuka N, Ehlers V. Adult patients' adherence to anti-retroviral treatment: a survey correlating pharmacy refill records and pill counts with immunological and virological indices. Int J Nurs Stud 2011;48(11):1323–9.
14. Senna G, Lombardi C, Canonica G, et al. How adherent to sublingual immunotherapy prescriptions are patients? the manufacturers' viewpoint. J Allergy Clin Immunol 2010;126:668–9.
15. Kiel M, Roder E, Gerth van Wijk P, et al. Real-life compliance and persistence among users of subcutaneous and sublingual allergen immunotherapy. J Allergy Clin Immunol 2013;132:353–60.

16. Hsu N, Reisacher W. A comparison of attrition rates in patients undergoing sublingual immunotherapy vs subcutaneous immunotherapy. Int Forum Allergy Rhinol 2012;2(4):280–4.
17. Marogna M, Spadolini I, Massolo A, et al. Long-lasting effects of sublingual immunotherapy according to its duration: a 15-year prospective study. J Allergy Clin Immunol 2010;126(5):969–75.
18. More D, Hagan L. Factors affecting compliance with allergen immunotherapy at a military medical center. Ann Allergy Asthma Immunol 2002;88:391–4.
19. Rhodes B. Patient dropouts before completion of optimal dose, multiple allergen immunotherapy. Ann Allergy Asthma Immunol 1999;82:281–6.
20. Hommers L, Ellert U, Scheidt-Nave C, et al. Factors contributing to conductance and outcome of specific immunotherapy: data from the German National Health Interview and Examination Survey 1998. Eur J Public Health 2007;17:278–84.
21. Lower T, Henry J, Mandik L, et al. Compliance with allergen immunotherapy. Ann Allergy 1993;70:480–2.
22. Pediatric allergies in America: a landmark survey of children with nasal allergies. 2008. Available at: http://www.mmcpub.com/scsaia/pediatric.pdf. Accessed August 16, 2010.
23. Hankin C, Cox L, Lang D, et al. Allergy immunotherapy among Medicaid-enrolled children with allergic rhinitis: patterns of care, resource use, and costs. J Allergy Clin Immunol 2008;121:227–32.
24. Asthma and Allergy Foundation of America, National Pharmaceutical Council. Ethnic disparities in the burden and treatment of asthma. Reston (VA): Asthma and Allergy Foundation of America; 2005.
25. Cox L, Hankin C, Lockey R. Allergy immunotherapy adherence and delivery route: location does not matter. J Allergy Clin Immunol Pract 2014;2(2):156–60.
26. Cox L, Nelson H, Lockey R. Allergen immunotherapy: a practice parameter third update. J Allergy Clin Immunol 2011;127(1):S1–55.
27. Committee on Quality of Health Care in America, Institute of Medicine. Crossing the quality chasm: a new health system for the 21st Century. Washington, DC: National Academic Press, 2001.
28. Bender B. Motivating patient adherence to allergic rhinitis treatments. Curr Allergy Asthma Rep 2015;15(3):10.
29. Makoul G. Essential elements of communication in medical encounters: the Kalamazoo consensus statement. Adac Med 2001;76(4):390–3.
30. DiMatteo M. The role of effective communication with children and their families in fostering adherence to pediatric regimens. Patient Educ Couns 2004;55:339–44.
31. Boulware L, Daumit G, Frick K, et al. An evidence-based review of patient-centered behavioral interventions for hypertension. Am J Prev Med 2001;1(21):221–32.
32. Bobbins L, Pfeiffer K, Maler K, et al. Treatment fidelity of motivational interviewing delivered by a school nurse to increase girls' physical activity. J Sch Nurs 2012;28(1):70–8.
33. Cook P, Bremer R, Ayala A, et al. Feasibility of motivational interviewing delivered by a glaucoma educator to improve medication adherence. Clin Ophthalmol 2010;4:1091–101.
34. Barkhof E, Meijer C, de Sonneville L, et al. The effect of motivational interviewing on medication adherence and hospitalization rates in nonadherent patients with multi-episode schizophrenia. Schizophr Bull 2014;39(6):1242–51.

35. Hedegaard U, Kjeldsen LJ, Pottegård A, et al. Multifaceted intervention including motivational interviewing to support medication adherence after stroke/transient ischemic attack: a randomized trial. Cerebrovasc Dis Extra 2014;4(3):221–34.
36. Bender B. Can healthcare organizations improve health behavior and treatment adherence? Popul Health Manag 2014;17:71–8.
37. Bender B. Nonadherence to COPD treatment: what have we learned and what do we do next? COPD 2012;9:209–10.
38. Borrelli B, Riekert K, Weinstien A. Brief motivational. J Allergy Clin Immunol 2007; 120(5):1023–30.
39. Wilson S, Strub P, Buist A, et al. Shared treatment decision making improves adherence and outcomes in poorly controlled asthma. Better Outcomes of Asthma Treatment (BOAT) Study Group. Am J Respir Crit Care Med 2010; 181(6):566–77.
40. Wensing M, Elwyn G, Edwards A, et al. Deconstructing patient centered communication and uncovering shared decision making: an observational study. BMC Med Inform Decis Mak 2002;2:2.
41. Freda M. Issues in patient education. J Midwifery Womens Health 2004;49(3): 1–8.
42. Knowles M. The modern practice of adult education. New York: Cambridge, The Adult Education Company; 1980.

Moving?

Make sure your subscription moves with you!

To notify us of your new address, find your **Clinics Account Number** (located on your mailing label above your name), and contact customer service at:

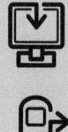

Email: journalscustomerservice-usa@elsevier.com

800-654-2452 (subscribers in the U.S. & Canada)
314-447-8871 (subscribers outside of the U.S. & Canada)

Fax number: 314-447-8029

Elsevier Health Sciences Division
Subscription Customer Service
3251 Riverport Lane
Maryland Heights, MO 63043

*To ensure uninterrupted delivery of your subscription, please notify us at least 4 weeks in advance of move.

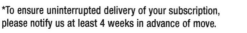

Printed and bound by CPI Group (UK) Ltd, Croydon, CR0 4YY

03/10/2024

01040494-0006